Advances in Surgical and Medical Interventions for Recalcitrant Chronic Rhinosinusitis

Jivianne T. Lee • Jakob L. Fischer
Peter H. Hwang • Joseph K. Han
Scott P. Stringer
Editors

Advances in Surgical and Medical Interventions for Recalcitrant Chronic Rhinosinusitis

Springer

Editors
Jivianne T. Lee, M.D.
Division of Rhinology & Endoscopic Sinus and Skull Base Surgery, Department of Head & Neck Surgery
University of California Los Angeles David Geffen School of Medicine
Los Angeles, CA, USA

Peter H. Hwang, M.D.
Division of Rhinology & Endoscopic Skull Base Surgery, Department of Otolaryngology-Head & Neck Surgery
Stanford University
Palo Alto, CA, USA

Scott P. Stringer, M.D.
Department of Otolaryngology-Head and Neck Surgery
Virginia Commonwealth University School of Medicine
Richmond, VA, USA

Jakob L. Fischer, M.D.
Department of Otolaryngology-Head & Neck Surgery
San Antonio Uniformed Services Health Education Consortium
San Antonio, TX, USA

Joseph K. Han, M.D.
Division of Rhinology & Endoscopic Sinus and Skull Base Surgery
East Virginia Medical School
Norfolk, VA, USA

ISBN 978-3-031-89190-8 ISBN 978-3-031-89191-5 (eBook)
https://doi.org/10.1007/978-3-031-89191-5

This Springer imprint is published by the registered company Springer Nature Switzerland AG
The registered company address is: Gewerbestrasse 11, 6330 Cham, Switzerland

Preface

In medical and surgical practice, we often encounter challenges that demand not only our knowledge but also our relentless dedication to innovation and excellence. Chronic rhinosinusitis, which remains an incompletely understood condition, impacts millions of patients on a daily basis and serves as a substantial burden to patients and healthcare providers alike. For those patients with recalcitrant chronic rhinosinusitis, this burden is even more severe; and their optimal management requires a thorough understanding of the broad spectrum of medical and surgical treatment options available to alleviate symptoms and improve quality of life. Through the collaborative efforts of experts worldwide, we have made significant strides in unraveling the mysteries of chronic rhinosinusitis. This textbook stands as a culmination of those efforts, offering a synthesis of evidence-based practices, innovative techniques, and nuanced strategies to optimize patient care.

In these pages, we offer a practical and comprehensive overview of the surgical and medical approaches to management of recalcitrant chronic rhinosinusitis. From foundational concepts to emerging algorithms, each chapter is designed to equip clinicians and surgeons of any specialty who may treat chronic rhinosinusitis with the most current knowledge to effectively address this complex condition. Narrated videos accompany surgical chapters to demonstrate cutting-edge procedures for treatment of refractory disease.

Interdisciplinary collaboration is emphasized throughout this textbook, recognizing the diverse expertise required for optimal patient care. We are honored to present the most up-to-date surgical techniques and medical therapies from some of the premier sinus surgeons, allergists, immunologists, and infectious disease specialists around the world.

We extend our gratitude to the contributors for their invaluable insights, and we hope that this textbook serves as a valuable resource for those navigating the challenges of chronic rhinosinusitis.

Los Angeles, CA, USA — Jivianne T. Lee, M.D.
San Antonio, TX, USA — Jakob L. Fischer, M.D.
Palo Alto, CA, USA — Peter H. Hwang, M.D.
Norfolk, VA, USA — Joseph K. Han, M.D.
Richmond, VA, USA — Scott P. Stringer, M.D.

Contents

Contributors

Bader M. Alim, M.D. Department of Otolaryngology—Head and Neck Surgery, Prince Mohammed Bin Abdul Aziz Hospital, National Guard Health Affairs, Medina, Saudi Arabia

Noel Ayoub, M.D. Division of Rhinology & Endoscopic Skull Base Surgery, Department of Otolaryngology-Head & Neck Surgery, Stanford University School of Medicine, Stanford, CA, USA

Claus Bachert, M.D., Ph.D. Department of Oto-Rhino-Laryngology, Münster University, Münster, Germany

First Affiliated Hospital, Sun Yat-sen University, International Airway Research Center, Guangzhou, China

Upper Airways Research Laboratory, Department of Oto-Rhino-Laryngology, Head and Skin, Ghent University, Ghent, Belgium

John V. Bosso, M.D. Division of Rhinology, Department of Otolaryngology, Perelman School of Medicine, University of Pennsylvania, Philadelphia, PA, USA

Alexander M. Choi, M.D. Department of Otolaryngology—Head and Neck Surgery, Baylor College of Medicine, Houston, TX, USA

John R. Craig, M.D. Department of Otolaryngology-Head and Neck Surgery, Henry Ford Health, Detroit, MI, USA

Greg E. Davis, M.D. Otolaryngology, Proliance Surgeons, Seattle and Puyallup, WA, USA

John M. DelGaudio, M.D. Department of Otolaryngology, Emory University, Atlanta, GA, USA

Angela M. Donaldson, M.D. Department of Otolaryngology Head and Neck Surgery, Mayo Clinic Florida, Jacksonville, FL, USA

Amy V. Dora, M.D. Infectious Diseases, VA Greater Los Angeles Healthcare System, Los Angeles, CA, USA

Jean Anderson Eloy, M.D. Department of Otolaryngology—Head and Neck Surgery, Rutgers New Jersey Medical School, Newark, NJ, USA

Department of Otolaryngology—Facial Plastic Surgery, Cooperman Barnabas Medical Center, Robert Wood Johnson Barnabas Health, Livingston, NJ, USA

Center for Skull Base and Pituitary Surgery, Neurological Institute of New Jersey, Rutgers New Jersey Medical School, Newark, NJ, USA

Department of Neurological Surgery, Rutgers New Jersey Medical School, Newark, NJ, USA

Department of Ophthalmology and Visual Science, Rutgers New Jersey Medical School, Newark, NJ, USA

Christina H. Fang, M.D. Department of Otorhinolaryngology—Head and Neck Surgery, Montefiore Medical Center, The University Hospital of Albert Einstein College of Medicine, Bronx, NY, USA

Akaansha Ganju, M.D. Department of Allergy and Immunology, Veterans Affairs Greater Los Angeles Healthcare System, Los Angeles, CA, USA

Philippe Gevaert, M.D. Department of Oto-Rhino-Laryngology, Münster University, Münster, Germany

Upper Airways Research Laboratory, Department of Oto-Rhino-Laryngology, Head and Skin, Ghent University, Ghent, Belgium

Matthew Bidwell Goetz, M.D. Infectious Diseases, VA Greater Los Angeles Healthcare System, Los Angeles, CA, USA

Clinical Medicine, David Geffen School of Medicine at UCLA, Los Angeles, CA, USA

Jordon G. Grube, D.O. Department of Otolaryngology—Albany Medical College, Albany Medical Center, Albany, NY, USA

Joseph K. Han, M.D., F.A.R.S., F.A.A.A.A.I. Division of Rhinology & Endoscopic Sinus and Skull Base Surgery, East Virginia Medical School, Norfolk, VA, USA

Richard J. Harvey, M.D., Ph.D. Rhinology and Skull Base, Applied Medical Research Centre, St Vincent's Hospital, Darlinghurst, NSW, Australia

Department of Otolaryngology, UNSW and Macquarie University, Sydney, NSW, Australia

Michael S. Hegazin, D.O. Department of Otolaryngology—Head and Neck Surgery, Rutgers New Jersey Medical School, Newark, NJ, USA

Juan Carlos Hernaiz-Leonardo, M.D. Department of Otolaryngology—Head and Neck Surgery, University of British Columbia, Vancouver, BC, Canada

Peter H. Hwang, M.D., F.A.C.S., F.A.R.S. Division of Rhinology & Endoscopic Skull Base Surgery, Department of Otolaryngology-Head & Neck Surgery, Stanford University School of Medicine, Stanford, CA, USA

Amin R. Javer, M.D. Department of Otolaryngology—Head and Neck Surgery, University of British Columbia, Vancouver, BC, Canada

Ashutosh Kacker, M.D. Department of Otolaryngology – Head & Neck Surgery, New York-Presbyterian/Weill Cornell Medicine, New York, NY, USA

Keonho Albert Kong, M.D. Department of Otolaryngology-Head and Neck Surgery, University of Mississippi Medical Center, Jackson, MS, USA

Anthony F. LaCava, M.D. Section of Allergy & Immunology, Division of Pulmonary, Allergy, & Critical Care Medicine, Perelman School of Medicine, University of Pennsylvania, Philadelphia, PA, USA

Devyani Lal, M.D. Department of Otolaryngology-Head & Neck Surgery, Mayo Clinic Arizona, Phoenix, AZ, USA

Daniel P. Lander, M.D. Department of Otolaryngology-Head & Neck Surgery, Washington University School of Medicine, St. Louis, MO, USA

Jivianne T. Lee, M.D., F.A.C.S., F.A.R.S. Divsion of Rhinology & Endoscopic Sinus and Skull Base Surgery, Department of Head and Neck Surgery, David Geffen School of Medicine at UCLA, Los Angeles, CA, USA

William Derek Leight, M.D. Ear, Nose and Throat Institute, Boys Town National Research Hospital, Boys Town, NE, USA

Stephen Leong, M.D. Vagelos College of Physicians & Surgeons, Columbia University Irving Medical Center, New York, NY, USA

Donald Arthur Leopold, M.D. Ear, Nose and Throat Institute, Boys Town National Research Hospital, Boys Town, NE, USA

Tran B. Locke, M.D. Department of Otolaryngology—Head and Neck Surgery, Baylor College of Medicine, Houston, TX, USA

Patricia A. Loftus, M.D. Department of Otolaryngology—Head and Neck Surgery, University of California San Francisco, San Francisco, CA, USA

Justin P. McCormick, M.D. Department of Head and Neck Surgery and Communication Sciences, Rutgers Robert Wood Johnson Medical School, New Brunswick, NJ, USA

Amar Miglani, M.D. Department of Otolaryngology-Head & Neck Surgery, Mayo Clinic Arizona, Phoenix, AZ, USA

Dafna Gershnabel Milk, M.D. Department of Otolaryngology Head and Neck Surgery, Eastern Virginia Medical School, Norfolk, VA, USA

Department of Otolaryngology Head and Neck Surgery, Meir Medical Center, Kfar Saba, Israel

Craig Miller, M.D. Otolaryngology, Virginia Mason Franciscan Health, Seattle, WA, USA

Zhang Nan, M.D., Ph.D. First Affiliated Hospital, Sun Yat-sen University, International Airway Research Center, Guangzhou, China

Upper Airways Research Laboratory, Department of Oto-Rhino-Laryngology, Head and Skin, Ghent University, Ghent, Belgium

Kazuhiro Omura, M.D. Department of Otorhinolaryngology, The Jikei University School of Medicine, Tokyo, Japan

Nobuyoshi Otori, M.D., Ph.D. Department of Otorhinolaryngology, The Jikei University School of Medicine, Tokyo, Japan

Neil N. Patel, M.D. Department of Otolaryngology—Head and Neck Surgery, University of California San Francisco, San Francisco, CA, USA

Prayag S. Patel, M.D. Department of Otolaryngology—Head & Neck Surgery, Maimonides Medical Center, Brooklyn, NY, USA

Nora W. Perkins, M.D., M.B.A. Albany ENT & Allergy Services, Albany, NY, USA

Shilpa M. Rao, M.D. Department of Otolaryngology-Head and Neck Surgery, University of Alabama in Birmingham, Birmingham, AL, USA

Daniel R. Romano, M.D. Department of Otolaryngology-Head & Neck Surgery, Washington University School of Medicine, St. Louis, MO, USA

Peta-Lee Sacks, M.D., Ph.D. Department of Otolaryngology, Macquarie University Hospital, Sydney, NSW, Australia

Firas Sbeih, MD Department of Otolaryngology, University of Florida, Jacksonville, FL, USA

John S. Schneider, M.D. Department of Otolaryngology-Head & Neck Surgery, Washington University School of Medicine, St. Louis, MO, USA

Kachorn Seresirikachorn, M.D. Department of Otolaryngology, Faculty of Medicine, Chulalongkorn University, Bangkok, Thailand

Daniel B. Spielman, M.D. Department of Otolaryngology, Emory University, Atlanta, GA, USA

Scott P. Stringer, M.D. Department of Otolaryngology-Head and Neck Surgery, Virginia Commonwealth University School of Medicine, Richmond, VA, USA

Jonathan Tyes, M.D. School of Medicine, University of Louisville, Louisville, KY, USA

Thibaut van Zele, M.D., Ph.D. Department of Oto-Rhino-Laryngology, Münster University, Münster, Germany

Upper Airways Research Laboratory, Department of Oto-Rhino-Laryngology, Head and Skin, Ghent University, Ghent, Belgium

Vivian Wang, M.D. Department of Allergy and Immunology, Veterans Affairs Greater Los Angeles Healthcare System, Los Angeles, CA, USA

Troy Woodard, M.D. Head and Neck Institute, Cleveland Clinic Foundation, Cleveland, OH, USA

Bradford A. Woodworth, M.D. Department of Otolaryngology-Head and Neck Surgery, University of Alabama in Birmingham, Birmingham, AL, USA

Gregory Fleming James Cystic Fibrosis Research Center, Birmingham, AL, USA

Michelle Yu, M.D. Department of Otolaryngology—Head & Neck Surgery, NewYork-Presbyterian/Weill Cornell Medicine/Columbia University Irving Medical Center, New York, NY, USA

Joseph Yusin, M.D. Department of Allergy and Immunology, Veterans Affairs Greater Los Angeles Healthcare System, Los Angeles, CA, USA

Part I

Introduction

Introduction to Recalcitrant Chronic Rhinosinusitis

1

Alexander M. Choi and Tran B. Locke

Key Points

- Chronic rhinosinusitis (CRS) is a multifactorial disease resulting from a complex interplay between extrinsic environmental exposures and intrinsic system factors resulting in chronic sinonasal inflammation.
- Multiple theories have been proposed to explain the pathogenesis of CRS, such as phenotypic descriptions based on presence of nasal polyposis and underlying inflammatory profile, but these inadequately describe the disease process.
- Current literature has moved towards classifying CRS based on endotype, the specific underlying cytokines, effectors, and biomarkers that may better explain the underlying pathogenesis of CRS and allow for personalized treatment regimens for impacted patients.

Introduction to Recalcitrant Chronic Rhinosinusitis

Chronic rhinosinusitis (CRS) is a disease process defined by at least 12 weeks of symptoms, consisting of at least two of the following: facial pain or pressure, anosmia, anterior/posterior rhinorrhea, and nasal congestion. In addition, patients must show objective evidence of mucosal inflammation on either nasal endoscopy or computed tomography (CT). CRS is classically divided into two clinical phenotypes, CRS with nasal polyps (CRSwNP) or CRS without nasal polyps (CRSsNP). The prevalence of CRS varies throughout the world. In Asian countries, prevalence from 2.6% to greater than 11% has been reported [1, 2]. European and U.S.

A. M. Choi · T. B. Locke (✉)
Department of Otolaryngology—Head and Neck Surgery, Baylor College of Medicine, Houston, TX, USA
e-mail: Alexander.Choi@bcm.edu; Tran.Locke@bcm.edu

J. T. Lee et al. (eds.), *Advances in Surgical and Medical Interventions for Recalcitrant Chronic Rhinosinusitis*,
https://doi.org/10.1007/978-3-031-89191-5_1

prevalence studies report a 6.9–27.1% prevalence in Europe and 4.8–12% prevalence in the U.S.A [3–5]. In addition, based on a large Korean database study, there is an overall higher prevalence of patients with CRSsNP (5.8%) compared to CRSwNP (2.6%) [6].

The incidence of CRS remains poorly defined. Two epidemiologic studies conducted in the U.S.A. and Canada used database evaluation to generate an estimated incidence of 1048 cases per 100,000 person-years, and 2.5 cases per 1000 individuals, both with variation based on geography and CRS phenotype [7, 8].

CRS is often treated in a multi-faceted approach, combining various medical therapies and surgical interventions. The reported outcomes of these therapies result in short- and long-term symptom reduction and improvement in quality of life in 85% of patients [9]. However, the remaining 15% of patients, who suffer from recalcitrant CRS, are plagued with chronic symptoms that require other medical regimens and revision surgeries.

CRS results in a significant economic healthcare burden. Based on cost analysis reports, the overall annual cost of CRS is $22 billion USD with $14 billion associated with direct costs. These direct costs include annual medication costs of $1547–$2700 per patient and $8200–$10,500 per endoscopic sinus surgery [10]. For those with recalcitrant CRS, it can be presumed that their costs would be greater as the pathogenesis of the disease is more complicated and less understood.

CRS is a multifactorial condition involving a complex interplay between extrinsic environmental exposures and intrinsic immune system factors, resulting in chronic inflammation in the sinonasal mucosa. This has fostered development of multiple theories to explain the pathogenesis of the disease process and why recalcitrant disease is difficult to treat.

The environmental exposures that are often a component to CRS include fungal infections, bacterial superantigen infections, biofilm formation, and microbiome changes. Host immune factors that are involved in the pathogenesis of CRS include defects in the epithelial barrier and dysregulation of the immune response [11].

Extrinsic Factors

Previously, it was thought that fungi played a central role in CRS. Studies evaluating fungal organisms in patients with CRS noted a 100% identification of fungi in the sinonasal cavities, specifically Alternaria species. However, further studies and randomized clinical trials evaluating antifungal therapy demonstrated minimal efficacy in treating CRS, disproving this hypothesis [12, 13]. Currently, fungal elements are considered a component of the CRS pathogenesis for select individuals as fungi contain proteases that can elicit cytokine activation and subsequent T helper (Th) type 2 response, remaining an essential component in allergic fungal sinusitis [14, 15].

Bacterial colonization of the sinonasal tract remains an understudied area. Historical data suggest that superantigen exotoxins produced by Staphylococcus aureus (S. aureus) elicit an inflammatory cascade conducive to nasal polyp formation and significant eosinophilic and type 2 immune response [16]. In addition, studies have isolated S. aureus in a large portion of nasal polyposis patients [17]. The superantigen exotoxin activates an immense immunologic response compared to the normal immune response prompting T lymphocyte proliferation and cytokine release. However, when evaluating control, CRSsNP, and cystic fibrosis (CF) patients, the effects of the superantigen were non-specific and did not elicit a Th2 response. Therefore, it is now hypothesized that the superantigen exotoxin amplifies the inflammatory changes already present in the nasal mucosa. This results in worse clinical symptoms and could serve as an indicator of recalcitrant CRS [11].

Biofilm formation is a microbial property that aids in the development of antibiotic resistance. Biofilms are organized structures comprised of bacteria within a protective external matrix, preventing the bacteria from being exposed to host defenses and antibiotics. Bacterial species capable of forming biofilms include S. aureus, P. aeruginosa, S. pneumoniae, H. influenzae, and M. catarrhalis. S. aureus is the most common offending agent in the sinonasal tract. Of the CRS patients undergoing sinus surgery, 42–75% had biofilm formation [18, 19]. The data supporting this hypothesis is scant but has not been identified without the presence of S. aureus superantigen exotoxin. Ultimately, this hypothesis highlights the phenotypic representation of CRS in the setting of superantigenic S. aureus infections [11].

Lastly, given the contributions of both fungal and bacterial infections, the sinonasal tract microbiome is ever changing. There remains a paucity of data regarding the microorganisms that normally inhabit the sinonasal cavity, but some studies have suggested differences in quantity and diversity in patients with CRS [20]. The literature regarding restoration of the natural symbiosis of the microbiome stems from the gastrointestinal literature and probiotic therapy. The International Sinonasal Microbiome Study (ISMS) 16S gene sequencing evaluation of the sinonasal microbiome identified three microbiotypes: Corynebacterium-dominant microbiotype, Staphylococcus-dominant microbiotype, and a mixed microbiotype. [21] While results remain untested, negative correlation between Corynebacterium and Staphylococcus suggest that Corynebacterium may have probiotic properties to bring about balance in dysbiosis [21–24]. Microbiotypes did not, however, correspond to a particular disease state or clinical traits, precluding its ability to serve as a biomarker. To complicate the pathogenesis of CRS further, there are geographic variations in microbiotype distributions. Asia and Australia were noted to have more Corynebacterium representation whereas Europe had more Staphylococcus representation. Currently, the reasons behind this variation remain too numerous and broad to classify and require further large-scale evaluation [21, 25].

Intrinsic Factors

The immune hypothesis theory proposes that defects in the physical barrier and innate immune response predispose individuals to CRS. This theory shifted the paradigm of CRS pathogenesis to genetic and epigenetic variations and abnormalities. This hypothesis was readily applicable to CF patients due to their impaired mucociliary clearance. However, studies have advocated that CRS patients also have increased transit time and increased risk for protease degradation and, thus, a weakened mechanical barrier [26, 27]. Additional studies have identified variations in host defense molecules which permit increased pathogen access and chronic inflammatory changes [28–31]. For instance, defects in the eicosanoid pathway are hypothesized as a cause of chronic inflammation due to the strong relationship between CRS and aspirin sensitivity. Although there is some evidence supporting symptomatic improvement with the use of leukotriene antagonists in CRSwNP, the evidence remains scarce and would require further assessment [32].

Alterations in the host immune response were previously implicated in the pathogenesis of CRS. As mentioned previously, CRS was classified into two clinical phenotypes, CRSwNP and CRSsNP, which was further broken down based on immune cell profile, namely eosinophilic profile for CRSwNP and neutrophilic for CRSsNP. Eosinophilic and non-eosinophilic profiles of those with CRSwNP remain nebulous. Studies conducted at various regions of Europe, Asia, and Australia have elucidated a predominantly eosinophilic inflammatory pattern of those in Europe and Australia with CRSwNP whereas, Asian populations with CRSwNP tend to have a neutrophilic profile. This bolsters the pattern of eosinophilic CRSwNP in Caucasians and neutrophilic CRSwNP in Asians, suggesting inherent genetic immunologic differences between diverse ethnicities [33–35]. To support this, Mahdavinia et al. evaluated a small cohort of 11 second-generation Asian patients with CRSwNP from Illinois and noted similar inflammatory backgrounds to native-born Asians with CRSwNP. [36] In contrast, histopathologic studies evaluating CRSwNP patients in Thailand and Korea in the 1990s and in the 2010s, who required sinus surgery, demonstrated an eosinophilic shift of nasal polyposis [37, 38]. This suggests that environmental factors play a substantial role in CRSwNP and that observing changes in immune patterns over time will emerge as an imperative part of understanding CRSwNP. Lastly, it reveals that a simple classification of eosinophilic vs. non-eosinophilic inflammation may not be adequate in CRS.

As a consequence of the uncertainty regarding inflammatory cell predominance, it is difficult to determine an overarching treatment algorithm that is applicable to the CRS population. Instead, the transition to individualized treatment regimens has been proposed based on a novel classification of endotypes [39]. The use of endotypes has become a stepping stone towards developing personalized treatment for those who suffer from CRS. Use of endotype classification has both prognostic and treatment implications allowing for prediction of success. This categorization has also driven the development and testing of biologic therapies that target specific cytokines to treat CRS.

The endotype classification is based on balance of the T-helper cell patterns of inflammation, namely, Th2 (type 2) vs. non-Th2. [Table 1.1] T-helper cells can determine the character of an immune response through the cytokines produced and the subsequent downstream differentiation or recruitment of other inflammatory

Table 1.1 Endotype classification of CRS

Endotype classification		
Endotype	Th2 (Type 2) inflammation	Non-Th2 inflammation
Primary cytokine	IL-4 IL-5 IL-13	Type 1: IL-12, IFN-γ Type 3: IL-17, IL-22
Cellular predominance	Eosinophils	Neutrophils

IL interleukin, *IFN* interferon, *Th* T-helper

cells. Type 1 endotype patients exhibit elevated interferon-gamma (IFN-γ). IFN-γ is a cytokine with pleiotropic immunologic modulation that is secreted by activated T cells and natural killer (NK) cells. It plays an essential component in neutrophil and macrophage activation for clearance of intracellular pathogens, including bacteria, viruses, and protozoa [40]. Type 3 endotypes have elevated IL-17 and IL-22, which are cytokines that support the innate barrier defenses on mucosal surfaces by promoting recruitment of neutrophils to clear extracellular infections and induce regeneration of epithelial surfaces after inflammation [41]. These two endotypes are generally neutrophilic dominant and are associated with CRSsNP. Conversely, type 2 endotypes are characterized by elevation of cytokines IL-4, IL-5, and IL-13, are eosinophilic dominant, and promote IgE differentiation. Type 2 endotype is associated with allergic disease, parasitic infections, and CRSwNP. [39, 42–44]

Understanding the underlying inflammatory pattern of a patient's CRS can assist in guiding both medical and surgical therapy. Biologic therapies specifically target IL-4, IL-5, IL-13, or IgE and have proven to be efficacious as an adjunct measure to standard medical therapy alongside surgical interventions [45–47].

While this is a simplistic summation of a complex disease, this serves as the foundation for endotype discussion. Further research has elucidated mixed endotype representations and elevation in cytokines and biomarkers. This suggests that rather than distinct categories of endotypes, CRS endotypes should be classified on a continuous spectrum [48, 49].

Due to its heterogeneity, recalcitrant CRS is a difficult disease process to treat. Despite appropriate medical therapy, alternative medical therapies, and multiple surgical interventions, CRS continues to greatly impair the quality of life of those affected. As more research is conducted, the complexity of CRS becomes more apparent. The previously listed hypotheses serve as disease modifiers that can accentuate the clinical presentation of the disease but do not explain the pathogenesis of CRS as a whole. The wide gamut of CRS presentation illuminates the incomplete understanding of the associated molecular pathways that define CRS and the need for more evaluation. The transition to endotype classification has paved the way for better characterization of the disease process and personalized treatment. The following chapters serve to highlight evidence based medical and surgical treatment options available for recalcitrant CRS.

References

1. Kim JH, Cho C, Lee EJ, Suh YS, Choi BI, Kim KS. Prevalence and risk factors of chronic rhinosinusitis in South Korea according to diagnostic criteria. Rhinology. 2016;54(4):329–35. https://doi.org/10.4193/Rhino15.157.
2. Kong IG, Kim DW. Pathogenesis of recalcitrant chronic rhinosinusitis: the emerging role of innate immune cells. Immune Netw. 2018; https://doi.org/10.4110/in.2018.18.e6.
3. Hastan D, Fokkens WJ, Bachert C, Newson RB, Bislimovska J, Bockelbrink A, et al. Chronic rhinosinusitis in Europe—an underestimated disease. A GA(2)LEN study. Allergy. 2011;66:1216–23.
4. Hirsch AG, Stewart WF, Sundaresan AS, Young AJ, Kennedy TL, Scott Greene J, et al. Nasal and sinus symptoms and chronic rhinosinusitis in a population-based sample. Allergy. 2017;72(274–81):22.
5. Sundaresan AS, Hirsch AG, Young AJ, Pollak J, Tan BK, Schleimer RP, et al. Longitudinal evaluation of chronic rhinosinusitis symptoms in a population based sample. J Allergy Clin Immunol Pract. 2018;6:1327–35.
6. Ahn JC, Kim JW, Lee CH, Rhee CS. Prevalence and risk factors of chronic rhinosinusitus, allergic rhinitis, and nasal septal deviation: results of the Korean National Health and Nutrition Survey 2008-2012. JAMA Otolaryngol Head Neck Surg. 2016;142:162–7.
7. Xu Y, Quan H, Faris P, et al. Prevalence and incidence of diagnosed chronic rhinosinusitis in Alberta, Canada. JAMA Otolaryngol Head Neck Surg. 2016; https://doi.org/10.1001/jamaoto.2016.2227.
8. Tan BK, Chandra RK, Pollak J, Kato A, Conley DB, Peters AT, et al. Incidence and associated premorbid diagnoses of patients with chronic rhinosinusitis. J Allergy Clin Immunol. 2013;131:1350–60.
9. Soler ZM, Mace J, Smith TL. Symptom-based presentation of chronic rhinosinusitis and symptom-specific outcomes after endoscopic sinus surgery. Am J Rhinol. 2008; https://doi.org/10.2500/ajr.2008.22.3172.
10. Smith KA, Orlandi RR, Rudmik L. Cost of adult chronic rhinosinusitis: a systematic review. Laryngoscope. 2015; https://doi.org/10.1002/lary.25180.
11. Lam K, Schleimer R, Kern RC. The etiology and pathogenesis of chronic rhinosinusitis: a review of current hypotheses. Curr Allergy Asthma Rep. 2015;15(7):41.
12. Ebbens FA, Scadding GK, Badia L, et al. Amphotericin B nasal lavages: not a solution for patients with chronic rhinosinusitis. J Allergy Clin Immunol. 2006;118:1149–56.
13. Weschta M, Rimek D, Formanek M, Polzehl D, Podbielski A, Riechelmann H. Topical antifungal treatment of chronic rhinosinusitis with nasal polyps: a randomized, double-blind clinical trial. J Allergy Clin Immunol. 2004; https://doi.org/10.1016/j.jaci.2004.03.038.
14. Shin SH, Lee SH, Jeong HS, Kita H. The effect of nasal polyp epithelial cells on eosinophil activation. Laryngoscope. 2003; https://doi.org/10.1097/00005537-200308000-00020.
15. Wu D, Wei Y, Bleier BS. Emerging role of proteases in the pathogenesis of chronic rhinosinusitis with nasal polyps. Front Cell Infect Microbiol. 2017;7:538.
16. Bachert C, Gevaert P, Holtappels G, Johansson SG, van Cauwenberge P. Total and specific IgE in nasal polyps is related to local eosinophilic inflammation. J Allergy Clin Immunol. 2001; https://doi.org/10.1067/mai.2001.112374.
17. Van Zele T, Gevaert P, Watelet JB, Claeys G, Holtappels G, Claeys C, van Cauwenberge P, Bachert C. Staphylococcus aureus colonization and IgE antibody formation to enterotoxins is increased in nasal polyposis. J Allergy Clin Immunol. 2004; https://doi.org/10.1016/j.jaci.2004.07.013.
18. Post JC, Stoodley P, Hall-Stoodley L, Ehrlich GD. The role of biofilms in otolaryngologic infections. Curr Opin Otolaryngol Head Neck Surg. 2004; https://doi.org/10.1097/01.moo.0000124936.46948.6a.
19. Calò L, Passàli GC, Galli J, Fadda G, Paludetti G. Role of biofilms in chronic inflammatory diseases of the upper airways. Adv Otorhinolaryngol. 2011; https://doi.org/10.1159/000324622.

20. Boase S, Foreman A, Cleland E, Tan L, Melton-Kreft R, Pant H, Hu FZ, Ehrlich GD, Wormald PJ. The microbiome of chronic rhinosinusitis: culture, molecular diagnostics and biofilm detection. BMC Infect Dis. 2013; https://doi.org/10.1186/1471-2334-13-210.
21. Bassiouni A, Paramasivan S, Shiffer A, Dillon MR, Cope EK, Cooksley C, Ramezanpour M, Moraitis S, Ali MJ, Bleier BS, Callejas C, Cornet ME, Douglas RG, Dutra D, Georgalas C, Harvey RJ, Hwang PH, Luong AU, Schlosser RJ, Tantilipikorn P, Tewfik MA, Vreugde S, Wormald PJ, Caporaso JG, Psaltis AJ. Microbiotyping the sinonasal microbiome. Front Cell Infect Microbiol. 2020; https://doi.org/10.3389/fcimb.2020.00137.
22. Ramsey MM, Freire MO, Gabrilska RA, Rumbaugh KP, Lemon KP. Staphylococcus aureus shifts toward commensalism in response to Corynebacterium species. Front Microbiol. 2016; https://doi.org/10.3389/fmicb.2016.01230.
23. Hardy BL, Dickey SW, Plaut RD, Riggins DP, Stibitz S, Otto M, et al. Corynebacterium pseudodiphtheriticum exploits Staphylococcus aureus virulence components in a novel polymicrobial defense strategy. MBio. 2019; https://doi.org/10.1128/mBio.02491-18.
24. Kiryukhina NV, Melnikov VG, Suvorov AV, Morozova YA, Ilyin VK. Use of Corynebacterium pseudodiphtheriticum for elimination of Staphylococcus aureus from the nasal cavity in volunteers exposed to abnormal microclimate and altered gaseous environment. Probiotics Antimicrob Proteins. 2013; https://doi.org/10.1007/s12602-013-9147-x.
25. Paramasivan S, Bassiouni A, Shiffer A, Dillon MR, Cope EK, Cooksley C, et al. The international sinonasal microbiome study (ISMS): a multi-centre, multi-national characterization of sinonasal bacterial ecology. Allergy. 2020; https://doi.org/10.1111/all.14276.
26. Antunes MB, Gudis DA, Cohen NA. Epithelium, cilia, and mucus: their importance in chronic rhinosinusitis. Immunol Allergy Clin N Am. 2009; https://doi.org/10.1016/j.iac.2009.07.004.
27. Zuckerman JD, Lee WY, DelGaudio JM, Moore CE, Nava P, Nusrat A, Parkos CA. Pathophysiology of nasal polyposis: the role of desmosomal junctions. Am J Rhinol. 2008; https://doi.org/10.2500/ajr.2008.22.3235.
28. Psaltis AJ, Bruhn MA, Ooi EH, Tan LW, Wormald PJ. Nasal mucosa expression of lactoferrin in patients with chronic rhinosinusitis. Laryngoscope. 2007; https://doi.org/10.1097/MLG.0b013e31812e01ab.
29. Seshadri S, Lin DC, Rosati M, Carter RG, Norton JE, Suh L, Kato A, Chandra RK, Harris KE, Chu HW, Peters AT, Tan BK, Conley DB, Grammer LC, Kern RC, Schleimer RP. Reduced expression of antimicrobial PLUNC proteins in nasal polyp tissues of patients with chronic rhinosinusitis. Allergy. 2012; https://doi.org/10.1111/j.1398-9995.2012.02848.x.
30. Ramanathan M Jr, Spannhake EW, Lane AP. Chronic rhinosinusitis with nasal polyps is associated with decreased expression of mucosal interleukin 22 receptor. Laryngoscope. 2007; https://doi.org/10.1097/MLG.0b013e31811edd4f.
31. Hulse KE, Chaung K, Seshadri S, Suh L, Norton JE, Carter RG, Kern RC, Conley DB, Chandra RK, Tan BK, Peters AT, Grammer LC 3rd, Harris KE, Torgerson TR, Kato A, Schleimer RP. Suppressor of cytokine signaling 3 expression is diminished in sinonasal tissues from patients with chronic rhinosinusitis with nasal polyps. J Allergy Clin Immunol. 2014; https://doi.org/10.1016/j.jaci.2013.08.015.
32. Wentzel JL, Soler ZM, DeYoung K, Nguyen SA, Lohia S, Schlosser RJ. Leukotriene antagonists in nasal polyposis: a meta-analysis and systematic review. Am J Rhinol Allergy. 2013; https://doi.org/10.2500/ajra.2013.27.3976.
33. Wang X, Zhang N, Bo M, Holtappels G, Zheng M, Lou H, Wang H, Zhang L, Bachert C. Diversity of T_H cytokine profiles in patients with chronic rhinosinusitis: a multicenter study in Europe, Asia, and Oceania. J Allergy Clin Immunol. 2016; https://doi.org/10.1016/j.jaci.2016.05.041.
34. Wang ET, Zheng Y, Liu PF, Guo LJ. Eosinophilic chronic rhinosinusitis in East Asians. World J Clin Cases. 2014; https://doi.org/10.12998/wjcc.v2.i12.873.
35. Yao Y, Yang C, Yi X, Xie S, Sun H. Comparative analysis of inflammatory signature profiles in eosinophilic and noneosinophilic chronic rhinosinusitis with nasal polyposis. Biosci Rep. 2020; https://doi.org/10.1042/BSR20193101.

36. Mahdavinia M, Suh LA, Carter RG, Stevens WW, Norton JE, Kato A, Tan BK, Kern RC, Conley DB, Chandra R, Lavin J, Peters AT, Grammer LC 3rd, Schleimer RP. Increased noneosinophilic nasal polyps in chronic rhinosinusitis in US second-generation Asians suggest genetic regulation of eosinophilia. J Allergy Clin Immunol. 2015; https://doi.org/10.1016/j.jaci.2014.08.031.
37. Katotomichelakis M, Tantilipikorn P, Holtappels G, De Ruyck N, Feng L, Van Zele T, Muangsomboon S, Jareonchasri P, Bunnag C, Danielides V, Cuvelier CA, Hellings PW, Bachert C, Zhang N. Inflammatory patterns in upper airway disease in the same geographical area may change over time. Am J Rhinol Allergy. 2013; https://doi.org/10.2500/ajra.2013.27.3922.
38. Kim SJ, Lee KH, Kim SW, Cho JS, Park YK, Shin SY. Changes in histological features of nasal polyps in a Korean population over a 17-year period. Otolaryngol Head Neck Surg. 2013; https://doi.org/10.1177/0194599813495363.
39. Staudacher AG, Peters AT, Kato A, Stevens WW. Use of endotypes, phenotypes, and inflammatory markers to guide treatment decisions in chronic rhinosinusitis. Ann Allergy Asthma Immunol. 2020; https://doi.org/10.1016/j.anai.2020.01.013.
40. Tau G, Rothman P. Biologic functions of the IFN-gamma receptors. Allergy. 1999; https://doi.org/10.1034/j.1398-9995.1999.00099.x.
41. Valeri M, Raffatellu M. Cytokines IL-17 and IL-22 in the host response to infection. Pathog Dis. 2016; https://doi.org/10.1093/femspd/ftw111.
42. Junttila IS. Tuning the cytokine responses: an update on Interleukin (IL)-4 and IL-13 receptor complexes. Front Immunol. 2018; https://doi.org/10.3389/fimmu.2018.00888.
43. Kato A, Schleimer RP, Bleier BS. Mechanisms and pathogenesis of chronic rhinosinusitis. J Allergy Clin Immunol. 2022; https://doi.org/10.1016/j.jaci.2022.02.016.
44. Tomassen P, Vandeplas G, Van Zele T, Cardell LO, Arebro J, Olze H, Förster-Ruhrmann U, Kowalski ML, Olszewska-Ziąber A, Holtappels G, De Ruyck N, Wang X, Van Drunen C, Mullol J, Hellings P, Hox V, Toskala E, Scadding G, Lund V, Zhang L, Fokkens W, Bachert C. Inflammatory endotypes of chronic rhinosinusitis based on cluster analysis of biomarkers. J Allergy Clin Immunol. 2016; https://doi.org/10.1016/j.jaci.2015.12.1324.
45. Gevaert P, Omachi TA, Corren J, Mullol J, Han J, Lee SE, Kaufman D, Ligueros-Saylan M, Howard M, Zhu R, Owen R, Wong K, Islam L, Bachert C. Efficacy and safety of omalizumab in nasal polyposis: 2 randomized phase 3 trials. J Allergy Clin Immunol. 2021; https://doi.org/10.1016/j.jaci.2020.05.032.
46. Bachert C, Sousa AR, Lund VJ, Scadding GK, Gevaert P, Nasser S, Durham SR, Cornet ME, Kariyawasam HH, Gilbert J, Austin D, Maxwell AC, Marshall RP, Fokkens WJ. Reduced need for surgery in severe nasal polyposis with mepolizumab: randomized trial. J Allergy Clin Immunol. 2017; https://doi.org/10.1016/j.jaci.2017.05.044.
47. Bachert C, Han JK, Desrosiers M, Hellings PW, Amin N, Lee SE, Mullol J, Greos LS, Bosso JV, Laidlaw TM, Cervin AU, Maspero JF, Hopkins C, Olze H, Canonica GW, Paggiaro P, Cho SH, Fokkens WJ, Fujieda S, Zhang M, Lu X, Fan C, Draikiwicz S, Kamat SA, Khan A, Pirozzi G, Patel N, Graham NMH, Ruddy M, Staudinger H, Weinreich D, Stahl N, Yancopoulos GD, Mannent LP. Efficacy and safety of dupilumab in patients with severe chronic rhinosinusitis with nasal polyps (LIBERTY NP SINUS-24 and LIBERTY NP SINUS-52): results from two multicentre, randomised, double-blind, placebo-controlled, parallel-group phase 3 trials. Lancet. 2019; https://doi.org/10.1016/S0140-6736(19)31881-1.
48. Gurrola J 2nd, Borish L. Chronic rhinosinusitis: endotypes, biomarkers, and treatment response. J Allergy Clin Immunol. 2017; https://doi.org/10.1016/j.jaci.2017.10.006.
49. Cardell LO, Stjärne P, Jonstam K, Bachert C. Endotypes of chronic rhinosinusitis: impact on management. J Allergy Clin Immunol. 2020; https://doi.org/10.1016/j.jaci.2020.01.019.

Part II

Surgical Procedures for Recalcitrant CRS

Revision Endoscopic Sinus Surgery: Maxillary, Ethmoid, and Sphenoid

2

John R. Craig

Key Points

- Revision endoscopic sinus surgery (ESS) should be considered in patients with objectively confirmed sinusitis who continue to suffer from sinonasal symptoms following prior ESS and appropriate medical therapy.
- Clinical features that may increase the risk of ESS failure should be considered when managing refractory chronic rhinosinusitis patients. These include nasal polyps, asthma, frontal sinus disease, and a history of prior ESS.
- Certain maneuvers such as complete ethmoid dissection, middle turbinate resection, and septoplasty may lead to improved ESS outcomes and should be considered during revision ESS.
- When revision ESS is appropriately selected and performed for chronic rhinosinusitis patients, it should lead to symptomatic improvements that are equivalent to primary ESS.

Indications

The indications for revision endoscopic sinus surgery (ESS) are generally the same as for primary ESS. After ESS, patients complaining of cardinal symptoms of CRS (nasal obstruction, anterior and posterior nasal drainage, smell loss, facial pressure) due to confirmed inflammatory and/or infectious sinus disease on nasal endoscopy or

Supplementary Information The online version contains supplementary material available at https://doi.org/10.1007/978-3-031-89191-5_2.

J. R. Craig (✉)
Department of Otolaryngology-Head and Neck Surgery, Henry Ford Health, Detroit, MI, USA
e-mail: Jcraig1@hfhs.org

J. T. Lee et al. (eds.), *Advances in Surgical and Medical Interventions for Recalcitrant Chronic Rhinosinusitis*,
https://doi.org/10.1007/978-3-031-89191-5_2

imaging modalities should be offered revision ESS when they fail one or more courses of appropriate medical management [1]. Revision ESS may also be necessary if patients develop iatrogenic sinus disease from scarring like mucoceles, regardless of symptoms.

Once patients meet criteria for revision ESS, surgeons must determine why the previous ESS failed, and which sinuses require revision surgery to alleviate patients' symptoms or prevent future complications from scarring of the sinonasal cavities. The next sections will discuss reported outcomes of primary and revision ESS, as well as patient-related and technical reasons for ESS failures. These reasons for ESS failure will then be considered when performing revision ESS.

Outcomes of Primary and Revision ESS

Most published ESS success rates relate to primary ESS. Multiple studies have shown improvement in cardinal sinusitis symptoms following ESS in 90–100% of chronic rhinosinusitis (CRS) cases, [2, 3] recurrent acute rhinosinusitis, [4] odontogenic sinusitis when the dental infectious source is controlled, [5] and paranasal sinus fungal balls [6]. Most literature on long-term ESS failure rates pertains to chronic rhinosinusitis with or without nasal polyps (CRSwNP, CRSsNP), with 4–19% of primary cases requiring revision ESS [7–10]. When necessary for CRS, revision ESS is performed on average about 2–5 years after primary ESS, but time to revision is shorter for patients with CRSwNP [8, 11–13]. There have been fewer publications on revision ESS outcomes, but studies to date have demonstrated similar degrees of symptomatic improvement in CRS patients when comparing primary to revision ESS [14–16]. Also important, a study based on all-payer claims databases showed equivalent rates of major complications after revision ESS (0.46%) compared to primary ESS (0.36%) [17]. However, some minor complications may be more common after revision ESS, like synechiae [18].

Risk Factors for ESS Failure

Multiple studies have demonstrated various patient-related and technical (surgical) factors that may place patients at risk for requiring revision ESS. One of the most frequently cited patient-related factors that contributes to revision ESS is CRSwNP, [8, 9]. Revision rates also increase in the setting of tissue eosinophilia, [19], eosinophilic mucin, [20] and aspirin sensitivity [13]. Additionally, allergic rhinitis [9, 21] and asthma [11] independently increase the risk of revision ESS for CRS. Other reported risk factors for revision ESS include female gender, [8, 9] older age [9], smoking, [12] frontal sinus disease, [9, 13] prior revision ESS, [9] bacterial biofilms, [1, 22, 23] immunodeficiency, [7, 24] cystic fibrosis, [25] and granulomatosis with polyangiitis [7]. Another possible source of ESS failure is odontogenic sinusitis when the infectious dental source is either overlooked or inadequately treated [5, 26, 27].

Regarding technical factors, multiple studies have shown that certain computed tomography (CT) or endoscopic findings are common in patients undergoing revision ESS, and presumably these anatomic or pathologic findings contributed to the ESS failures. Common CT and endoscopic findings in patients undergoing revision ESS include residual ethmoid sinus partitions (50–96%), osteitis or neo-osteogenesis (66%), nasal polyps (20–60%), synechiae (20–56%) (Fig. 2.1), middle turbinate (MT) scarring/lateralization (8–78%) (Fig. 2.2), residual uncinate plus maxillary recirculation (4–52%) (Fig. 2.3), and maxillary, sphenoid, or frontal sinus stenosis (15–48%) [28–33]. While it is reasonable to presume these findings contribute to ESS failures, future studies should correlate these findings with sinonasal symptoms to understand which findings are most important to address with revision ESS.

Two features that have been associated with worse symptomatic outcomes after ESS include synechiae and osteitis. Sinus synechiae can occur anywhere in the sinonasal cavities after ESS. The location and extent of synechiae may be a factor in the severity of persistent symptoms after ESS and the need for subsequent revision ESS [18]. Another common finding in CRS patients who have had prior ESS is osteitis (neo-osteogenesis) of sinus walls or partitions, [34–36] especially in the ethmoid sinus [37]. Osteitis has been correlated with worsened objective measures of disease severity on CT, endoscopy, and olfactory scores, [38] and may worsen postoperative outcomes after ESS [34, 39]. One literature review concluded that osteitic bone should be removed during ESS when feasible, [38] but more research is necessary to determine the prognostic significance and optimal management of osteitis in CRS.

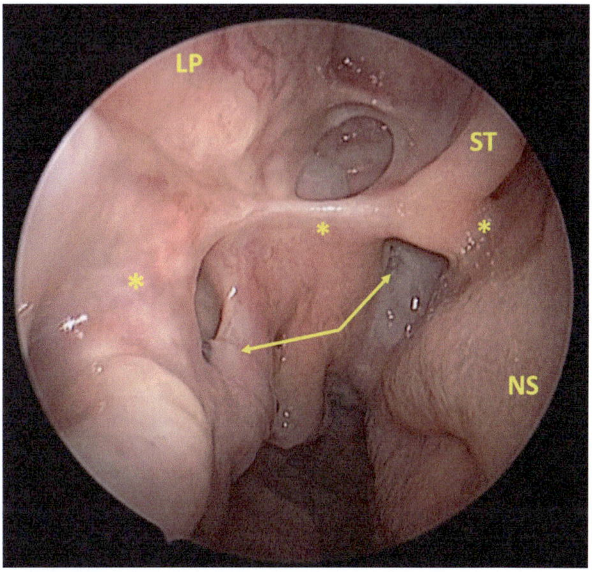

Fig. 2.1 Endoscopic view of right-sided sinus cavities after prior endoscopic sinus surgery, demonstrating multiple synechiae (yellow asterisks), and thick mucus that may be related to possible recirculation or stenotic ostia (yellow arrows). *LP* lamina papyracea, *ST* superior turbinate, *NS* nasal septum

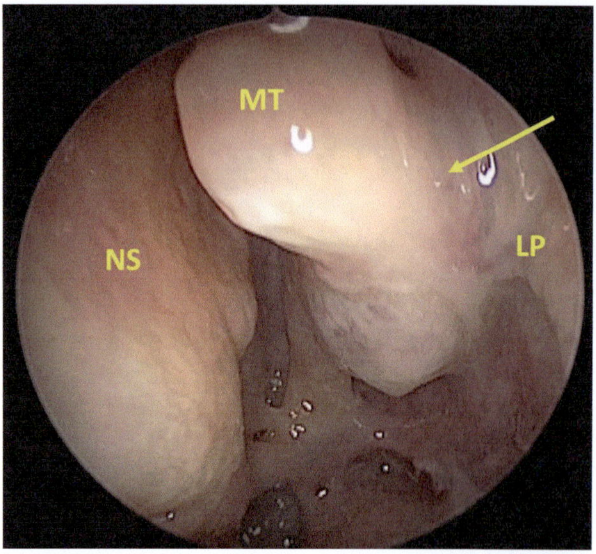

Fig. 2.2 Endoscopic view of left-sided sinus cavities after prior endoscopic sinus surgery, demonstrating a partially resected middle turbinate (MT) with the superior portion having scarred to the lamina papyracea (LP) (yellow arrow). Scarring in this region can cause frontal sinus outflow obstruction and either frontal sinusitis or mucocele. *NS* nasal septum

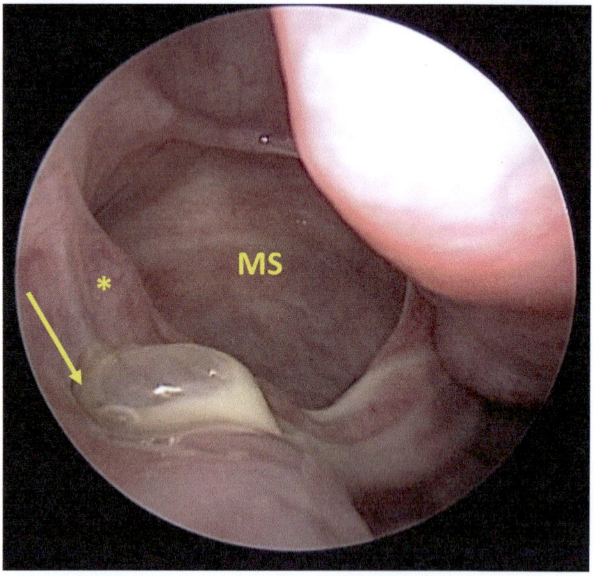

Fig. 2.3 Endoscopic view of prior right-sided endoscopic maxillary antrostomy, with evidence of recirculation due to either incomplete dissection of the anterior aspect of the antrostomy leaving residual uncinate tissue, or scarring in this region after complete antrostomy (yellow asterisk). Mucopurulence is seen draining from the natural ostium (yellow arrow) back into the maxillary sinus (MS), and posteriorly through the middle meatus into the nasopharynx

Surgical Techniques to Address Risk Factors for ESS Failure

Multiple studies have demonstrated that certain surgical techniques improve symptomatic results and prolong time to revision ESS. These studies have generally been conducted in the setting of primary ESS for CRS, but this data will be extrapolated to revision ESS for this chapter.

In patients with CRSwNP, one of the most common conditions requiring revision ESS, the decision to perform more extensive ESS results in decreased polyp recurrence rates, lower revision ESS rates, and longer times to revision ESS when compared to the conventional functional ESS. Extensive ESS refers to wide openings being created into each sinus with complete removal of ethmoid sinus and frontal recess partitions with middle turbinate resection (MTR) [40–43]. The end result is creating a common cavity between all the sinus cavities to improve topical saline and drug delivery, disease monitoring, and sinus debridements (Fig. 2.4) [1]. Surgeons should consider more extensive ESS in CRSwNP patients for both primary and revision cases. It remains to be studied whether extensive ESS is more effective during revision ESS in conditions other than CRS, but may be necessary in some cases if it can be performed safely.

Middle turbinate resection (MTR) is a frequent point of debate during ESS. Partial and subtotal MTR during ESS for CRSwNP have been shown to be safe, with extremely low rates of postoperative epistaxis, frontal sinus stenosis, cerebrospinal fluid leaks, empty nose syndrome, and hyposmia/anosmia [44–48]. While there is mixed evidence in the literature with regard to efficacy of MTR during ESS for CRSwNP, multiple studies have shown a preponderance of benefit with improved sinonasal quality-of-life (QOL) [43], olfaction, [41, 48, 49] sinus topical irrigation delivery, [50] decreased polyp recurrence, [21, 40–42] decreased need for revision ESS, [40, 42, 43] and longer times to revision ESS [12, 43]. Conversely, some studies have shown no significant differences in QOL improvements with MTR versus MT preservation during primary ESS for CRS [49, 51, 52]. Interestingly, Scangas,

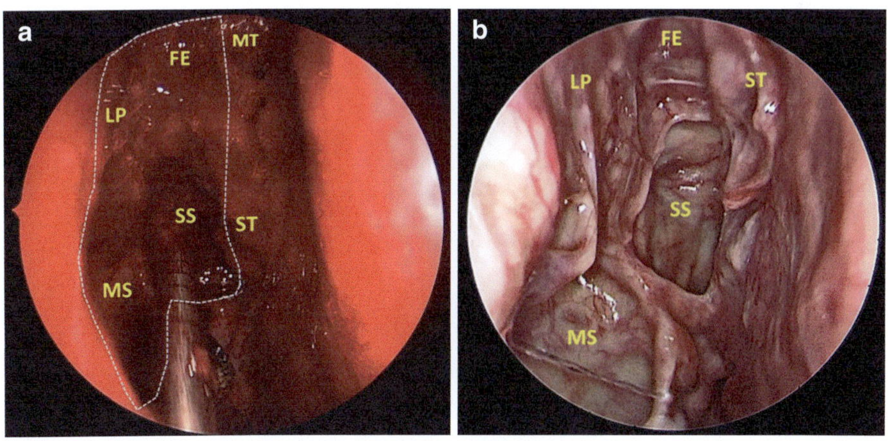

Fig. 2.4 Endoscopic view of sinus cavities **a**, immediately, and **b**, 6 months postoperatively after extensive right-sided endoscopic sinus surgery. The maxillary (MS), ethmoid, and sphenoid sinuses (SS) appear to communicate as a common cavity, after wide maxillary antrostomy and sphenoidotomy, and removing all ethmoid partitions between the superior turbinate (ST) and lamina papyracea (LP), and superiorly to the fovea ethmoidalis (FE). The middle turbinate was subtotally resected, with a small remnant left superiorly along the cribriform plate (not seen in **b** with the 0° view)

et al. showed that while bilateral MTR did not improve QOL after primary ESS, it did improve sinonasal QOL after revision ESS [52]. Given the high prevalence of MT scarring and lateralization at the time of revision ESS for CRS, and improved outcomes after primary and revision ESS for CRSwNP, there is good reason to perform MTR at the time of revision ESS for CRS, especially for CRswNP.

There are also some considerations that have mixed evidence to date, but may improve surgical outcomes. Should patients undergo septoplasty during ESS? A recent matched case-control study showed that in patients undergoing revision ESS, having an untreated deviated nasal septum was an independent predictor of worsened disease severity, and therefore could contribute to ESS failures [53]. While some studies have shown no significant differences in QOL in patients getting ESS versus ESS plus septoplasty, [54] more studies have shown reductions in revision ESS when septoplasty is performed with ESS [55, 56]. The recent international consensus statement on rhinosinusitis recommended concurrent septoplasty during ESS when the septum is notably deviated, given a preponderance of published literature demonstrating improved nasal obstruction, improved ESS access (Fig. 2.5), and possibly a reduced need for revision ESS [1].

Another consideration during revision ESS is whether inferior turbinate reduction (ITR) should be performed. Soudry, et al. conducted a multi-center prospective cohort study of patients undergoing primary or revision ESS with or without bilateral ITR. While ITR did not result in differences in overall QOL metrics, it did lead to improved nasal obstruction scores [57]. In summary, if patients have prominent nasal obstruction and clinically evident septal deviation or inferior turbinate

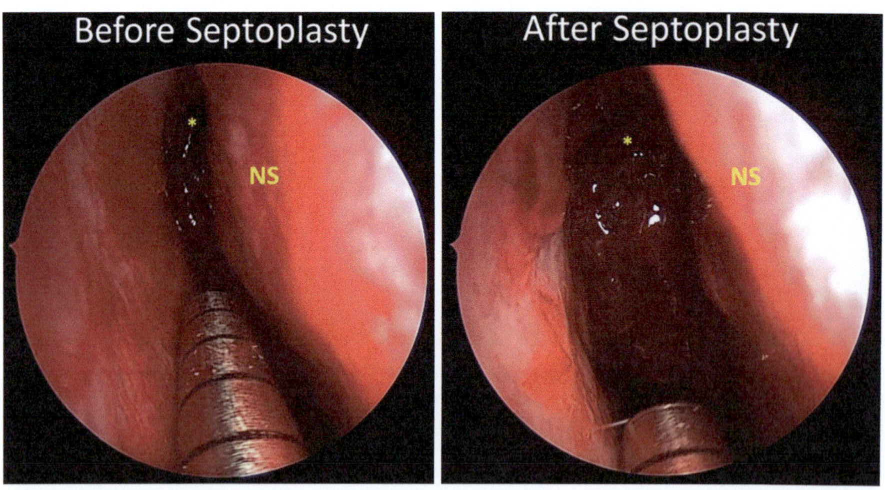

Fig. 2.5 Endoscopic views of the right nasal cavity during revision endoscopic sinus surgery, demonstrating the improvement in medial-to-lateral dimension between the nasal septum (NS) (**a**) and the lateral nasal wall after endoscopic septoplasty (**b**). This greatly improved surgical access to the ethmoid sinus and frontal recess regions. Additionally, this improved the patient's nasal airflow on this side

hypertrophy, septoplasty and/or ITR may provide additional benefit when performed with ESS. Regardless of symptoms, these techniques may improve intraoperative access for sinus dissection, and postoperative access for sinus disease monitoring and debridements.

One final point to discuss is the use of image-guided surgery, which has become commonly used by many surgeons during ESS. While evidence has been mixed with regard to whether image-guided surgery improves outcomes and decreases complications, the recent international consensus on rhinosinusitis presented multiple studies showing its benefits, especially in advanced or revision ESS, and recommended it as a viable option during ESS [1].

Surgical Technique

All patients should undergo preoperative CT evaluation to identify anatomic reasons for persistent disease, locations of persistent disease, and anatomy that may be high-risk for complications and for surgical failure intra-operatively [58]. Specific attention should be paid to anatomy that can contribute to persistent disease or limit access to all sinuses and ostia, areas of residual bony partitions with or without osteitis/neo-osteogenesis, lateralization of middle turbinates, and deviated nasal septum. High-risk anatomy to consider includes orbital and/or skull base dehiscences, high maxillary:ethmoid high ratio, low-lying anterior ethmoid arteries, dehiscences of the optic nerve or carotid artery, and the presence of Onodi (sphenoethmoid) cells.

Intra-operatively, the head of the bed should be elevated, either by placing the patient in reverse Trendelenburg or placing the patient in a head-up flexed position to approximately 20° from the horizontal, to improve hemostasis during the case [59]. Decongesting the nasal cavities should be performed early and can be performed with either topical epinephrine 1:1000, oxymetazoline, or cocaine on nasal pledgets. Once adequate time has been allowed for nasal decongestion, approximately 5–10 min, nasal endoscopy is performed. The goals of this initial endoscopy are to assess for areas of obstruction or previous treatment failure. First, surgeons should assess the septum and inferior turbinates; if they are preventing access to the middle meatus, sphenoethmoid recess, or frontal recess, surgeons should consider septoplasty +/− inferior turbinate outfracture or reduction. Next, the sinus drainage pathways should be assessed for areas of current disease, specifically for scarring, purulence, edema, or polyps. If purulence is present, cultures should be obtained for targeted antibiotics in the perioperative period.

The middle turbinate should also be assessed. Surgeons should consider MTR for CRSwNP, or in other cases where the MT is felt to be high risk for scarring and lateralization. MTR can be performed prior to opening sinuses to improve surgical access, leaving a remnant superiorly as a landmark for the medial extent of ethmoidectomy and for identifying skull base. Alternatively, MTR can be performed after finishing ESS, if surgeons prefer to leave the MT completely intact as landmark during surgery. If septoplasty is necessary for surgical access to the sinuses, it can be performed up front, or one side of sinuses can be completed on the less obstructed side, then the septoplasty can be performed before performing ESS on the narrower nasal cavity side.

Once access has been addressed, a wide maxillary antrostomy is performed. This included a complete uncinectomy and removal of the maxillary fontanelle mucosa, creating an opening from the inferior turbinate insertion inferiorly to the maxillary sinus roof superiorly, and from the nasolacrimal canal anteriorly to the palatine bone posteriorly. It is ideal to complete the anterior extent of the antrostomy under either 45° or 70° endoscopic visualization to ensure optimal tissue removal at the anterosuperior corner of the antrostomy to minimize the risk of scarring and recirculation (Fig. 2.6) [60]. This can be done during the initial antrostomy, or after completing the frontal sinusotomy later in the case when an angled scope is being used.

After completing the maxillary antrostomy, a total ethmoidectomy is performed. All bony partitions, polyps, and fibro-osseous scar tissue are removed to the boundaries of the anterior and posterior ethmoid sinuses. The lamina papyracea is identified laterally early during the anterior ethmoid dissection, and all ethmoid partitions are removed to this boundary posteriorly until reaching the sphenoid sinus face. Initially it is wise to complete the dissection low in the posterior ethmoid cavity at approximately the level of maxillary sinus roof, to minimize the chance of skull base injury [61]. The sphenoidotomy can be completed before completing ethmoid partition removal along the ethmoid roof, as opening the sphenoid face superiorly facilitates identification of the skull base.

For the sphenoidotomy, surgeons should first identify the superior turbinate along the medial aspect of the posterior ethmoid dissection, adjacent to the nasal septum. One can draw an imaginary line from the maxillary sinus roof over to the nasal septum (Fig. 2.7) which gives the approximate height of the sphenoid ostium,

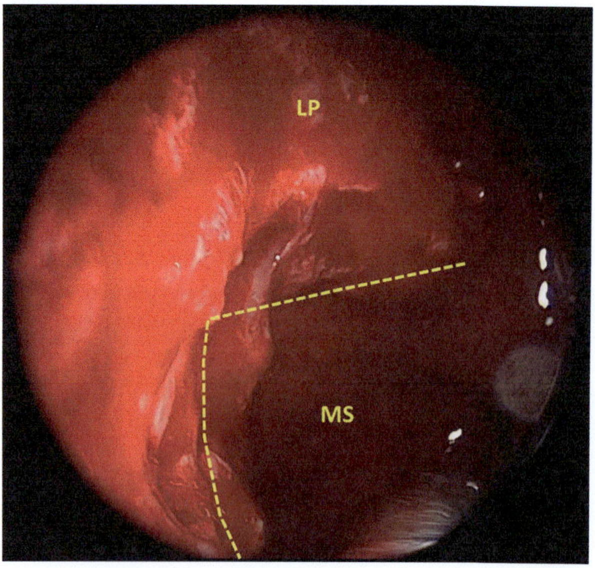

Fig. 2.6 Endoscopic view with a 70° endoscope showing the anterior extent of a completed maxillary antrostomy. The goal is to achieve a crisp, usually acute, angle at the anterosuperior corner of the antrostomy. In this case, there was fibrous tissue at the anterosuperior corner that could not be removed further, but this opening remained perfectly patent and functional (dotted yellow line). *MS* maxillary sinus, *LP* lamina papyracea

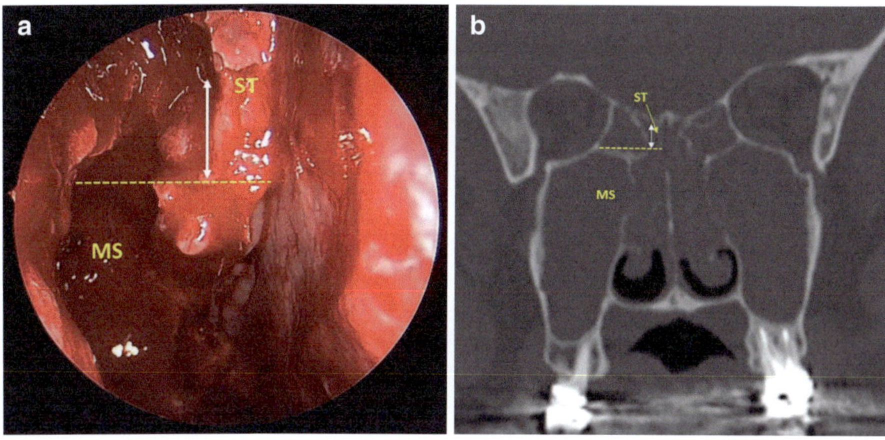

Fig. 2.7 Using the maxillary sinus floor as a fixed landmark to facilitate posterior ethmoid and sphenoid sinus dissections. (**a**) an imaginary horizontal line is drawn from the maxillary sinus roof over to the nasal septum, and this helps the surgeon appreciate that the skull base will be above this line, and therefore it should be safe dissecting posteriorly at or below this level. Additionally, the sphenoid sinus ostium is generally identified posterior and/or medial to the superior turbinate, at approximately the level of this horizontal line. (**b**) coronal CT correlation in this patient with the horizontal line being drawn from the maxillary sinus roof to the nasal septum. This highlights that in patients with a tall maxillary sinus (high maxillary: ethmoid sinus height ratio), the cribriform plate can be quite close to the level of the maxillary sinus roof in the posterior ethmoid sinus. Therefore, surgeons must be careful dissecting superiorly in the posterior ethmoid sinus, especially medially near the lateral lamella of the cribriform plate (white double arrows represent the height to the skull base from the medial aspect of the horizontal line). *MS* maxillary sinus, *ST* superior turbinate

and the posterior wall of the maxillary sinus is typically in the same coronal plane as the sphenoid sinus face. At the level of the maxillary sinus roof, the inferior 1/3 to 1/2 of the superior turbinate is removed until reaching the anterior face of the sphenoid sinus. The sphenoid ostium is then usually seen, and can be cannulated with blunt probing instruments. The ostium can then be widened to allow for insertion of through-cutting forceps and Kerrison Rongeurs to remove the anterior face of the sphenoid sinus from the nasal septum medially to the medial orbital wall laterally, and from the choanal rim inferiorly to the skull base superiorly. The posterior septal branch of the sphenopalatine artery may be encountered during removal of the sphenoid face inferiorly. It can be avoided by first dissecting the mucosa off the sphenoid face inferiorly, but if injured, it is easy to control with suction monopolar cautery, and this should not significantly increase the risk of postoperative epistaxis or stenosis [62] (Video 2.1).

At this point, the fovea ethmoidalis should be apparent at its junction with the planum sphenoidale. This point generally indicates the lowest point of the skull base and dissection of the ethmoid roof can then be performed more safely in a posterior to anterior direction. Under 30°, 45°, or 70° endoscopic visualization, ethmoid bony partitions are removed to their insertions along the fovea ethmoidalis superiorly, lamina papyracea laterally, and middle and superior turbinates medially, until reaching the frontal recess. Be careful to avoid injuries to the skull base, orbit, and anterior ethmoid artery. Frontal sinus dissection is covered in Chaps. 7, 9, 10, and 11 of this text and will not be covered in this chapter. In general, the largest frontal sinusotomy that adequately evacuates all frontal sinus disease and optimizes post-operative postoperative ostial patency is recommended during revision ESS. This could involve Draf IIA, IIB, or III depending on patient factors and sinus ostial scarring.

The final result of this surgery should be a common cavity between all the sinuses on one side, from the middle and superior turbinates medially to the lamina papyracea laterally, and from the inferior aspect of the maxillary antrostomy inferiorly to the skull base superiorly (Fig. 2.4). Consider sinus packings or stents at the end of ESS, like chitosan-based or steroid-impregnated absorbable packings, steroid-eluting stents, or silastic stents. It is beyond the scope of this chapter to discuss the literature on these materials, but these packing options have been recognized as options to improve ESS outcomes by decreasing risks of synechiae formation and ostial stenosis [1].

Other Operative Points

Hemostasis should be maintained throughout surgery to optimize surgical field visualization and decrease the risk of major complications. Topical epinephrine 1:1000 on wrung-out nasal cotton pledgets suffices to achieve hemostasis during ESS and should not result in dangerous hemodynamic parameter changes [63–65]. On the contrary, submucosally injected epinephrine 1:100,000 provides no improvement in surgical field visualization over topical epinephrine 1:1000 on pledgets alone [65] and is more likely to cause hemodynamic parameter changes during ESS [63]. Therefore, surgeons should consider using only topical epinephrine 1:1000 on wrung-out pledgets during ESS. Additionally, surgeons should aim to leave healthy mucoperiosteum intact along the bony boundaries of the sinus cavities and ostia to facilitate wound healing and minimize osteitis/neo-osteogenesis, scar formation, and sinus stenosis. Due to higher rates of neo-osteogenesis during revision ESS, surgeons may also need high-speed diamond burs to remove the osteitic bone.

Tips and Pearls

- Assess for patient-related and technical reasons for prior ESS failure.
- Address the disease plus the anatomy that explain patients' symptoms.
- Topical epinephrine 1:1000 applied via wrung-out cotton pledgets alone is sufficient for hemostasis, without the need for injectable epinephrine.
- Create a common cavity between all the sinuses on each side by removing bony partitions and debris to the bony boundaries of each sinus cavity.
  - Use fixed bony landmarks to facilitate dissection and avoid critical structures.
  - MTR is generally beneficial and safe.

- Remove osteitic bone when feasible.
- Consider concurrent septoplasty +/− ITR to improve surgical access as well as nasal obstruction outcomes.

References

1. Orlandi RR, Kingdom TT, Smith TL, Bleier B, DeConde A, Luong AU, et al. International consensus statement on allergy and rhinology: rhinosinusitis 2021. Int Forum Allergy Rhinol. 2021;11:213–739. https://doi.org/10.1002/alr.22741.
2. DeConde AS, Mace JC, Alt JA, Soler ZM, Orlandi RR, Smith TL. Investigation of change in cardinal symptoms of chronic rhinosinusitis after surgical or ongoing medical management. Int Forum Allergy Rhinol. 2015;5:36–45. https://doi.org/10.1002/alr.21410.
3. Senior BA, Kennedy DW, Tanabodee J, Kroger H, Hassab M, Lanza D. Long-term results of functional endoscopic sinus surgery. Laryngoscope. 1998;108:151–7. https://doi.org/10.1097/00005537-199802000-00001.
4. Costa ML, Psaltis AJ, Nayak JV, Hwang PH. Medical therapy vs surgery for recurrent acute rhinosinusitis. Int Forum Allergy Rhinol. 2015;5:667–73. https://doi.org/10.1002/alr.21533.
5. Craig JR, Tataryn RW, Aghaloo TL, Pokorny AT, Gray ST, Mattos JL, et al. Management of odontogenic sinusitis: multidisciplinary consensus statement. Int Forum Allergy Rhinol. 2020;10:901–12. https://doi.org/10.1002/alr.22598.
6. Fadda GL, Allevi F, Rosso C, Martino F, Pipolo C, Cavallo G, et al. Treatment of paranasal sinus fungus ball: a systematic review and meta-analysis. Ann Otol Rhinol Laryngol. 2021;130:1302–10. https://doi.org/10.1177/00034894211002431.
7. Miglani A, Divekar RD, Azar A, Rank MA, Lal D. Revision endoscopic sinus surgery rates by chronic rhinosinusitis subtype. Int Forum Allergy Rhinol. 2018;8:1047–51. https://doi.org/10.1002/alr.22146.
8. Stein NR, Jafari A, DeConde AS. Revision rates and time to revision following endoscopic sinus surgery: a large database analysis. Laryngoscope. 2018;128:31–6. https://doi.org/10.1002/lary.26741.
9. Smith KA, Orlandi RR, Oakley G, Meeks H, Curtin K, Alt JA. Long-term revision rates for endoscopic sinus surgery. Int Forum Allergy Rhinol. 2019;9:402–8. https://doi.org/10.1002/alr.22264.
10. Hopkins C, Slack R, Lund V, Brown P, Copley L, Browne J. Long-term outcomes from the English national comparative audit of surgery for nasal polyposis and chronic rhinosinusitis. Laryngoscope. 2009;119:2459–65. https://doi.org/10.1002/lary.20653.
11. Gill AS, Smith KA, Meeks H, Oakley GM, Curtin K, LeClair L, et al. Asthma increases long-term revision rates of endoscopic sinus surgery in chronic rhinosinusitis with and without nasal polyposis. Int Forum Allergy Rhinol. 2021;11:1197–206. https://doi.org/10.1002/alr.22779.
12. Wu AW, Ting JY, Platt MP, Tierney HT, Metson R. Factors affecting time to revision sinus surgery for nasal polyps: a 25-year experience. Laryngoscope. 2014;124:29–33. https://doi.org/10.1002/lary.24213.
13. Mendelsohn D, Jeremic G, Wright ED, Rotenberg BW. Revision rates after endoscopic sinus surgery: a recurrence analysis. Ann Otol Rhinol Laryngol. 2011;120:162–6. https://doi.org/10.1177/000348941112000304.
14. Bhattacharyya N. Clinical outcomes after revision endoscopic sinus surgery. Arch Otolaryngol Head Neck Surg. 2004;130:975–8. https://doi.org/10.1001/archotol.130.8.975.
15. Prasad S, Fong E, Ooi EH. Systematic review of patient-reported outcomes after revision endoscopic sinus surgery. Am J Rhinol Allergy. 2017;31:248–55. https://doi.org/10.2500/ajra.2017.31.4446.

16. Litvack JR, Griest S, James KE, Smith TL. Endoscopic and quality-of-life outcomes after revision endoscopic sinus surgery. Laryngoscope. 2007;117:2233–8. https://doi.org/10.1097/MLG.0b013e31814539e8.
17. Krings JG, Kallogjeri D, Wineland A, Nepple KG, Piccirillo JF, Getz AE. Complications of primary and revision functional endoscopic sinus surgery for chronic rhinosinusitis. Laryngoscope. 2014;124:838–45. https://doi.org/10.1002/lary.24401.
18. Henriquez OA, Schlosser RJ, Mace JC, Smith TL, Soler ZM. Impact of synechiae after endoscopic sinus surgery on long-term outcomes in chronic rhinosinusitis. Laryngoscope. 2013;123:2615–9. https://doi.org/10.1002/lary.24150.
19. Tosun F, Arslan HH, Karslioglu Y, Deveci MS, Durmaz A. Relationship between postoperative recurrence rate and eosinophil density of nasal polyps. Ann Otol Rhinol Laryngol. 2010;119:455–9. https://doi.org/10.1177/000348941011900705.
20. Younis RT, Ahmed J. Predicting revision sinus surgery in allergic fungal and eosinophilic mucin chronic rhinosinusitis. Laryngoscope. 2017;127:59–63. https://doi.org/10.1002/lary.26248.
21. Marchioni D, Alicandri-Ciufelli M, Mattioli F, Marchetti A, Jovic G, Massone F, et al. Middle turbinate preservation versus middle turbinate resection in endoscopic surgical treatment of nasal polyposis. Acta Otolaryngol. 2008;128:1019–26. https://doi.org/10.1080/00016480701827541.
22. Singhal D, Psaltis AJ, Foreman A, Wormald PJ. The impact of biofilms on outcomes after endoscopic sinus surgery. Am J Rhinol Allergy. 2010;24:169–74. https://doi.org/10.2500/ajra.2010.24.3462.
23. Zhang Z, Linkin DR, Finkelman BS, O'Malley BW Jr, Thaler ER, Doghramji L, et al. Asthma and biofilm-forming bacteria are independently associated with revision sinus surgeries for chronic rhinosinusitis. J Allergy Clin Immunol. 2011;128:221–3.e1. https://doi.org/10.1016/j.jaci.2011.02.022.
24. Samargandy S, Grose E, Chan Y, Monteiro E, Lee JM, Yip J. Medical and surgical treatment outcomes in patients with chronic rhinosinusitis and immunodeficiency: a systematic review. Int Forum Allergy Rhinol. 2021;11:162–73. https://doi.org/10.1002/alr.22647.
25. Krajewska J, Zub K, Słowikowski A, Zatoński T. Chronic rhinosinusitis in cystic fibrosis: a review of therapeutic options. Eur Arch Otorhinolaryngol. 2022;279:1–24. https://doi.org/10.1007/s00405-021-06875-6.
26. Longhini AB, Branstetter BF, Ferguson BJ. Unrecognized odontogenic maxillary sinusitis: a cause of endoscopic sinus surgery failure. Am J Rhinol Allergy. 2010;24:296–300. https://doi.org/10.2500/ajra.2010.24.3479.
27. Albu S, Baciut M. Failures in endoscopic surgery of the maxillary sinus. Otolaryngol Head Neck Surg. 2010;142:196–201. https://doi.org/10.1016/j.otohns.2009.10.038.
28. Schaitkin B, May M, Shapiro A, Fucci M, Mester SJ. Endoscopic sinus surgery: 4-year follow-up on the first 100 patients. Laryngoscope. 1993;103:1117–20. https://doi.org/10.1288/00005537-199310000-00007.
29. Ramadan HH. Surgical causes of failure in endoscopic sinus surgery. Laryngoscope. 1999;109:27–9. https://doi.org/10.1097/00005537-199901000-00006.
30. Chambers DW, Davis WE, Cook PR, Nishioka GJ, Rudman DT. Long-term outcome analysis of functional endoscopic sinus surgery: correlation of symptoms with endoscopic examination findings and potential prognostic variables. Laryngoscope. 1997;107:504–10. https://doi.org/10.1097/00005537-199704000-00014.
31. Musy PY, Kountakis SE. Anatomic findings in patients undergoing revision endoscopic sinus surgery. Am J Otolaryngol. 2004;25:418–22. https://doi.org/10.1016/j.amjoto.2004.06.002.
32. Khalil HS, Eweiss AZ, Clifton N. Radiological findings in patients undergoing revision endoscopic sinus surgery: a retrospective case series study. BMC Ear Nose Throat Disord. 2011;11:4. https://doi.org/10.1186/1472-6815-11-4.
33. Baban MIA, Mirza B, Castelnuovo P. Radiological and endoscopic findings in patients undergoing revision endoscopic sinus surgery. Surg Radiol Anat. 2020;42:1003–12. https://doi.org/10.1007/s00276-020-02427-5.

34. Telmesani LM, Al-Shawarby M. Osteitis in chronic rhinosinusitis with nasal polyps: a comparative study between primary and recurrent cases. Eur Arch Otorhinolaryngol. 2010;267:721–4. https://doi.org/10.1007/s00405-009-1146-x.
35. Sacks PL, Snidvongs K, Rom D, Earls P, Sacks R, Harvey RJ. The impact of neo-osteogenesis on disease control in chronic rhinosinusitis after primary surgery. Int Forum Allergy Rhinol. 2013;3:823–7. https://doi.org/10.1002/alr.21192.
36. Georgalas C, Videler W, Freling N, Fokkens W. Global Osteitis Scoring Scale and chronic rhinosinusitis: a marker of revision surgery. Clin Otolaryngol: Official Journal of ENT-UK; Official Journal of Netherlands Society for Oto-Rhino-Laryngology & Cervico-Facial Surgery. 2010;35:455–61. https://doi.org/10.1111/j.1749-4486.2010.02218.x.
37. Lee JT, Kennedy DW, Palmer JN, Feldman M, Chiu AG. The incidence of concurrent osteitis in patients with chronic rhinosinusitis: a clinicopathological study. Am J Rhinol. 2006;20:278–82. https://doi.org/10.2500/ajr.2006.20.2857.
38. Bhandarkar ND, Sautter NB, Kennedy DW, Smith TL. Osteitis in chronic rhinosinusitis: a review of the literature. Int Forum Allergy Rhinol. 2013;3:355–63. https://doi.org/10.1002/alr.21118.
39. Bhandarkar ND, Mace JC, Smith TL. The impact of osteitis on disease severity measures and quality of life outcomes in chronic rhinosinusitis. Int Forum Allergy Rhinol. 2011;1:372–8. https://doi.org/10.1002/alr.20068.
40. Jankowski R, Pigret D, Decroocq F, Blum A, Gillet P. Comparison of radical (nasalisation) and functional ethmoidectomy in patients with severe sinonasal polyposis. A retrospective study. Rev Laryngol Otol Rhinol (Bord). 2006;127:131–40.
41. Chen FH, Deng J, Hong HY, Xu R, Guo JB, Hou WJ, et al. Extensive versus functional endoscopic sinus surgery for chronic rhinosinusitis with nasal polyps and asthma: a 1-year study. Am J Rhinol Allergy. 2016;30:143–8. https://doi.org/10.2500/ajra.2016.30.4271.
42. Masterson L, Tanweer F, Bueser T, Leong P. Extensive endoscopic sinus surgery: does this reduce the revision rate for nasal polyposis? Eur Arch Otorhinolaryngol. 2010;267:1557–61. https://doi.org/10.1007/s00405-010-1233-z.
43. Zhang L, Zhang Y, Gao Y, Wang K, Lou H, Meng Y, et al. Long-term outcomes of different endoscopic sinus surgery in recurrent chronic rhinosinusitis with nasal polyps and asthma. Rhinology. 2020;58:126–35. https://doi.org/10.4193/Rhin19.184.
44. Pinther S, Deeb R, Peterson EL, Standring RT, Craig JR. Complications are rare from middle turbinate resection: a prospective case series. Am J Rhinol Allergy. 2019;33:657–64. https://doi.org/10.1177/1945892419860299.
45. Law RH, Ahmed AM, Van Harn M, Craig JR. Middle turbinate resection is unlikely to cause empty nose syndrome in first year postoperatively. Am J Otolaryngol. 2021;42:102931. https://doi.org/10.1016/j.amjoto.2021.102931.
46. Miller AJ, Bobian M, Peterson E, Deeb R. Bleeding risk associated with resection of the middle turbinate during functional endoscopic sinus surgery. Am J Rhinol Allergy. 2016;30:140–2. https://doi.org/10.2500/ajra.2016.30.4273.
47. Tan NC, Goggin R, Psaltis AJ, Wormald PJ. Partial resection of the middle turbinate during endoscopic sinus surgery for chronic rhinosinusitis does not lead to an increased risk of empty nose syndrome: a cohort study of a tertiary practice. Int Forum Allergy Rhinol. 2018; https://doi.org/10.1002/alr.22127.
48. Choby GW, Hobson CE, Lee S, Wang EW. Clinical effects of middle turbinate resection after endoscopic sinus surgery: a systematic review. Am J Rhinol Allergy. 2014;28:502–7. https://doi.org/10.2500/ajra.2014.28.4097.
49. Soler ZM, Hwang PH, Mace J, Smith TL. Outcomes after middle turbinate resection: revisiting a controversial topic. Laryngoscope. 2010;120:832–7. https://doi.org/10.1002/lary.20812.
50. Kidwai SM, Parasher AK, Khan MN, Eloy JA, Del Signore A, Iloreta AM, et al. Improved delivery of sinus irrigations after middle turbinate resection during endoscopic sinus surgery. Int Forum Allergy Rhinol. 2017;7:338–42. https://doi.org/10.1002/alr.21894.
51. Byun JY, Lee JY. Middle turbinate resection versus preservation in patients with chronic rhinosinusitis accompanying nasal polyposis: baseline disease burden and surgical outcomes

between the groups. J Otorhinolaryngol Head Neck Surg = Le Journal d'oto-rhino-laryngologie et de chirurgie cervico-faciale. 2012;41:259–64.
52. Scangas GA, Remenschneider AK, Bleier BS, Holbrook EH, Gray ST, Metson RB. Does the timing of middle turbinate resection influence quality-of-life outcomes for patients with chronic rhinosinusitis? Otolaryngol Head Neck Surg. 2017;157:874–9. https://doi.org/10.1177/0194599817706929.
53. Fu T, Lee D, Yip J, Jamal A, Lee JM. Impact of septal deviation on recurrent chronic rhinosinusitis after primary surgery: a matched case-control study. Otolaryngol Head Neck Surg. 2019;160:922–7. https://doi.org/10.1177/0194599818815106.
54. Rudmik L, Mace J, Ferguson BJ, Smith TL. Concurrent septoplasty during endoscopic sinus surgery for chronic rhinosinusitis: does it confound outcomes assessment? Laryngoscope. 2011;121:2679–83. https://doi.org/10.1002/lary.22361.
55. Rudmik L, Xu Y, Alt JA, Deconde A, Smith TL, Schlosser RJ, et al. Evaluating surgeon-specific performance for endoscopic sinus surgery. JAMA Otolaryngol Head Neck Surg. 2017;143:891–8. https://doi.org/10.1001/jamaoto.2017.0752.
56. Chang CC, Tai CJ, Ng TY, Tsou YA, Tsai MH. Can FESS combined with submucosal resection (SMR)/septoplasty reduce revision rate? Otolaryngol Head Neck Surg. 2014;151:700–5. https://doi.org/10.1177/0194599814543778.
57. Soudry E, Mace J, Smith TL, Hwang PH. Role of inferior turbinate reduction in the quality of life of patients undergoing endoscopic sinus surgery for chronic rhinosinusitis. Int Forum Allergy Rhinol. 2019;9:926–33. https://doi.org/10.1002/alr.22356.
58. Error M, Ashby S, Orlandi RR, Alt JA. Single-blinded prospective implementation of a preoperative imaging checklist for endoscopic sinus surgery. Otolaryngol Head Neck Surg. 2018;158:177–80. https://doi.org/10.1177/0194599817731740.
59. Gan EC, Habib AR, Rajwani A, Javer AR. Five-degree, 10-degree, and 20-degree reverse Trendelenburg position during functional endoscopic sinus surgery: a double-blind randomized controlled trial. Int Forum Allergy Rhinol. 2014;4:61–8. https://doi.org/10.1002/alr.21249.
60. Kennedy DW, Adappa ND. Endoscopic maxillary antrostomy: not just a simple procedure. Laryngoscope. 2011;121:2142–5. https://doi.org/10.1002/lary.22169.
61. Harvey RJ, Shelton W, Timperley D, Debnath NI, Byrd K, Buchmann L, et al. Using fixed anatomical landmarks in endoscopic skull base surgery. Am J Rhinol Allergy. 2010;24:301–5. https://doi.org/10.2500/ajra.2010.24.3473.
62. Kam J, Ahmad A, Williams A, Peterson EL, Craig JR. Postoperative epistaxis and sphenoid sinus ostial stenosis after posterior septal branch injury during sphenoidotomy. Int Forum Allergy Rhinol. 2019;9:842–9. https://doi.org/10.1002/alr.22345.
63. Peleman JR, Tarwade P, Han X, Penning DH, Craig JR. Hemodynamic changes with 1:1000 epinephrine on wrung-out pledgets before and during sinus surgery. Ann Otol Rhinol Laryngol. 2021;130:490–6. https://doi.org/10.1177/0003489420959107.
64. Gunaratne DA, Barham HP, Christensen JM, Bhatia DD, Stamm AC, Harvey RJ. Topical concentrated epinephrine (1:1000) does not cause acute cardiovascular changes during endoscopic sinus surgery. Int Forum Allergy Rhinol. 2016;6:135–9. https://doi.org/10.1002/alr.21642.
65. Tangbumrungtham N, Hwang PH, Maul X, Borchard NA, Dholakia SS, Patel ZM, et al. The effect of topical epinephrine 1:1000 with and without infiltration of 1% lidocaine with epinephrine 1:100,000 on endoscopic surgical field visualization: a double-blind randomized controlled study. Int Forum Allergy Rhinol. 2020;10:147–52. https://doi.org/10.1002/alr.22468.

Mega-antrostomy/Endoscopic Medial Maxillectomy for Recalcitrant Chronic Maxillary Rhinosinusitis

3

Noel Ayoub and Peter H. Hwang

Key Points

- Endoscopic maxillary mega antrostomy (EMMA) is a minimally invasive, mucosal-preserving technique that enhances access to the maxillary sinus, permits dependent drainage, and improves endoscopic surveillance.
- EMMA can be performed for recalcitrant chronic rhinosinusitis, or in select cases during primary surgery, such as for patients with cystic fibrosis or primary ciliary dyskinesia.
- Existing data supports the use of EMMA in select patients with improved quality of life, reduced disease burden, and low need for revision surgery.
- EMMA is also an overall safe procedure, although there are potential risks.

Background

Methods to access the maxillary sinus endoscopically have evolved over the years [1–9]. A traditional endoscopic maxillary antrostomy involves removal of the uncinate process and widening of the natural os of the maxillary sinus [10]. Drawbacks of this procedure include limited access to the anterior, lateral, and inferior walls of the maxillary sinus. In 1996, Coleman et al. described the extended middle meatal

Supplementary Information The online version contains supplementary material available at https://doi.org/10.1007/978-3-031-89191-5_3.

N. Ayoub · P. H. Hwang (✉)
Division of Rhinology & Endoscopic Skull Base Surgery, Department of Otolaryngology-Head & Neck Surgery, Stanford University School of Medicine, Stanford, CA, USA
e-mail: nfa@stanford.edu; hwangph@stanford.edu

J. T. Lee et al. (eds.), *Advances in Surgical and Medical Interventions for Recalcitrant Chronic Rhinosinusitis*,
https://doi.org/10.1007/978-3-031-89191-5_3

antrostomy, also called the endoscopic modified medial maxillectomy (EMMM), which included widening of the maxillary antrostomy posteriorly to the posterior wall of the maxillary sinus, inferiorly to the inferior meatus while remaining posterior to Hasner's valve, and with removal of the inferior turbinate [5]. Many other variations have been described, some of which involve removal of the entire inferior turbinate or transection of the nasolacrimal duct (NLD) [3–7]. Some surgeons advocate for a complete inferior turbinectomy to improve access, while most others (including the authors) aim to preserve the anterior 1/3 to ½ of the inferior turbinate to minimize iatrogenic insult and promote mucosal preservation [11]. We also preserve the NLD in endoscopic maxillary mega antrostomy (EMMA).

For the purposes of this discussion, the EMMA will be defined as an endoscopic procedure that includes a maxillary antrostomy with widening of the antrostomy posteriorly to the posterior wall of the maxillary sinus, inferiorly to the floor of the nasal cavity, and anteriorly along the lateral wall of the inferior meatus to Hasner's valve. This extended antrostomy is facilitated by resection of the posterior ½ to 2/3 of the inferior turbinate.

The goal of this mucosal-sparing technique is to increase the size of the maxillary antrostomy enough to promote gravity-dependent drainage of the sinus, improve access for saline irrigations and topical medications, optimize nasal hygiene, and enhance postoperative clinic observation and surveillance.

Anatomy and Key Landmarks

Uncinate process The uncinate process is a sickle-shaped thin bone that represents a medial projection of the ethmoid bone. Situated posterior to the maxillary line, the uncinate process forms the anterior border of the hiatus semilunaris and thus contributes to the ostiomeatal complex (OMC).

Inferior turbinate The inferior turbinate is one of three paired nasal conchae. Unlike the middle, superior, and supreme turbinates that are medial extensions of the ethmoid bone, the inferior turbinate is a separate bone. The inferior turbinate functions to humidify and warm inspired air. Extensive resection of the inferior turbinate increases the risk for paradoxical nasal obstruction (empty nose syndrome), but preservation of the anterior 1/3 to ½ of the inferior turbinate is considered sufficient to prevent empty nose syndrome.

Nasolacrimal duct (NLD) The nasolacrimal sac begins in the space between the nasal and lacrimal bones, about 8 mm above the axilla of the middle turbinate. The inferior aspect of the sac travels posteriorly about 11 mm and forms the NLD [12]. The NLD then descends anterior to the true maxillary os and empties into the inferior meatus at Hasner valve.

Maxillary line Intraoperatively, the maxillary line can be used as a rough landmark for the location of the NLD [12]. The maxillary line is a curvilinear eminence found at the junction of the lacrimal bone and the frontal process of the maxilla. The NLD is closest to the true maxillary os at the midpoint of the maxillary line.

Maxillary os The true maxillary os is the natural opening into the maxillary sinus. The os can be found along the inferior 1/3 of the maxillary line.

Posterior fontanelle The posterior fontanelle is an area along the posteromedial aspect of the medial wall of the maxillary sinus. This is typically covered by mucosa but can be patent and thus allow for direct communication between the nasal cavity and the maxillary sinus, especially in patients with inflammatory sinus disease. Widening the posterior fontanelle without connecting it to the true maxillary os can lead to recirculation.

Greater palatine canal The greater palatine canal houses the greater and lesser palatine nerves and is situated on average 2.8 mm anterior to the posterior wall of the maxillary sinus with a dehiscence rate of 38% [13]. Injury to this structure can lead to palatal numbness, most often temporary.

Innervation The posterior superior alveolar branch of the maxillary nerve is the main source of sensory innervation to the maxillary sinus [14]. The anterior and middle superior alveolar branches and the infraorbital nerve also contribute to maxillary sinus innervation. The infraorbital nerve may be seen intraoperatively traversing the maxillary sinus as it passes from the infraorbital canal along the orbital floor to the infraorbital foramen along the face of the maxilla.

Blood supply The primary blood supply of the inferior turbinate is the descending branch of the sphenopalatine artery. This branch enters the inferior turbinate about 1–1.5 cm from its posterior border.

Preoperative Considerations

Patients should undergo careful review by endoscopic and radiologic examination to evaluate for evidence of prior surgery, including retained uncinate, persistent infraorbital ethmoid cells, and discontinuity between the surgical antrostomy and natural os. An inferior meatal window may be present in patients with a history of Caldwell-Luc procedure or LeFort I maxillary advancement.

The consent process should include a discussion of uncommon risks specific to maxillary mega-antrostomy: bleeding related to branches of the sphenopalatine artery, numbness along the palate and/or incisors, epiphora due to injury to and stenosis of the nasolacrimal duct, and persistent mucostasis despite patency of the mega-antrostomy.

At a minimum, we recommend the surgeon has the following equipment available to ensure adequate widening of the EMMA: maxillary ball probe, curved suction, backbiters forceps, 45° through-cutting forceps, down-biting antrum punch, curved endoscopic scissors, microdebrider with straight and angled attachments (40- and/or 60-degree attachments), monopolar suction cautery, and endoscopic drill.

Surgical Indications

Initial surgical indications for EMMA were focused on resection of tumors, including malignant tumors and benign but locally aggressive neoplasms (e.g., inverted papilloma) [3]. EMMA improved endoscopic access to the maxillary sinus to resect these lesions to reduce the need for a Caldwell-Luc or open maxillectomy.

The indications for EMMA have broadened over time to include inflammatory disorders of the maxillary sinus. The main indications for a mega-antrostomy in a patient with chronic rhinosinusitis include recalcitrant maxillary sinusitis despite prior surgery, anticipated need to access sinus for topical therapy and surveillance, and primary or acquired mucociliary dysfunction. EMMA for CRS is most often performed as a salvage surgical intervention. However, this procedure can, in select cases, be performed during primary surgery. Primary EMMA is typically reserved for patients with sinusitis related to primary disorders of mucociliary clearance, including cystic fibrosis and primary ciliary dyskinesia. Less common indications for EMMA include odontogenic cysts, mucoceles, fungus balls, allergic fungal sinusitis, and mucus recirculation between an inferior meatal window and middle meatal antrostomy.

Surgical Technique (Video 3.1)

The procedure is performed endoscopically under general anesthesia. General principles of the procedure include sufficient widening of the maxillary antrostomy, mucosal preservation, avoidance of injury to the nasolacrimal duct, and preservation of the anterior portion of the inferior turbinate. The initial procedure details vary depending on whether the patient had a prior maxillary antrostomy or is surgically naïve (e.g., patient with CF).

If the patient is surgically naïve, the procedure begins with a traditional endoscopic maxillary antrostomy. Uncinectomy is performed from posterior to anterior using backbiting and through-cutting instruments. A 30-degree nasal endoscope is then used to visualize the lateral nasal wall and identify the maxillary os. Once the true os is identified, it can be dilated gently with a maxillary ball probe or curved suction. A microdebrider and through-cut instruments can then be used to widen the antrostomy posteriorly.

When mega-antrostomy is being performed as revision surgery, the prior antrostomy should be inspected with the angled endoscope, with particular attention to the os. Residual uncinate process and/or scarring that may be obstructing the ostial outflow or causing recirculation are removed. Because the mega-antrostomy is a mucosal sparing procedure, it is expected that the maxillary sinus mucosa will still direct mucus towards the natural os, even with the extended antrostomy. If not previously done so, the antrostomy is extended posteriorly with through-cut forceps towards the posterior wall of the maxillary sinus.

Next, the posterior ½ to 2/3 of the inferior turbinate is resected in order to expose the inferior aspect of the medial wall of the maxillary sinus as it forms the lateral wall of the inferior meatus. Using curved endoscopic scissors, the inferior turbinate is first transected full-thickness with a vertically oriented cut, positioning the scissors at the ventral aspect of the turbinate and aiming the tip of the scissors towards the maxillary ostium (Fig. 3.1). The planned incision can be marked by crimping the turbinate with a curved surgical clamp, which may reduce bleeding, although this step is not routinely used by the senior author. Next, the posterior segment of the inferior turbinate is detached from the lateral wall of the nasal cavity by using a straight endoscopic scissor to cut the attachment of the turbinate to the medial wall of the maxillary sinus (Fig. 3.2). Extension of the scissor cut posteriorly across the posterior stump of the inferior turbinate fully releases the posterior inferior turbinate, which is removed from the surgical field. The final cut across the posterior stump of the inferior turbinate often exposes the inferior turbinate artery, which should be cauterized, along with the residual turbinate stump, with monopolar suction cautery to decrease the risk of postoperative epistaxis.

Next, down-biting through-cutting antral punches are used to resect the medial wall of the maxillary sinus and extend the antrostomy down to the level of the nasal floor. Some surgeons favor drilling thicker portions of the medial maxillary wall and rotating local mucosal flaps to cover exposed areas of bone, but this is not routinely performed by the senior author. If additional anterior exposure is required, the mega-antrostomy can be extended anteriorly along the nasal floor using a backbiting forceps, remaining inferior to Hasner's valve (Fig. 3.3). This additional anterior-inferior limb of the mega-antrostomy can be brought forward as far anteriorly as the medial maxillary buttress.

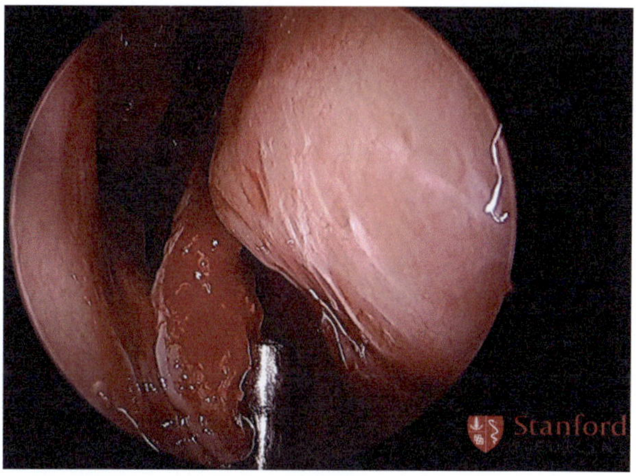

Fig. 3.1 Curved endoscopic scissors are used to resect the posterior ½ to 2/3 of the inferior turbinate. Medialization of the turbinate prior to transection can reduce the risk of injury to the lateral nasal wall and Hasner's valve

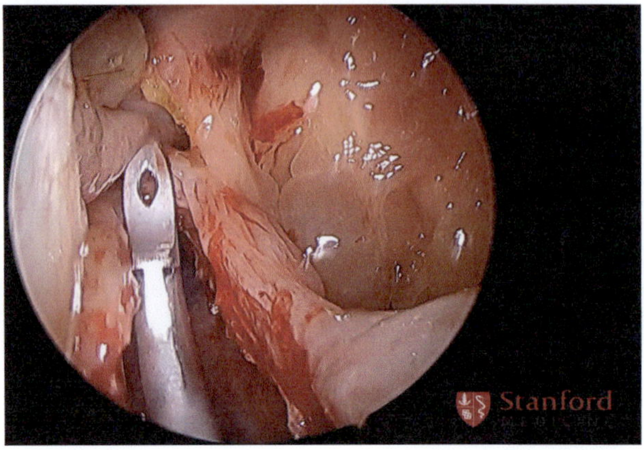

Fig. 3.2 The posterior stump of the inferior turbinate is transected, which often results in bleeding from the inferior turbinate branch of the sphenopalatine artery

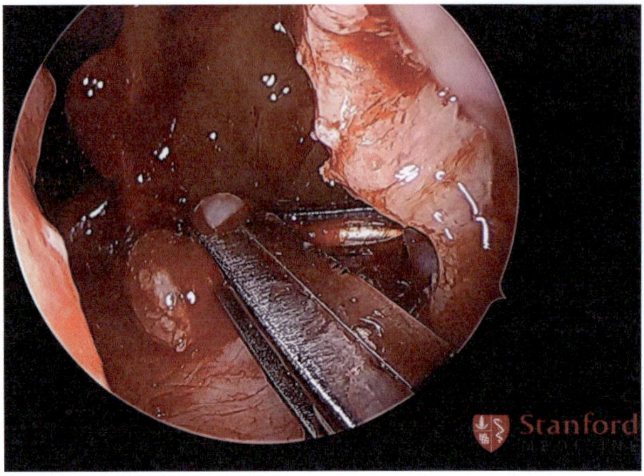

Fig. 3.3 After the medial wall of the maxillary sinus is resected to the floor of the nasal cavity, the antrostomy can be extended anteriorly, taking care to remain inferior to Hasner's valve

After securing hemostasis with electrocautery and topical vasoconstrictors, the procedure is concluded without placement of any absorbable or non-absorbable nasal packing.

Reported Outcomes

There is a growing body of literature showing the benefits and overall safety of this procedure; however, prospective data is limited. There was a 2020 systematic review that included two level 2 evidence studies and four level 4 studies [15].

Cho et al. showed a significant improvement in symptoms and endoscopy scores after EMMA, with >80% of patients showing a reduction in the need for antibiotic and oral steroid use [16]. Long-term follow-up (mean 6.9 years) in a subsequent paper by the same research group showed maintenance of the symptomatic benefits of EMMA, with 72% of patients describing complete or significant improvement in symptoms and 28% a partial improvement [17]. No patient in that review described exacerbation of any sinonasal symptoms.

Wang, et al., in a retrospective analysis of 46 patients with recalcitrant maxillary sinusitis who underwent EMMA, showed a complete resolution of sinonasal symptoms in 80% of patients over a mean 35-month follow-up period [18]. Within a subgroup of 15 patients who had undergone prior Caldwell-Luc, 73% experienced symptomatic improvement after EMMA. No patients required revision surgery. Similarly, Woodworth et al. reviewed 19 patients with chronic maxillary sinusitis, 14 of whom had undergone prior Caldwell-Luc, and showed resolution of hyperplastic mucosa in 95% of patients after a mean 19.5-month follow-up [19]. Thulasidas et al. reported no recurrence of disease in all 24 patients who underwent EMMA over a mean follow-up of 14.6 months [20].

In a review of 551 medial maxillectomies, Wong, et al. showed a 25% incidence of mucostasis 3 months postoperatively, but this incidence decreased to 10.2% at the last postoperative visit, suggesting an improved rate of sustained mucostasis over time [21]. Patients in that review had a 5% incidence of revision sinus surgery after EMMA. Given the widened maxillary antrostomy, the risks of restenosis are arguably lower.

EMMA has also been proposed as an initial or subsequent procedure for patients with predilection for sinonasal inflammatory disease [22]. In a subset of patients with cystic fibrosis, Virgin et al. reported significant improvement in SNOT-22 score and Lund-Kennedy score one year after surgery [23]. The frequency of pulmonary exacerbation-associated hospital admissions also decreased in the year after surgery. There was a 9.1% reoperation rate in this group of patients with cystic fibrosis.

In a cadaveric study, Govindaraju, et al. showed that more extended maxillary sinus antrostomies, including EMMA, were associated with greater postoperative irrigation penetration, visualization, and instrument reach [1]. EMMA has also been shown to improve air entry into the maxillary sinus. Through computational fluid dynamics modeling, Siu et al. showed a positive linear correlation between the maxillary antrostomy size and the rate of airflow into the maxillary sinus [24].

Potential Complications

Potential complications specific to EMMA include bleeding from the posterior stump of the partially resected inferior turbinate, injury to the nasolacrimal duct, and paradoxical nasal obstruction (i.e., empty nose syndrome) due to partial resection of the inferior turbinate [25]. However, the actual incidence of complications of EMMA is low. A systematic review by Loftus, et al. reported a total of 4 complications out of 211 (1.9%) included patients. These included nasolacrimal duct obstruction ($n = 2$), epistaxis requiring return to the operating room ($n = 1$), and hypoplastic maxillary sinus ($n = 1$) [19–21].

Preservation of a portion of the anterior aspect of the inferior turbinate may decrease the incidence of certain complications. Using computational fluid dynamics modeling, Saibene et al. found greater flow rates and fluid velocities at the maxillary sinus after EMMA compared to modified EMMA with preservation of the inferior turbinate, suggesting a greater disruption in normal nasal airflow dynamics after EMMA [26]. The authors postulated that this difference could contribute to the more persistent postoperative crusting and reduced nasal air conditioning seen after EMMA. Gras-Cabrerizo et al. discussed a technique to preserve the inferior turbinate during EMMA [27]. The authors initially make an incision at the head and body of the inferior turbinate, then perform the medial maxillectomy. At the end of the procedure, the head and body of the middle turbinate are sutured back to each other. Using acoustic rhinometry, Gras-Cabrerizo showed maintenance of normal nasal resistance with this technique.

Tips and Pearls

- Maintain the anterior 1/3 to ½ of the inferior turbinate undisturbed to decrease the risk of empty nose syndrome.
- When performing the inferior turbinate partial resection, first medialize the inferior turbinate. This helps decrease the risk of inadvertent injury to the lateral nasal wall and Hasner valve.
- Cauterize the posterior stump of the inferior turbinate to decrease the risk of postoperative epistaxis from the inferior turbinate branch of the sphenopalatine artery.
- Perform only limited postoperative debridement of the posterior inferior turbinate stump at the first postoperative visit, as early removal of the crust may lead to epistaxis.
- If the nasolacrimal duct is injured, a complete inferior transection of the duct decreases the risk of postoperative nasolacrimal duct stenosis when compared to incision without complete transection.
- The surgeon can consider upfront EMMA for patients with chronic ciliary dysfunction (e.g., cystic fibrosis or primary ciliary dyskinesia).

References

1. Govindaraju R, Prepageran N. The role of endoscopic medial maxillectomy in sinus disease. Curr Opin Otolaryngol Head Neck Surg. 2021;29(1):1–8.
2. Ashman A, Psaltis AJ, Wormald PJ, et al. Extended endoscopic approaches to the maxillary sinus. J Laryngol Otol. 2020;134:473–80.
3. Kamel RH. Transnasal endoscopic medial maxillectomy in inverted papilloma. Laryngoscope. 1995;105:847–53.
4. Tepedino MS, Miotello Ferrao AC, Morais Higa HC, et al. Reversible endoscopic medial maxillectomy: endonasal approach to diseases of the maxillary sinus. Int Arch Otorhinolaryngol. 2020;24:E247–52.

5. Coleman JR Jr, Duncavage JA. Extended middle meatal antrostomy: the treatment of circular flow. Laryngoscope. 1996;106:1214–7.
6. Nakayama T, Asaka D, Okushi T, et al. Endoscopic medial maxillectomy with preservation of inferior turbinate and nasolacrimal duct. Am J Rhinol Allergy. 2012;26:405–8.
7. Sessions RB, Humphreys DH. Technical modifications of the medial maxillectomy. Arch Otolaryngol. 1983;109:575–7.
8. Ghosh A, Pal S, Srivastava A, et al. Modification of endoscopic medial maxillectomy: a novel approach for inverted papilloma of the maxillary sinus. J Laryngol Otol. 2015;129:159–63.
9. Jurado-Ramos A, Jodas JG, Romero FR, et al. Endoscopic medial maxillectomy as a procedure of choice to treat inverted papillomas. Acta Otolaryngol. 2009;129:1018–25.
10. Kennedy DW, Adappa ND. Endoscopic maxillary antrostomy: not just a simple procedure. Laryngoscope. 2011;121(10):2142–5.
11. Thamboo A, Ayoub N, Maul X, et al. The inferior turbinate: role in normal respiration and airway obstruction. Curr Otorhinolaryngol Rep. 2021;9:383–8.
12. Chastain JB, Cooper MH, Sindwani R. The maxillary line: anatomic characterization and clinical utility of an important surgical landmark. Laryngoscope. 2005;115(6):990–2.
13. Greater palatine canal: Ayoub N, Thamboo A, Hwang PH, Walgama ES. Radioanatomic Study of the Greater Palatine Canal relevant to endoscopic endonasal surgical landmarks. Otolaryngol Head Neck Surg 2017;157(4):731–736.
14. Iwanaga J, Wilson C, Lachkar S, Tomaszewski KA, Walocha JA, Tubbs RS. Clinical anatomy of the maxillary sinus: application to sinus floor augmentation. Anat Cell Biol. 2019;52(1):17–24.
15. Loftus CA, Yoo F, Desiato VM, Schlosser RJ, Soler ZM. Treatment of recalcitrant maxillary sinusitis with endoscopic modified medial maxillectomy: a systematic review of safety and efficacy. Am J Rhinol Allergy. 2020;34(1):127–33.
16. Cho DY, Hwang PH. Results of endoscopic maxillary mega-antrostomy in recalcitrant maxillary sinusitis. Am J Rhinol. 2008;22:658–62.
17. Costa ML, Psaltis AJ, Nayak JV, Hwang PH. Long-term outcomes of endoscopic maxillary mega-antrostomy for refractory chronic maxillary sinusitis. Int Forum Allergy Rhinol. 2015;5:60–5.
18. Wang EW, et al. Modified endoscopic medial maxillectomy for recalcitrant chronic maxillary sinusitis. Int Forum Allergy Rhinol. 2011;1(6):493–7.
19. Woodworth BA, Parker RO, Schlosser RJ. Modified endoscopic medial maxillectomy for chronic maxillary sinusitis. Am J Rhinol. 2006;20:317–9.
20. Thulasidas P, Vaidyanathan V. Role of modified endoscopic medial maxillectomy in persistent chronic maxillary sinusitis. Int Arch Otorhinolaryngol. 2014;18:159–64.
21. Wong EH, Cavada MN, Orgain CA, et al. The modified medial maxillectomy as a radical or extended,-yet still functional,-technique in sinus surgery. Am J Rhinol Allergy. 2023;37(4):476–84.
22. Illing EA, Woodworth BA. Management of the upper airway in cystic fibrosis. Curr Opin Pulm Med. 2014;20(6):623–31.
23. Virgin FW, et al. Extensive surgical and comprehensive postoperative medical management for cystic fibrosis chronic rhinosinusitis. Am J Rhinol Allergy. 2012;26(1):70–5.
24. Siu J, Dong J, Inthavong K, Shang Y, Douglas RG. Quantification of airflow in the sinuses following functional endoscopic sinus surgery. Rhinology. 2020;58(3):257–65.
25. Talmadge J, Nayak JV, Yao W, Citardi MJ. Management of postsurgical empty nose syndrome. Facial Plast Surg Clin North Am. 2019;27(4):465–75.
26. Saibene AM, Felisati G, Pipolo C, Bulfamante AM, Quadrio M, Covello V. Partial preservation of the inferior turbinate in endoscopic medial maxillectomy: a computational fluid dynamics study. Am J Rhinol Allergy. 2020;34(3):409–16.
27. Gras-Cabrerizo JR, Martel-Martin M, Montserrat-Gili JR, et al. Endoscopic medial maxillectomy with preservation of inferior turbinate: assessing results by acoustic rhinometry. J Craniofac Surg. 2019;30(4):996–9.

4 Endoscopic Denker's Approach

Justin P. McCormick and Jivianne T. Lee

Key Points

- Chronic rhinosinusitis is a complex inflammatory disease with a surgical revision rate of up to 15–20%.
- The modified endoscopic Denker's approach is classically described for addressing tumors involving the anterior or lateral wall of the maxillary sinus, but also is an option for the management of recalcitrant chronic rhinosinusitis.
- This surgical technique utilizes an endonasal maxillotomy without the need for separate external incisions.
- The modified endoscopic Denker's approach allows for complete exposure of the anterior and medial maxilla and may be a useful adjunct procedure in patients with severe recalcitrant chronic rhinosinusitis.

Supplementary Information The online version contains supplementary material available at https://doi.org/10.1007/978-3-031-89191-5_4.

J. P. McCormick
Department of Head and Neck Surgery and Communication Sciences, Rutgers Robert Wood Johnson Medical School, New Brunswick, NJ, USA

J. T. Lee (✉)
Division of Rhinology & Endoscopic Sinus and Skull Base Surgery, Department of Head and Neck Surgery, David Geffen School of Medicine at UCLA, Los Angeles, CA, USA
e-mail: JTLee@mednet.ucla.edu

J. T. Lee et al. (eds.), *Advances in Surgical and Medical Interventions for Recalcitrant Chronic Rhinosinusitis*,
https://doi.org/10.1007/978-3-031-89191-5_4

Background

Chronic rhinosinusitis (CRS) is an inflammatory disease of the paranasal sinuses which causes symptoms of nasal obstruction, thick nasal drainage, smell dysfunction, and facial pain or pressure for a time period of greater than 12 weeks [1]. The management of CRS begins with medical therapy which can include a combination of large volume saline irrigations, intranasal corticosteroids, oral corticosteroids, and/or antibiotics depending on the phenotype/endotype of the CRS, typically for a 3–4 week period [1]. The response rate to medical therapy alone is quite varied and has been reported to be 37.5–90% [2, 3]. When patients fail to respond to appropriate medical therapy, which can be defined as persistence of symptoms with findings of sinonasal inflammation on radiography or endoscopy, they can be offered sinus surgery.

The goals of endoscopic sinus surgery (ESS) have been similar since its introduction in the 1980s. ESS seeks to reestablish sinus ventilation and improve access for delivery of topical medications [4]. Despite adequate ESS and post-operative medical management, a subset of patients will develop recurrent or refractory symptoms. Several large database studies have reported overall revision rates after ESS of 15–20% [5–7]. Reasons for primary surgical failure have been suggested to include postoperative scarring, neo-osteogenesis, inadequate postoperative management, or incomplete primary surgical extirpation. After initial surgical failure, extended approaches may be required to improve access for long-term topical therapies. The maxillary sinus has several extended approaches that may be employed to address recalcitrant chronic maxillary sinusitis [8].

A standard middle meatal maxillary antrostomy involves resecting the uncinate process to expose the natural ostium of the maxillary sinus, followed by widening of the natural ostium. The appropriate maxillary ostium size is a topic of debate; however, it is the preference of the authors to perform a wide maxillary antrostomy during primary ESS to facilitate in-office monitoring and management. The primary maxillary antrostomy may involve extending the natural ostium from the nasolacrimal duct anteriorly to the posterior wall of the maxillary sinus, and opening the sinus superiorly to the orbital floor and inferiorly to the attachment of the inferior turbinate. There are several extended surgical approaches to the maxillary sinus. The endoscopic maxillary mega-antrostomy involves resection of the mid-portion of the inferior turbinate, and extends the antrostomy inferiorly to the floor of the nasal cavity [9]. The modified endoscopic medial maxillectomy, which involves more aggressive resection of the inferior turbinate and extends the antrostomy anterior and inferior to Hasner's valve to expose the more anterior aspect of the maxillary sinus. The Caldwell-Luc approach utilizes an intraoral incision to perform an anterior maxillotomy allowing access to the far anterior-lateral aspect of the maxillary sinus [10]. Recently, an endoscopic modification to the standard Denker's approach has been described to address tumors of the maxillary sinus; however, it may also be adapted to address recalcitrant maxillary sinusitis, as the standard Denker's approach has been used previously [11].

Surgical Technique

The standard Denker's approach involves a sublabial incision that exposes a wide area of the anterior maxillary wall. An anterior maxillotomy is then performed and extended laterally to the infraorbital foramen and superiorly to the orbital rim. The lateral nasal wall is then incised and resected to the floor of the nasal cavity, including resection of the inferior turbinate. This allows exposure of the ethmoid sinuses where complete sphenoethmoidectomy can be performed, and the middle turbinate is resected. The nasolacrimal duct is then identified and sharply transected near the lacrimal sac. Once the sinuses have been widely opened, forceps are used to the remove the mucosa of sinus cavities [12].

Recently the Denker's approach has been modified to allow for similar access via a completely endoscopic approach (Table 4.1) [11]. An endoscopic medial maxillectomy is performed. Electrocautery with a guarded needle tip [Megadyne, Draper, UT] is used to make a mucosal incision at the junction of the nasal floor and lateral nasal wall through the periosteum. The incision is then extended along the head of the inferior turbinate at the edge of the pyriform aperture. Then, a subperiosteal dissection is performed with a suction freer elevator [Olympus ENT, Southborough, MA] to expose the anterior aspect of the maxilla, the infraorbital foramen, and its neurovascular bundle. A high-speed drill is utilized to create a bony window into the anterior wall of the maxillary sinus, taking care to stay inferior to the infraorbital foramen and preserve the anterior superior alveolar nerve. Further drilling of the pyriform aperture is performed to connect the anterior maxillotomy to the inferior portion of the endoscopic medial maxillectomy. This exposure allows access to the anterior-lateral, and anterior-inferior medial portion of the maxillary sinus (Fig. 4.1). At the end of the procedure, the nasolacrimal duct is identified and is sharply obliquely transected to prevent stenosis (Video 4.1).

Table 4.1 Steps to perform the modified endoscopic Denker's approach

Step 1	Perform an endoscopic medial maxillectomy by completing a standard maxillary antrostomy and then excising the middle portion of the inferior turbinate allowing the medial maxillary sinus wall to be resected to the nasal floor.	
Step 2	Using monopolar electrocautery, make a mucosal incision at the pyriform aperture extending from the floor of the nose to the superior portion of the inferior turbinate	(Fig. 4.2)
Step 3	Using a suction elevator, dissect in a subperiosteal plane along the anterior aspect of the maxilla until the infraorbital neurovascular bundle is identified	(Fig. 4.3)
Step 4	A high speed drill is used to create a bony window into the anterior wall of the maxillary sinus, taking care to stay inferior to the infraorbital foramen	(Fig. 4.4)
Step 5	Further drilling of the medial aspect of the pyriform aperture is performed to connect the anterior maxillotomy to the inferior portion of the endoscopic medial maxillectomy	(Fig. 4.5)
Step 6	The nasolacrimal duct is then identified within the mucosal of the lateral nasal wall, and the lumen is cut obliquely to prevent stenosis	(Fig. 4.6)

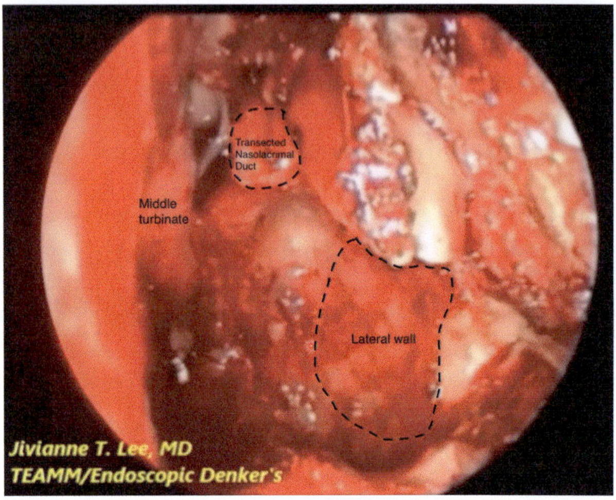

Fig. 4.1 Completion of the endoscopic Denker's approach allows for full visualization of all walls of the maxillary sinus

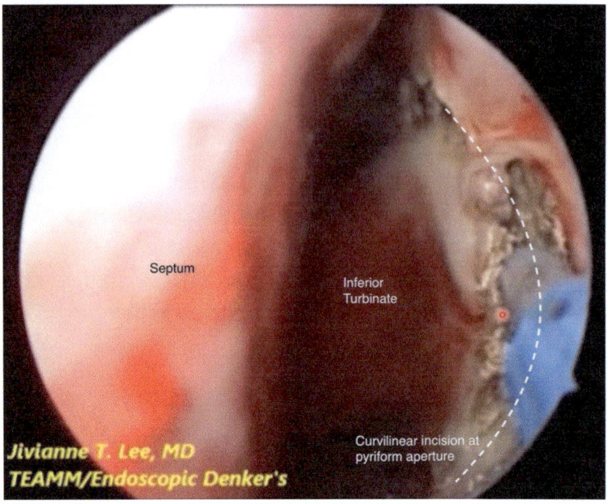

Fig. 4.2 To begin the endoscopic Denker's approach, a mucosal incision is made with a monopolar cautery at the pyriform aperture

Role of the Denker's Approach in Recalcitrant CRS

The Denker's approach for treatment-resistant maxillary sinusitis was first reported in the 1990s by a group in the Netherlands. Kerrebijn et al [12] reviewed their series of 56 patients with treatment resistant chronic rhinosinusitis with nasal polyps (CRSwNP). All patients underwent the standard Denker's approach and had at least 36 months of follow-up. Long term results after radical surgery demonstrated resolution of nasal discharge in 82% of patients, restored sense of smell in 89% of patients, and resolution of headaches in 87% of patients. Despite these positive

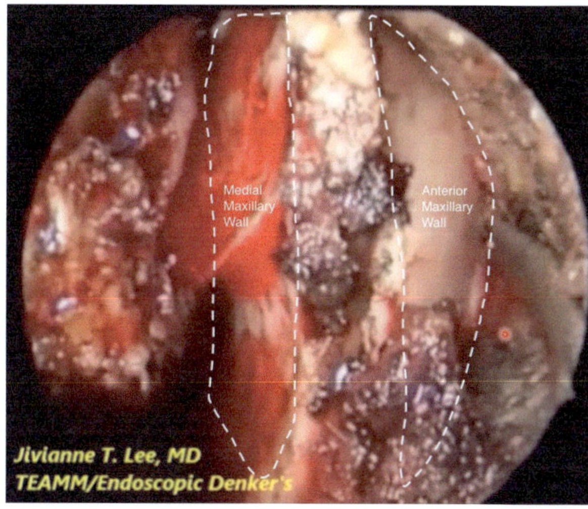

Fig. 4.3 A suction freer elevator is used to elevate the anterior maxillary soft tissues off of the anterior wall of the maxillary sinus in a subperiosteal plane

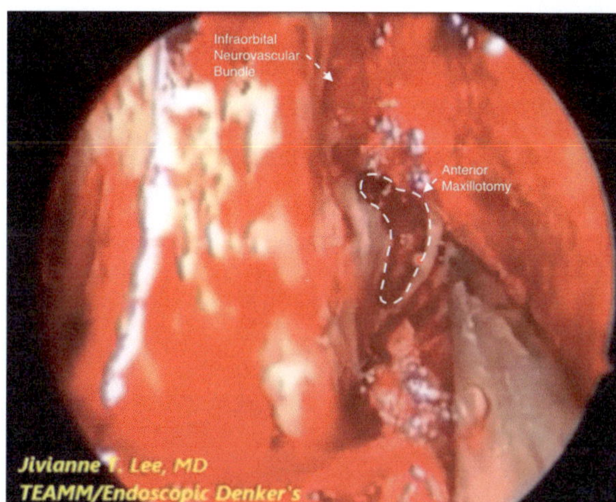

Fig. 4.4 An anterior maxillotomy is performed taking care to avoid trauma to infraorbital neurovascular bundle

subjective findings, recurrent polyposis was noted in 80% of patients. The authors report that all patients were treated with nasal saline irrigations, but do not comment on the use of intranasal corticosteroids post-operatively.

Wreesman et al [13] reviewed their series of 82 patients who underwent the Denker's procedure over a 10-year period. Sixty-three patients (77%) completed and returned surveys exploring their sinonasal symptoms prior to, and after, the Denker's procedure. Prior to surgery, the majority of patients complained of nasal obstruction, reduced olfaction, headache, and facial fullness despite prior medical and surgical therapy. After the Denker's surgery, patients reported nearly a 50% reduction in nasal obstruction, rhinorrhea, and facial fullness, but contrary to the prior study, olfaction was not significantly restored. Subgroup analysis of patients

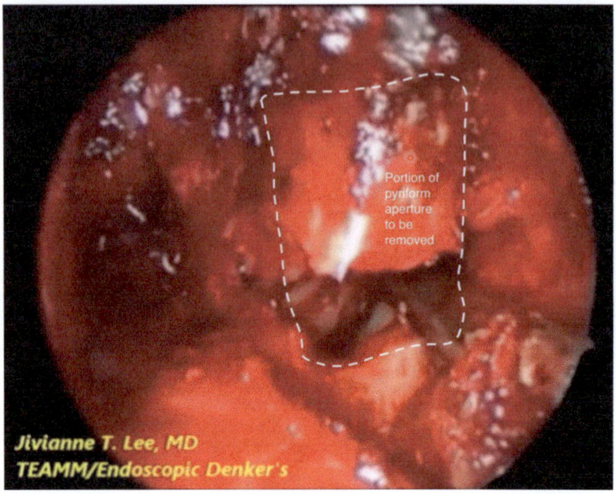

Fig. 4.5 The pyriform aperture is drilled out to allow for wide exposure of the entire maxillary sinus

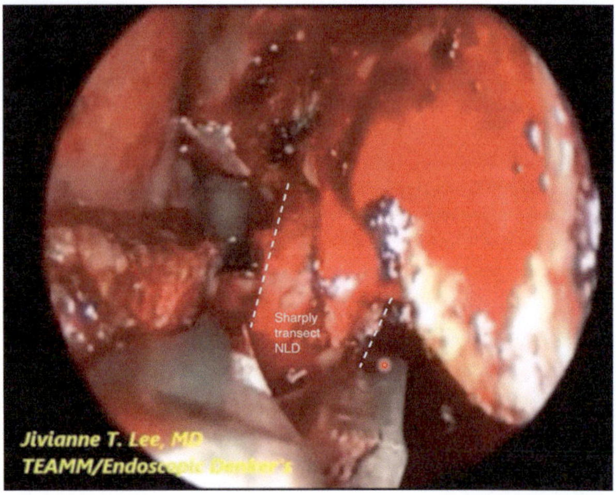

Fig. 4.6 At the conclusion of the procedure the nasolacrimal duct (NLD) is identified and sharply transected

with asthma demonstrated significant reduction of lower airway symptoms as well after the Denker's surgery.

In 2006, the same group conducted a prospective survey-based study on a group of refractory CRS patients who underwent the Denker's procedure [14]. The included patients had undergone three prior ESS procedures, in addition to medical therapy including topical saline irrigations, antibiotics, and topical and/or oral corticosteroids. Similar to the prior study, patients reported severe congestion, nasal obstruction, rhinorrhea, and olfactory disturbance prior to surgery. After the

Denker's surgery, a majority of patients reported significant improvement in nasal congestion (73%), rhinorrhea (70%), and nasal obstruction (60%). Again, there was no significant change in olfactory function. Over a 2-year follow-up period of this cohort, no patient required revision surgery after the Denker's procedure. A follow-up to this study was published in 2007, reporting on the effect of radical surgery on general quality of life and pain in CRS patients [15]. The results of this study suggest that after the Denker's procedure, patients have less impairment in work and other daily activities as a result of their physical health problems. Additionally, patients tend to experience less pain after radical surgery based on results of the McGill pain questionnaire. Table 4.2 summarizes the included studies and their findings.

Table 4.2 Studies investigated the Denker's approach for refractory maxillary sinusitis

Author Date	Number of patients	Indication for surgery	Outcomes	Complications
Kerrebijn et al. 1996	56	Recurrent sinusitis and nasal polyposis Failure of prior surgery to resolve symptoms	Complete resolution of nasal discharge ($n = 46$, 82%) Restored olfaction ($n = 50$, 89%) Recurrent polyposis ($n = 45$, 80%) patients. Authors note recurrent polyposis was typically small and along the ethmoid roof	Nasolacrimal duct stenosis requiring DCR ($n = 6$, 11%) Dacryocystitis treated with antibiotics ($n = 2$) Meningitis ($n = 1$)
Wreesman et al. 2001	82	Refractory chronic rhinosinusitis and/or nasal polyposis Failure of established functional sinus surgery	84% reported overall reduction in sinonasal symptoms 50% reduction in feeling of fullness 47% reduction in nasal obstruction 47% reduction in rhinorrhea Olfaction did not improve significantly 34% required revision after the Denker's procedure, most commonly for recurrent polyps	*Did not report complications

(continued)

Table 4.2 (continued)

Author Date	Number of patients	Indication for surgery	Outcomes	Complications
Videler et al. 2006	23	Refractory chronic rhinosinusitis +/− nasal polyposis Failure of at least 3 prior endoscopic sinus surgeries	70% reported overall reduction in sinonasal symptoms 74% reported improved congestion 70% reported improved post nasal drip 60% reported improved nasal obstruction Olfaction did not improve significantly No revision surgery required in 2 year follow up period	Oroantral fistula without clinical symptoms ($n = 1$)
Videler et al. 2007	23	Refractory chronic rhinosinusitis +/− nasal polyposis Failure of at least 3 prior endoscopic sinus surgeries	Improvement in 7 of 8 SF-36 domains at 2 years, though only role limitations due to physical problems is significant Significant reduction in sensory pain and total pain based on McGill pain questionnaire	*Did not report complications

Reported Outcomes

The introduction of the modified endoscopic Denker's approach (MED) permits similar access and visualization of the maxillary sinus as the standard Denker's approach, without the need for a sublabial incision. Within the literature, the MED has been primarily used for management of maxillary sinus and infratemporal fossa tumors [11]. However, the MED may prove valuable in the management of refractory maxillary sinus CRS.

Nasalization or radical ethmoidectomy has been described for patients with extensive polyposis in order to decrease the likelihood of early recurrence. Nasalization entails removing all ethmoid bony lamellae and mucosa, in addition to the middle turbinate, and making a wide maxillary antrostomy and sphenoidotomy. Surgeons have reported a lower incidence of polyp recurrence, greater symptom improvement, and less need for revision surgery after nasalization [16]. Patients undergoing the so-called full-reboot procedure which involves clearance of all polyps and mucosa, as well as a Draf III frontal sinusotomy, were noted to have significantly reduced polyp recurrence rate, and symptom scores were also significantly reduced based on the SNOT-22 questionnaire [17]. The MED is a means by which full clearance of disease within the maxillary sinus may be achieved. Opponents of radical surgery express valid concern for delayed wound healing, potential for increased scar formation, and increased complications as a result of more aggressive surgery. In patients who underwent the reboot procedure however, there was no evidence of abnormal scarring. and biopsy of the new mucosa at 28 months post-op showed normal ciliated respiratory epithelium.

With the exception of Kerrebijn et al [12], most studies reporting on outcomes of the Denker's approach for CRS did not comment on complications associated with this procedure. However, more recent studies investigating the MED for maxillary sinus tumors more thoroughly described potential complications (Table 4.3) [18, 19]. Reported complications of the MED include the standard complications of endoscopic sinus surgery, as well as temporary numbness of the cheek or palate, epiphora, and alar collapse. These complications tend to be self-resolving, with epiphora being the complication to most likely need secondary intervention [11]. The MED was utilized successfully in 22 patients with maxillary sinus inverted papilloma [18]. Across a mean follow-up of 2 years, only 1 patient recurred, with the recurrence developing along the infraorbital nerve after prior conservative resection to maintain facial sensation. Three patients in this series developed epiphora; however, only one required dacryocystorhinostomy (DCR), while the others resolved spontaneously within 3 months after surgery. Additionally, only one patient

Table 4.3 Studies investigating the modified endoscopic Denker's approach for maxillary sinus tumors

Author Date	Number of patients	Indication for surgery	Outcomes	Complications
Lee et al. 2020	22	Maxillary sinus inverted papilloma attached to anterior or lateral maxillary sinus wall	4.5% recurrence rate ($n = 1$), tumor attachment at infraorbital nerve. Bony canal was preserved at initial resection to avoid risk of facial numbness	4.5% epiphora rate requiring DCR ($n = 1$). Two other patients had spontaneous resolution of post-operative epiphora within 3 months post-op 1 patient with transient parethesia of the lip
McCormick et al. 2022	58 35 benign 23 malignant	Maxillary sinus tumors, both benign and malignant	19% overall recurrence rate ($n = 11$). 5.7% local recurrence rate for benign tumors ($n = 2$) 26.1% local recurrence rate for malignant tumors ($n = 6$)	13.8% overall complication rate 6.9% epiphora rate requiring DCR ($n = 4$). Spontaneous resolution of post-op epiphora occurred in 57% of cases 5.2% with long-term facial numbness/ paresthesia 1 patient with nasal vestibular stenosis following adjuvant radiation therapy

had transient upper lip numbness that resolved within 3 months of surgery. A larger, multicenter study evaluated outcomes following the MED for management of both benign and malignant maxillary sinus tumors [19]. Similar to the prior study, the recurrence rate for benign tumors was 5.7%. Malignant tumors, however, had a recurrence rate of 26.1%. The overall complication rate in this series was 13.8%. The most common reported complications were facial numbness and epiphora. Facial numbness was noted to be more likely to resolve spontaneously, as 78% of patients who initially reported facial numbness ultimately recovered full sensation. Epiphora seems to be less likely to resolve spontaneously, as four out of seven patients who initially reported epiphora at follow-up visits ultimately required DCR. The overall rate of epiphora requiring DCR in this tumor series (6.9%) is less than what Kerrebijn et al [12] reported in their refractory CRS series (11%), which may be related to advanced technology and refinement of surgical techniques throughout the modern endoscopic age.

As the indications for endoscopic surgery continue to expand and evolve, modifications of previously described open approaches may enhance access and visualization from an endoscopic standpoint. While further research will need to be conducted to validate the utility of these approaches, it is useful for the endoscopic surgeon to have a vast armamentarium of techniques to adequately manage the subset of patients with refractory disease. The MED is yet another method by which surgeons may access and treat the maxillary sinus in these difficult cases.

References

1. Orlandi RR, Kingdom TT, Smith TL, et al. International consensus statement on allergy and rhinology: rhinosinusitis 2021. Int Forum Allergy Rhinol. 2021;11:213–739.
2. Young LC, Stow NW, Zhou L, Douglas RG. Efficacy of medical therapy in treatment of chronic rhinosinusitis. Allergy Rhinol (Providence). 2012;3:e8–e12.
3. Subramanian HN, Schechtman KB, Hamilos DL. A retrospective analysis of treatment outcomes and time to relapse after intensive medical treatment for chronic sinusitis. Am J Rhinol. 2002;16:303–12.
4. Kennedy DW, Zinreich SJ, Rosenbaum AE, Johns ME. Functional endoscopic sinus surgery. Theory and diagnostic evaluation. Arch Otolaryngol. 1985;111:576–82.
5. Hopkins C, Slack R, Lund V, Brown P, Copley L, Browne J. Long-term outcomes from the English national comparative audit of surgery for nasal polyposis and chronic rhinosinusitis. Laryngoscope. 2009;119:2459–65.
6. Hunter TD, DeConde AS, Manes RP. Disease-related expenditures and revision rates in chronic rhinosinusitis patients after endoscopic sinus surgery. J Med Econ. 2018;21:610–5.
7. Smith KA, Orlandi RR, Oakley G, Meeks H, Curtin K, Alt JA. Long-term revision rates for endoscopic sinus surgery. Int Forum Allergy Rhinol. 2019;9:402–8.
8. McCormick JP, Hicks MD, Grayson JW, Woodworth BA, Cho DY. Endoscopic Management of Maxillary Sinus Diseases of Dentoalveolar origin. Oral Maxillofac Surg Clin North Am. 2020;32:639–48.
9. Cho DY, Hwang PH. Results of endoscopic maxillary mega-antrostomy in recalcitrant maxillary sinusitis. Am J Rhinol. 2008;22:658–62.

10. Kim E, Duncavage J. Caldwell-Luc procedure. Oper Tech Otolaryngol Head Neck Surg. 2010;21:163–5.
11. Lee JT, Suh JD, Carrau RL, Chu MW, Chiu AG. Endoscopic Denker's approach for resection of lesions involving the anteroinferior maxillary sinus and infratemporal fossa. Laryngoscope. 2017;127:556–60.
12. Kerrebijn JD, Drost HE, Spoelstra HA, Knegt PP. If functional sinus surgery fails: a radical approach to sinus surgery. Otolaryngol Head Neck Surg. 1996;114:745–7.
13. Wreesmann VB, Fokkens WJ, Knegt PP. Refractory chronic sinusitis: evaluation of symptom improvement after Denker's procedure. Otolaryngol Head Neck Surg. 2001;125:495–500.
14. Videler WJ, Wreesmann VB, van der Meulen FW, Knegt PP, Fokkens WJ. Repetitive endoscopic sinus surgery failure: a role for radical surgery? Otolaryngol Head Neck Surg. 2006;134:586–91.
15. Videler WJ, van Drunen CM, van der Meulen FW, Fokkens WJ. Radical surgery: effect on quality of life and pain in chronic rhinosinusitis. Otolaryngol Head Neck Surg. 2007;136:261–7.
16. Jankowski R, Pigret D, Decroocq F, Blum A, Gillet P. Comparison of radical (nasalisation) and functional ethmoidectomy in patients with severe sinonasal polyposis. A retrospective study. Rev Laryngol Otol Rhinol (Bord). 2006;127:131–40.
17. Alsharif S, Jonstam K, van Zele T, Gevaert P, Holtappels G, Bachert C. Endoscopic sinus surgery for Type-2 CRS wNP: an Endotype-based retrospective study. Laryngoscope. 2019;129:1286–92.
18. Lee JT, Yoo F, Wang M, Vengerovich G, Suh JD. Modified endoscopic Denker approach in management of inverted papilloma of the anterior maxillary sinus. Int Forum Allergy Rhinol. 2020;10:533–8.
19. McCormick JP, Suh JD, Wang EW, et al. Modified endoscopic Denker's approach for Management of Anterior Maxillary Sinus Tumors: multicenter series of 58 cases. Am J Rhinol Allergy. 2022;36:763.

The Reboot Procedure for Severe Chronic Rhinosinusitis with Nasal Polyps

5

Claus Bachert, Zhang Nan, Philippe Gevaert, and Thibaut van Zele

Key Points

- Chronic rhinosinusitis with nasal polyps (CRSwNP) is characterized by persistent mucosal disease that is multifactorial in nature and may persist despite surgical and medical therapy.
- There is evidence that some patients demonstrate long-term immunologic memory that may lead to persistent type 2 inflammation and recurrent or recalcitrant sinonasal disease.

C. Bachert (✉)
Department of Oto-Rhino-Laryngology, Münster University, Münster, Germany

First Affiliated Hospital, Sun Yat-sen University, International Airway Research Center, Guangzhou, China

Upper Airways Research Laboratory, Department of Oto-Rhino-Laryngology, Head and Skin, Ghent University, Ghent, Belgium
e-mail: Claus.Bachert@Ugent.be; Claus.Bachert@ukmuenster.de

Z. Nan
First Affiliated Hospital, Sun Yat-sen University, International Airway Research Center, Guangzhou, China

Upper Airways Research Laboratory, Department of Oto-Rhino-Laryngology, Head and Skin, Ghent University, Ghent, Belgium
e-mail: Nan.Zhang@Ugent.be

P. Gevaert · T. van Zele
Department of Oto-Rhino-Laryngology, Münster University, Münster, Germany

Upper Airways Research Laboratory, Department of Oto-Rhino-Laryngology, Head and Skin, Ghent University, Ghent, Belgium
e-mail: Philippe.Gevaert@Ugent.be; Thibaut.VanZele@Ugent.be

J. T. Lee et al. (eds.), *Advances in Surgical and Medical Interventions for Recalcitrant Chronic Rhinosinusitis*,
https://doi.org/10.1007/978-3-031-89191-5_5

- The reboot procedure seeks to provide broad access to the paranasal sinuses and remove dysfunctional sinonasal mucosa and polypoid tissue to allow the regrowth of functional mucosa.

Background

Chronic rhinosinusitis with nasal polyposis (CRSwNP) is classically considered a type 2 inflammatory disease process of the paranasal sinuses characterized by nasal polyp growth that may be refractory to medical and/or surgical management [1, 2]. Although nasal polyps are called "nasal," they typically originate from the sinuses and are secondarily prolapsing into the nose. Nasal polyps in the majority of cases are derived from the ethmoidal and maxillary sinus mucosa, but also may grow out from frontal and sphenoid sinus mucosa. They very rarely develop from nasal mucosa including the turbinates. I personally have seen nasal polyps originating in the nose only in specific cases such as patients with Woakes syndrome (massive polyp grow from the nose, sinuses and middle ear mucosa, leading to the broadening of the midface in younger subjects caused by the polyp pressure [3].

The reboot procedure aims to remove the sinus mucosa from the maxillary, ethmoidal, frontal and (if necessary) sphenoidal sinuses bilaterally. The goal is to allow for the complete re-epithelialization of the paranasal sinuses by nasal mucosa which has a low potential of developing nasal polyps [4].

The Role of Type 2 Inflammation in CRSwNP, Diagnosis, and Outcomes

Chronic rhinosinusitis (CRS), affecting up to 15% of the adult population in Europe and the USA, may be differentiated in two large groups, CRS with and without (Latin: sine) nasal polyps (CRSw/sNP) [5]. The differentiation is based on nasal endoscopy and CT scanning, which also allows for estimations regarding the extent of paranasal sinus disease. However, these clinical techniques do not allow providers to differentiate the underlying pathogenesis of the patient's inflammation. Approximately 80% of CRSwNP and 50% of CRSsNP are type 2 "eosinophilic" inflammatory reactions. Type 2 inflammation has been associated with comorbid asthma, increased disease recurrence after treatment including surgery, and more severe symptoms, and a differentiation of inflammatory types therefore is considered important [6, 7]. Furthermore, modern biologic approaches for CRSwNP primarily target type 2 cytokines and may have limited efficacy in the non-type 2 population [8–11].

Traditionally, CRSwNP is considered the more difficult to treat subgroup on a long-term basis. Polyp recurrence is common, impacting as many as 78% of patients according to one 12 year postoperative control study of CRSwNP patients treated surgically [12]. However, recurrence rates vary based on the inflammatory type and severity of inflammation at the time of surgery, the surgical technique, the post-operative care, and the length of the observation period. These factors are strongly interrelated and should be considered to correctly understand the situation of the individual patient (Fig. 5.1).

In this chapter, we focus on type 2 inflammatory CRSwNP with the aim of achieving long-term control with the first or a subsequent surgical procedure (in those patients who already had unsuccessful former surgery) without the primary intention to use biologic agents. This implies several questions for further decisions:

1. Is the patient suffering from type 2 disease?
2. Is the patient surgery-naïve or did she/he had former sinus surgery?
3. Has the patient received repeated oral/systemic (glucocorticoids) GCS treatments over the past year?
4. Would a biologic treatment be an option to consider, and if so, as single treatment or combined with surgery?

These questions are interrelated and each may dictate different approaches in patient management. Surgical intervention and/or biopsy of polyp tissue can provide clear signs of the presence of type 2 inflammation, e.g., through the description of eosinophils in the tissue. The authors recommend routine histologic evaluation of nasal polyp tissues obtained either in clinic or intra-operatively as it provides valuable information that may guide future treatment. In the authors' experience, a once proven type 2 inflammation remains type 2, whenever polyps should recur. Should even a small polyp regrow, it will be characterized by type 2 inflammation again. In these patients, a reboot procedure may be an option to break the cycle of repetitive inflammation related to type 2 inflammation and provide an opportunity for fresh mucosalization that may not undergo this same inflammatory pathway. If pathology is unavailable, clinical signs may also indicate the presence of type 2 disease. These signs are included in Table 5.1.

Recalcitrant CRSwNP can be defined based on the nasal polyposis score (0–8 bilaterally) and on subjective symptom severity scales [5]. Severe CRSwNP is defined as bilateral chronic rhinosinusitis with nasal polyps (CRSwNP) with a nasal polyp score (NPS) of ≥4 points and persistent symptoms including loss of

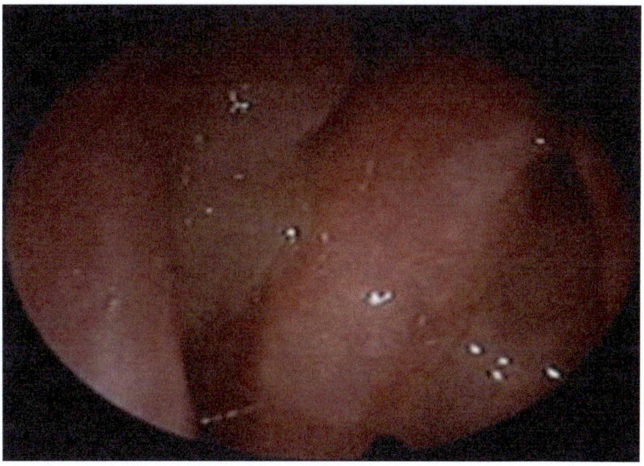

Fig. 5.1 Nasal endoscopy in a patient with nasal polyps (CRSwNP) medial and lateral to the middle turbinate

Table 5.1 Clinical signs for presence of type 2 inflammatory disease

Eosinophils found in sinus specimen
Comorbid asthma (may be before or after CRSwNP diagnosis)
Aspirin or other non-steroidal anti-inflammatory sensitivity
Recurrence of nasal polyposis after surgery
Serum eosinophilia (>150 cells/mL of intermediate association, >300 cells/mL strongly associated)
Clinically relevant allergic rhinitis or other allergic comorbidities (weak association)

smell and/or taste, nasal obstruction, rhinorrhea and/or post-nasal drip, and facial pain/pressure despite medical therapy. Uncontrolled CRSwNP is defined as persistent or recurring rhinosinusitis symptoms despite long-term (intranasal corticosteroids) INCS, at least one course of systemic corticosteroids in the preceding 2 years (or having a medical contraindication to receiving systemic corticosteroids) and/or previous sinonasal surgery (or having a contraindication/unwillingness to undergo surgery).

Indications and Surgical Considerations for Reboot Procedure

In patients who have failed previous surgical intervention for type 2 CRSwNP and report uncontrolled or severe recalcitrant CRSwNP, the reboot procedure can be considered as an additional surgical option. Additional considerations for the reboot procedure are included in Table 5.2.

When former surgery is reported, an estimation of the kind and extent of this operation should be deduced from available reports, nasal endoscopy, and eventually CT scanning. Which sinuses have been approached (were the frontal and sphenoid sinuses included?), and has a "ventilation and drainage" approach or a "mucosal" approach been performed? Have the sinuses been opened and clearly thickened mucosa been removed (partially) or did the surgeon aim to (almost) completely remove the sinus mucosa, as described under the terms "nasalization" [13] or "reboot" [14]? Are those openings still functional, and can the sinuses be inspected with the endoscope? What is the condition of the sinus mucosa in the various sinuses? Healthy, thickened, are there secretions and crusts? The ultimate aim of surgical intervention is to provide an open ostium and a non-inflamed relatively thin sinus mucosa without colored secretions in all sinuses (Fig. 5.2).

If these sinus conditions are not achieved and the patient still has symptoms derived from remaining pan-sinus disease, a reboot surgery approach in severe CRSwNP should be considered. The authors also advocate consideration of the reboot procedure as a primary procedure in patients who suffer from severe uncontrolled bilateral type 2 CRSwNP disease.

Table 5.2 Potential indications for reboot procedure in patients with CRSwNP

Involvement of equal to or more than two sinuses on both sides
Comorbid asthma
Comorbid aspirin sensitivity (NSAID)
Increased blood eosinophils
Failure of previous surgical intervention with return of nasal polyposis

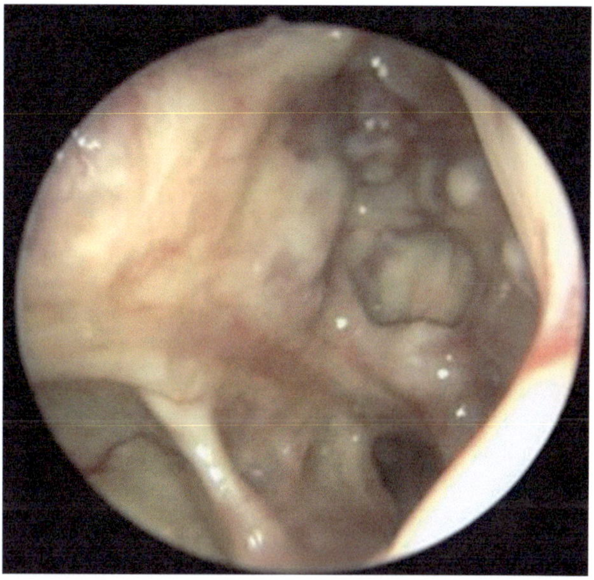

Fig. 5.2 View into the ethmoid after Reboot surgery; maxillary and sphenoid sinuses accessible, no polyps visible

Surgical Principles and Considerations

For the reboot procedure, standard techniques for endoscopic sinus surgery should be applied, with an emphasis on broad openings of each of the sinuses. Once this is obtained, the inflamed mucosa of the sinuses should be removed. Typically, the inflamed mucosa of the sinuses is easily removable with the typical instruments for sinus surgery including grasping instruments like the antrum grasping forceps "Heuwieser" or Blakesley's forceps. The principles of reboot surgery are listed in Table 5.3.

Removal of mucosa may lead to some bleeding from the underlying bone upon immediate removal. This tends to improve quickly but may also be aided by the application of topical vasoconstrictors and/or foam-based hemostatic agents. Nasal packing may be necessary for additional hemostasis.

After completion of the surgery, the nasal re-mucosalization will extend from the edges of the stripped mucosa in the nose into the sinuses within just a few days, and often can be observed to cover most of the maxillary and ethmoidal sinuses after

Table 5.3 Principles of reboot surgery

(a) Broadly opening of the ethmoid, maxillary, frontal and sphenoid sinuses
(b) Completely removing the sinus mucosa of the maxillary and ethmoid sinuses
(c) Completely removing the sinus mucosa of the sphenoid and frontal sinuses. In cases where these sinuses demonstrate normal mucosa, the mucosa can be spared
(d) Preservation of the nasal mucosa of the inferior turbinate, middle turbinate (if without polyp growth), superior turbinate, the lateral nasal mucosa of the pre-maxillary and pre-ethmoidal regions, the olfactory cleft mucosa

just 1 week. After 2 weeks, the total surgical field is often fully re-mucosalized with a thin, but functional mucosa. It is important in this period of wound healing to avoid infections. The authors will often provide doxycycline 200 mg initially, then 100 mg/day, given prophylactically for up to 4 weeks to minimize the risk of infection. These patients should be closely observed to ensure sinus stenosis does not occur. The authors advocate for early and frequent use of topical sinus irrigations twice daily and debridement of the sinuses at 1 and 2 weeks post-operatively. Any early stenosis should be promptly dilated and scar bands cut. We see the patients post-operatively for cleaning and control of pain up to once a week for the first 4 week. The post-operative wound healing period is mostly completed within 8–12 weeks.

Only occasionally, the frontal sinus ostia have to be enlarged with the help of bougies or balloons, or small single polyps from any sinus have to be removed within that time. At the end of this period, all sinuses should be accessible, free of infection and edema formation. Temporary hyposmia is anticipated but does improve. Within 6–12 months, >80% of the formerly anosmic subjects regain smell. To avoid CRSwNP recurrence and to support the smell potential, topical steroid rinses are continued after surgery twice daily for up to 3 years and once daily thereafter, provided the mucosa remains free of polyp burden.

Another approach is the combination of surgery with biologic drugs such as Omalizumab, Mepolizumab, Dupilumab, or Benralizumab [8–11]. The indication for biologics is discussed in Chap. 25 of this book; however, when Reboot surgery is planned and the sinus mucosa is completely removed, a combination with biologics may not be needed.

Reported Outcomes

The authors' own data show that markers of Type-2 inflammation in secretions decrease post-operatively, and smell improves within one to 3 months and is maintained at a functional level over a follow-up of 6 months or longer (up to 5 years documented). Recurrence of nasal polyps rarely occurs, and if so, mostly localized areas of minor disease may occur. In these cases, small polyps can be removed in local anesthesia. The need for revision surgery for CRSwNP is low (below 10% over 5 years).

Tips and Pearls

- Create a relatively large enough ostium such that you can visualize the complete sinus cavities and visibly verify complete removal of the sinus mucosa.
- For removal of the maxillary floor sinus mucosa, the "Heuwieser" bended grasping forceps or frontal instruments may be helpful.
- The frontal sinus ostium enlargement anteriorly and medially can be achieved with the Bachert frontal sinus punch, which can be used to remove the bony frontal sinus floor.
- Blakesley's with different angles (up to 90°) are helpful for the maxillary ostium and the anterior ethmoid approach to the frontal sinus.
- The inferior turbinate as well as the middle turbinate should be maintained as much as possible, as they only seldomly develop nasal polyps and serve the humidification of the ambient air post-operatively.
- Strictly avoid stripping of mucosa in the olfactory cleft or removal of the superior turbinate to minimize the risk of postoperative hyposmia.

References

1. Bachert C, Wagenmann M, Hauser U, Rudack C. IL-5 is upregulated in human nasal polyp tissue. J Allergy Clin Immunol. 1997;99:837–42.
2. Tomassen P, Vandeplas G, van Zele T, Cardell LO, Arebro J, Olze H, Förster-Ruhrmann U, Kowalski ML, Olszewska-Ziąber A, Holtappels G, De Ruyck N, Wang XD, Van Drunen C, Mullol J, Hellings P, Hox V, Toskala E, Scadding G, Lund V, Zhang L, Fokkens W, Bachert C. Inflammatory endotypes of chronic rhinosinusitis based on cluster analysis of biomarkers. J Allergy Clin Immunol. 2016;137(5):1449–56.
3. De Loof M, De Leenheer EMR, Holtappels G, Bachert C. Cytokine profile of nasal and middle ear polyps in a patient with Woakes' syndrome and eosinophilic otitis media. BMJ Case Rep. 2016;2016:bcr2016215054. https://doi.org/10.1136/bcr-2016-215054.
4. Alsharif S, Jonstam K, van Zele T, Gevaert P, Holtappels G, Bachert C. Endoscopic sinus surgery for Type-2 CRSwNP: an Endotype-based retrospective study. Laryngoscope. 2019;129(6):1286–92.
5. Bachert C, Han JK, Wagenmann M, Hosemann W, Lee SE, Backer V, Mullol J, Gevaert P, Klimek L, Prokopakis E, Knill A, Cavaliere C, Hopkins C, Hellings P. EUFOREA expert board meeting on uncontrolled severe chronic rhinosinusitis with nasal polyps (CRSwNP) and biologics: definitions and management. J Allergy Clin Immunol. 2021;147(1):29–36.
6. Bachert C, Zhang N, Holtappels G, De Lobel L, van Cauwenberge P, Shixi L, Lin P, Bousquet J, van Steen K. Presence of IL-5 protein and IgE-antibodies to staphylococcal enterotoxins in nasal polyps is associated with co-morbid asthma. JACI. 2010;126:962–8.
7. Bachert C, Zhang N, Holtappels G, Tomassen P, Liu S, Lin P, Bousquet J. Nasal polyp endotypes: IL-5 and asthma co-morbidity. J Allergy Clin Immunol. 2011.
8. Gevaert P, Omachi T, Corren J, Mullol J, Han J, Lee SE, Kaufman D, Ligueros-Saylan M, Howard M, Zhu R, Owen R, Wong K, Islam L, Bachert C. Efficacy and safety of omalizumab in nasal polyposis: two randomized 1 phase III trials. JACI. 2020;146:595–605.
9. Han JK, Bachert C, Fokkens W, Desrosiers M, Wagenmann M, Lee SE, Smith SG, Martin N, Mayer B, Yancey SW, Sousa AR, Chan R, Hopkins C, SYNAPSE study investigators. Mepolizumab for chronic rhinosinusitis with nasal polyps (SYNAPSE): a randomised, double-blind, placebo-controlled, phase 3 trial. Lancet. Respir Med. 2021;9(10):1141–53.
10. Bachert C, Han JK, Desrosiers M, Hellings PW, Amin N, Lee SF, Mullol J, Greos LS, Bosso JV, Laidlaw TM, Cervin A, Maspero JF, Hopkins C, Olze H, Canonica GW, Paggiaro P, Cho

SH, Fokkens W, Fujieda S, Zhang M, Lu Y, Fan C, Draikiwicz S, Kamat SA, Khan A, Pirozzi GL, Patel N, Graham N, Ruddy M, Staudinger H, Weinreich CD, Stahl N, Yancopoulos GD, Mannent LP. Dupilumab efficacy and safety in severe chronic rhinosinusitis with nasal polyps in the multicentre, randomised, double-blind, placebo-controlled, parallel group phase 3 trials LIBERTY NP SINUS-24 and LIBERTY NP SINUS-52. Lancet. 2019;394(10209):1638–50.

11. Bachert C, Han JK, Desrosiers MY, Gevaert P, Heffler E, Hopkins C, Tversky JR, Barker P, Cohen D, Emson C, Martin UJ, Shih VH, Necander S, Kreindler JL, Jison M, Werkström V. Efficacy and safety of Benralizumab in chronic rhinosinusitis with nasal polyps: a randomized, placebo-controlled trial. J Allergy Clin Immunol. 2021;S0091–6749(21):01459–7.
12. Calus L, Van Bruaene N, Bosteels C, Dejonckheere S, Van Zele T, Holtappels G, Bachert C, Gevaert P. Twelve-year follow-up study after endoscopic sinus surgery in patients with chronic rhinosinusitis with nasal polyposis. Clin Transl Allergy. 2019;9:30.
13. Jankowski R, Rumeau C, Nguyen DT, Gallet P. Updating nasalisation: from concept to technique and results. Eur Ann Otorhinolaryngol Head Neck Dis. 2018;135(5):327–34.
14. Costa Gomes S, Cavaliere C, Masieri S, Van Zele T, Gevaert P, Holtappels G, Zhang N, Ramasamy P, Voegels RL, Bachert C. Reboot surgery for CRSwNP: recurrence and smell kinetics. Eur Arch Otorrinolaringol. 2022;279:5691.

Sphenoid Drill-out for Recalcitrant Chronic Sphenoid Rhinosinusitis

6

William Derek Leight and Donald Arthur Leopold

Key Points

- The management of chronic sphenoid rhinosinusitis (CSR) recalcitrant to medical therapy is time consuming and difficult.
- Sphenoid drill-out is a safe and effective technique that allows large volume irrigation to the sphenoid analogous to a Draf III with a procedure time and degree of invasiveness similar to a Draf IIb.
- It is a versatile technique that can be combined with other extended approaches to the frontal and maxillary sinuses, as well as previously described extended sphenoid surgery techniques, such as mini-nasoseptal flap or nasoseptal rescue flap.
- The technique is a natural transition for most sinus surgeons who perform endoscopic approaches to the pituitary.
- The sphenoid drill-out should be reserved for recalcitrant disease and revision surgery, or in cases of difficult primary disease with high likelihood of recurrence due to anatomic factors.

Donald Arthur Leopold passed away during the composition of this chapter.

Supplementary Information The online version contains supplementary material available at https://doi.org/10.1007/978-3-031-89191-5_6.

W. D. Leight (✉) · D. A. Leopold
Ear, Nose and Throat Institute, Boys Town National Research Hospital, Boys Town, NE, USA
e-mail: William.Leight@boystown.org

J. T. Lee et al. (eds.), *Advances in Surgical and Medical Interventions for Recalcitrant Chronic Rhinosinusitis*,
https://doi.org/10.1007/978-3-031-89191-5_6

Background

Chronic sphenoid rhinosinusitis (CSR) recalcitrant to medical and surgical therapy may result from advanced chronic infectious or inflammatory disease, anatomic factors, or inadequate initial surgical/postoperative management of primary chronic sphenoid rhinosinusitis. It is often multifactorial [1]. Persistent inflammatory disease in the sphenoid more commonly results from systemic factors leading to sphenoid sinusitis in the setting of chronic pansinusitis (Fig. 6.1) and occasionally from local factors resulting in isolated chronic sphenoid rhinosinusitis (Fig. 6.2).

In cases of revision sinus surgery, the sphenoid will be involved approximately 30–50% of the time [2, 3]. The goal of surgical management in recalcitrant chronic sphenoid rhinosinusitis is to improve sphenoid function and mucociliary clearance by removing irreversibly inflamed mucosa, neo-osteogenic bone, and scar. In most cases of refractory chronic sphenoid inflammation, long-term topical therapy will be required, and optimizing the sphenoid for maximal high volume, low pressure saline irrigation is therefore also key in long term management [4]. While a traditional type I, II, or III sphenoidotomy [5] is highly effective in the management of most cases of primary surgery for chronic sphenoid rhinosinusitis, extended procedures are sometimes needed for advanced disease [6].

The sphenoid drill-out is a modification of the traditional bilateral sphenoidotomy that allows for the creation of a single common sphenoid cavity by removal of the rostrum, posterior nasal septum and sphenoid intersinus septum in order to maximize irrigation volume and topical drug delivery (Fig. 6.3). In the surgical hierarchy of chronic sphenoid rhinosinusitis, it lies between traditional sphenoidotomy and sphenoid marsupialization, which requires extensive drilling of the clivus to fully eliminate the need for mucociliary transport [7]. Although it is conceptually similar to a Draf III in the frontal sinus in that a single common cavity is created, in the degree of invasiveness and time required, it is more similar to a Draf IIb. This allows it to be readily performed in the same setting as extended approaches to the maxillary and frontal sinuses [8, 9].

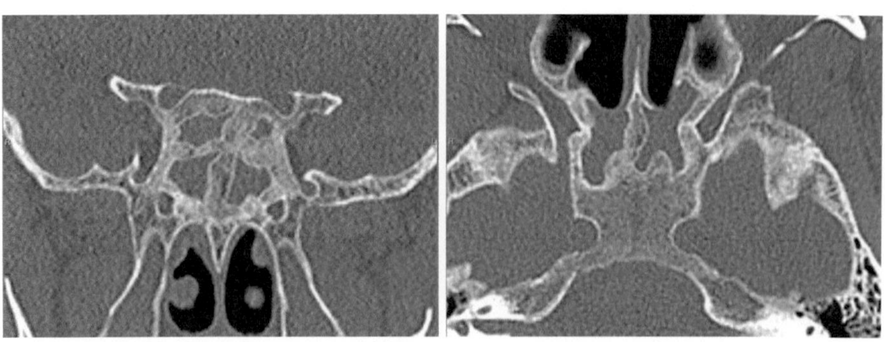

Fig. 6.1 Coronal and axial computed tomography (CT) images of a patient with aspirin exacerbated respiratory disease after 3 previous surgeries

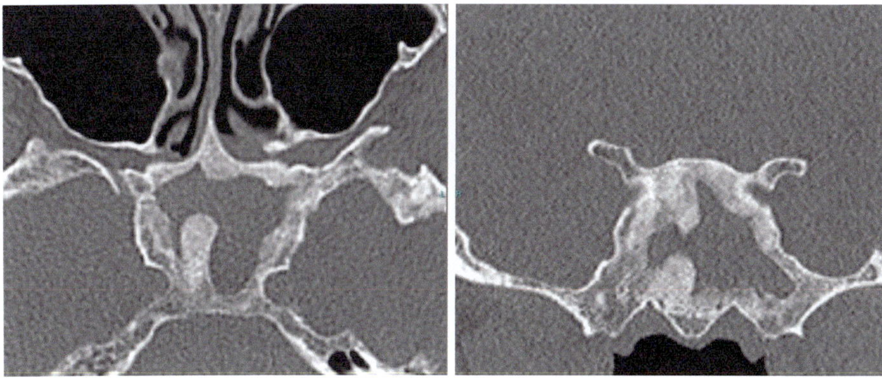

Fig. 6.2 Coronal and axial CT images of a patient with an isolated sphenoid sinus mycetoma without prior surgical intervention. Notice intense inflammatory changes and neo-osteogenesis and absence of a portion of sphenoid intersinus septum despite no prior surgery

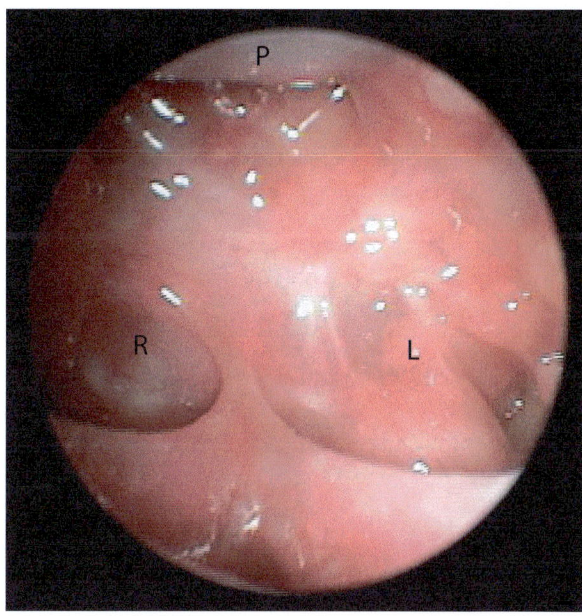

Fig. 6.3 Long-term postoperative result from a patient who has undergone sphenoid drill-out. Notice absence of rostrum and intersinus septum as right (R) and left (L) sphenoid cavity can be appreciated together in the same field as the planum sphenoidale (P) using a 0-degree endoscope

Surgical Indications

Sphenoid drill-out should be considered primarily for surgical salvage. Patients requiring sphenoid drill-out have typically had one or more prior sphenoidotomies. Only rarely should it be performed in the primary surgical setting [8, 9]. Patients typically have impaired mucociliary clearance and advanced mucosal disease (Table 6.1). Advanced chronic rhinosinusitis with and without nasal polyps

Table 6.1 Indications for sphenoid drill-out

1. Recalcitrant sphenoid sinusitis in the presence of:
(a) Isolated sphenoid sinusitis with neo-osteogenesis and/or aggressive synechiae formation
(b) Recurrent sphenoid mycetoma
(c) Sphenoid mycetoma with severe neo-osteogenesis
(d) Chronic rhinosinusitis with and without nasal polyposis
(e) Eosinophilic mucin chronic rhinosinusitis with nasal polyposis
(f) Aspirin exacerbated respiratory disease (AERD)
(g) Eosinophilic granulomatosis with polyangiitis (EGPA)
(h) Granulomatosis with polyangiitis (GPA)
(i) Recurrent allergic fungal rhinosinusitis
(j) Cystic fibrosis
(k) Primary ciliary dyskinesia
2. Neoplasia
3. Recurrent sphenoid mucocele with neo-osteogenesis or bone erosion

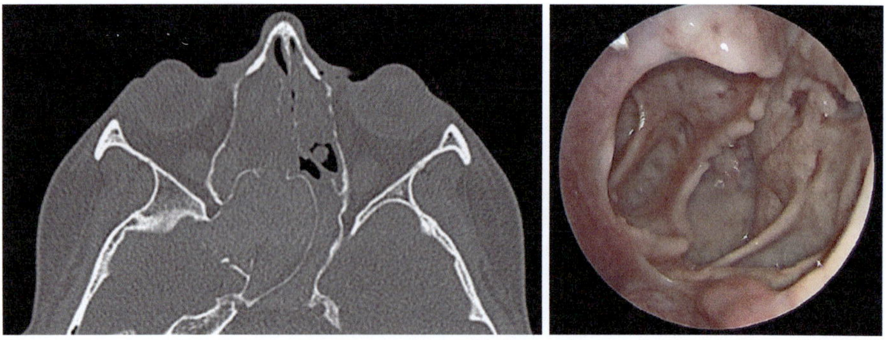

Fig. 6.4 On the left, axial CT image from a patient with AFRS after two previous surgeries. Note extensive inflammatory disease, bony remodeling, high density infiltrates, and multiple areas of skull base dehiscence. On the right, 0-degree endoscopic view of same patient 5 years after a sphenoid drill-out procedure

(CRSwNP, CRSsNP), eosinophilic mucin chronic rhinosinusitis with nasal polyps (eCRSwNP), allergic fungal rhinosinusitis (AFRS) (Fig. 6.4), aspirin exacerbated respiratory disease (AERD) (Fig. 6.1), cystic fibrosis, sphenoid mycetoma (Fig. 6.2), sphenoid mucocele (Fig. 6.5), and eosinophilic granulomatous polyangiitis (EGPA) with CRS are some of the conditions that are more likely to require a sphenoid drill-out.

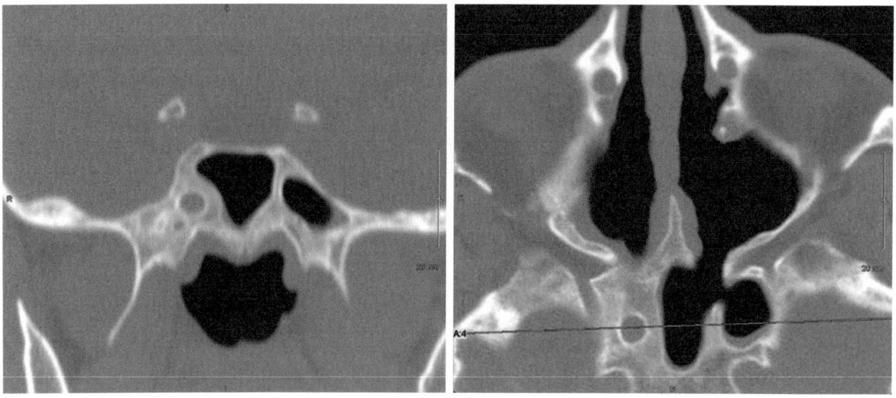

Fig. 6.5 Coronal CT image revealing a mucocele surrounded by severe osteoneogenesic bone in the right sphenoid

Surgical Technique

The technique has similar elements to an endoscopic approach to lesions of the sella. Stereotactic computed tomography (CT) guidance is recommended due to the enhanced difficulty usually encountered in terms of anatomic landmarks, inflammatory change, scar, neo-osteogenesis, increased blood loss, and presence of vital neurovascular structures in the region. 1% lidocaine with 1:100,000 epinephrine is injected into the lateral nasal wall just anterior to the sphenopalatine foramen, as well as into the posterior nasal septum. In the absence of other mitigating factors, the less diseased sphenoid is addressed first. This allows for better access and visualization when addressing the more severely diseased sinus later.

Any revision surgery that needs to be accomplished in the maxillary and ethmoid sinuses is performed first. If a Draf III is planned, the entire sphenoid drill-out is performed prior to addressing the frontal sinuses. Most commonly, a trans-ethmoid approach to the sphenoid is used, as most of these cases are done in the setting of refractory pansinusitis; however a trans-nasal approach is possible.

If present, the superior turbinate or its remnant is partially resected. The natural or surgical ostium of the sphenoid is identified if present. If small, a stapes curette or J-curette are typically used to gently enlarge the ostium initially. A wide sphenoidotomy is then performed with a variety of Kerrison rongeurs using a standard push-pull technique. These are ideal instruments for revision sphenoid surgery, as they allow for forceful removal of thickened bone and mucosa in a controlled fashion that minimizes risk to nearby structures. Having a wide array of rongeurs of different angles and sizes can greatly aid this portion of the dissection. As the initial sphenoidotomy is being performed, care is taken to identify the important landmarks of the sphenoid including the sella, carotid artery, optico-carotid recess, optic nerve, and lateral recess (if present) with V2 and vidian nerves.

The initial boundaries of the dissection are the lateral wall of the sphenoid, intersinus septum, and planum sphenoidale. The inferior portion of the dissection is complicated by the branches of the sphenoidal segment of the posterior septal artery. There are several possible variations when addressing the inferior sphenoid rostrum, posterior nasal septectomy, and sphenoid intersinus septectomy. As originally described, the sphenoid drill-out is then performed by excising the sphenoid rostrum inferiorly, down toward the sphenoid floor, in a type III fashion as described by Simmen et al. [5]. Frequently, a diamond drill and/or kerrisons are required for this portion. A branch of the posterior septal artery may be encountered, requiring bipolar or monopolar cautery for control.

Next, the posterior septal mucosa is incised at the vomerorostral suture and a posterior septectomy is performed using a diamond drill, kerrisons, and backbiters. The septectomy is usually approximately 1 cm for chronic inflammatory disease, although can be made larger if required. The intersinus septum is then removed using a combination of through-cutting instruments and drills. Care must be taken at this point to avoid any grasping and torquing of the intersinus septum of the sphenoid, as it frequently inserts on the carotid canal in the posterolateral portion of the sinus, and could potentially cause vascular injury to the carotid, or possibly CSF leak at the planum. The intersinus septum is then carefully removed as close as possible to the planum, the face of the sella, and the clival recess. The initial steps are then repeated on the contralateral side. Next, the intersinus septum is then carefully removed down towards the sphenoid floor using a diamond drill. This can require up to a 70 degree angled drill, and a 30 degree endoscope, and is typically best accomplished through a binarial approach (Fig. 6.6). Once this is accomplished, the remainder of the sphenoid borders may be drilled if necessary, and any other pathology may be addressed (Fig. 6.7).

Other variations have been proposed to preserve the posterior septal artery through the creation of a mini-nasoseptal flap [10] prior to extending the sphenoidotomy inferiorly. This allows for the inward rotation of the flap over the sphenoidotomy and onto the sphenoid floor at the conclusion of the procedure. This is a good option if extensive drilling is required in the sphenoid that will leave a significant amount of exposed bone. Another possible variation is to perform a modification of the nasoseptal rescue flap [11], where mucosa of the inferior rostrum of the sphenoid is separated from the bone using a cottle elevator. Then, using down-biting kerrisons or up-biting through-cutting forceps held in an inverted position, the more inferior portion of the sphenoid rostrum can be removed without injuring the vascular pedicle. If this variation is chosen, a conservative posterior septectomy must be performed, in order to minimize the possibility of damage to the inferior branch of the posterior septal artery in its septal segment. It has been shown that this is typically the dominant branch [12]. Its preservation would allow for a nasoseptal flap to be raised if required in the future (Video 6.1, Fig. 6.8).

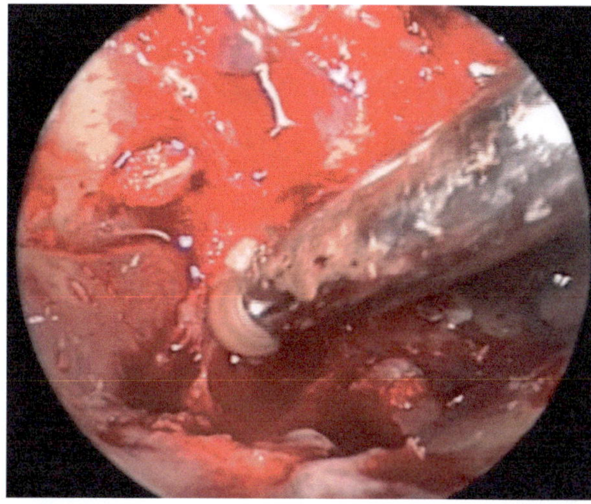

Fig. 6.6 Intraoperative photo showing inferior portion of sphenoid intersinus septectomy using 30 degree endoscope and 70 degree diamond drill

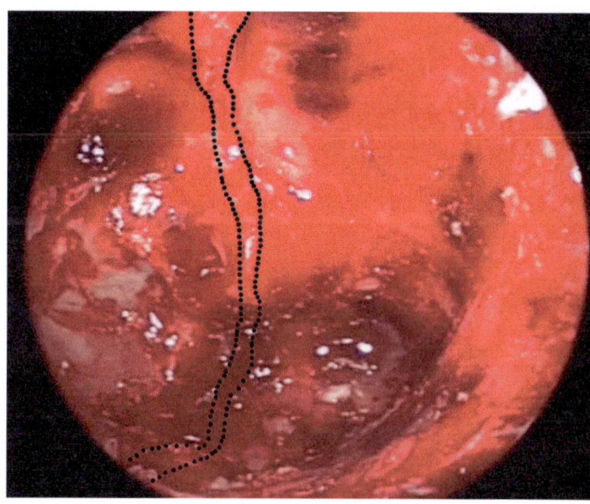

Fig. 6.7 Intraoperative photo showing final common sphenoid cavity after drill-out. Dotted lines mark insertion of intersinus septum which has been removed

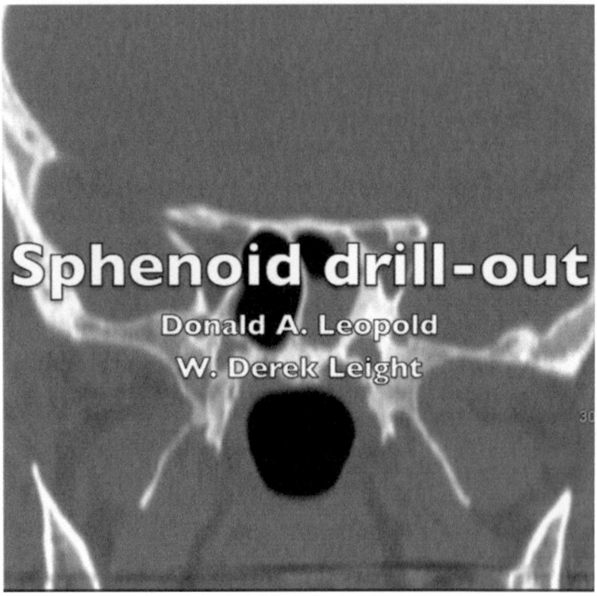

Fig. 6.8 Screenshot of Video 6.1

Reported Outcomes

Two studies have reported outcomes on the sphenoid drill-out procedure. Leight et al. reported on a retrospective case series involving nine patients. Patients averaged 2.6 prior sphenoidotomies. A concomitant Draf III was performed in 8/9 cases. 8/9 patients achieved a stable, healthy common sphenoid cavity at an average of 17 months postoperatively. One patient required a revision drill-out procedure. Lund-Kennedy scores were significantly reduced postoperatively [9].

Van Zele et al. completed a prospective study on the outcome of sphenoid drill-out in 10 patients. Patients averaged 2.1 prior sphenoidotomies. A concomitant Draf III was performed in 3/10 cases. All 10 patients achieved a stable, healthy common sphenoid cavity without evidence of scar at an average of 14 months postoperatively. No patients required a revision drill-out [8]. Importantly, no patient in either study experienced complications due to damage to the surrounding neurovascular structures.

The sphenoid drill-out is a useful procedure that combines a simple technique routinely employed in skull base surgery with the principles of revision sinus surgery for chronic inflammatory disease. The result is a tool which enables the sinus surgeon to effectively address the majority of cases involving recalcitrant chronic sphenoid rhinosinusitis in a safe and expeditious manner.

Tips and Pearls

- Study preoperative imaging carefully in three axes, to understand where critical landmarks of the sphenoid (onodi cells, natural/surgical ostia, carotid canal, planum sphenoidale, optic nerve, lateral recess, V2, vidian, sella, clival recess) are in relation to one another and review areas of bony dehiscence, particularly in cases of onodi cells, mucocele or allergic fungal rhinosinusitis.
- Review CT for the course of the sphenoid intersinus septum, which frequently inserts on the carotid canal. Avoid rocking/torquing the septum when excising to prevent carotid injury.
- Onodi cell divisions should be removed in a similar fashion to intersinus septum. If present, assess for a dehiscent optic nerve.
- Image guidance is recommended to facilitate confirmation of key anatomical landmarks in salvage surgery for severe chronic inflammatory disease.
- Kerrison rongeurs are versatile instruments that allow for removal of severely thickened bone of the rostrum in a safe, efficient fashion.
- Identify key landmarks within the sphenoid as early as possible to help maximize the dimensions of the surgical cavity.
- If a mini-nasoseptal flap is planned, harvest the flap prior to performing the inferior portion of the sphenoidotomy.
- If no mini-nasoseptal flap is planned, a conservative initial septectomy will likely preserve the dominant inferior branch of the posterior septal artery for later use if necessary.
- Drilling the posterior septum thinly with a diamond burr makes the posterior septectomy easier to perform, requiring less force to enter the contralateral side.
- Cutting burrs should be avoided in the sphenoid sinus.
- Use binarial access early and often to facilitate drilling the intersinus septum.
- Despite presumptive "sump effect" in many of these cases, mucosal preservation remains key to salvage as much mucociliary transport as possible.
- Early and frequent postoperative saline irrigation is important for optimal wound healing.

In Memoriam Donald Arthur Leopold passed away during the composition of this chapter. That he undertook this opportunity in the face of severe illness provides a perfect illustration of his indomitable spirit, inexhaustible energy, exuberant curiosity, joie de vivre, and his genuine, deep love of all things Otolaryngology. He was the consummate gentleman surgeon. He gave of himself and his time liberally in the pursuit of caring for others. While thousands of patients benefited from his willing heart and skillful hands, countless office staff, nurses, medical students, undergraduates, residents, fellows, and colleagues were touched by his generous spirit. The breadth and depth of his influence cannot be known. On behalf of all who were trained by him, thank you Dr. Leopold.

Conflicts of Interest None.

Conflicts of Interest W. Derek Leight is a consultant for Medtronic.

References

1. Orlandi RR, Kingdom TT, Smith TL, et al. International consensus statement on allergy and rhinology: rhinosinusitis 2021. Int Forum Allergy Rhinol. 2021;11:213–739.
2. Musy PY, Kountakis SE. Anatomic findings in patients undergoing revision endoscopic sinus surgery. Am J Otolaryngol Head Neck Med Surg. 2004;25:418–22.
3. Baban MIA, Mirza B, Castelnuovo P. Radiological and endoscopic findings in patients undergoing revision endoscopic sinus surgery. Surg Radiol Anat. 2020;42:1003–12.
4. Grayson JW, Cavada M, Wong E, Lien B, Duvnjak M, Campbell R, Kalish L, Sacks R, Harvey RJ. Effects of sphenoid surgery on nasal irrigation delivery. Int Forum Allergy Rhinol. 2019;9:971–6.
5. Simmen D, Jones N. Sphenoidal sinusotomy (I, II, III). In: Simmen D, Jones N, editors. Manual of endoscopic sinus and Skull Base surgery. 2nd ed. Stuttgart: Georg Thieme Verlag; 2014. p. 154–5.
6. Lee J, Yip J. Extended sphenoid sinus Antrostomy and radical sphenoidectomy. In: Chiu A, Palmer J, Adappa N, editors. Atlas of endoscopic sinus and Skull Base surgery, second. Philadelphia: Elsevier; 2019. p. 133–40.
7. Donald PJ. Sphenoid marsupialization for chronic sphenoidal sinusitis. 2000.
8. van Zele T, Pauwels B, Dewaele F, Gevaert P, Bachert C. Prospective study on the outcome of the sphenoid drill out procedure. Rhinology. 2018;56:178–82.
9. Leight WD, Leopold DA. Sphenoid "drill-out" for chronic sphenoid rhinosinusitis. Int Forum Allergy Rhinol. 2011;1:64–9.
10. Thompson CF, DeConde AS, Chiu AG, Lee JM, Suh JD. Mini-nasoseptal flap for recalcitrant sphenoid sinusitis. Am J Rhinol Allergy. 2013;27:144–7.
11. Rivera-Serrano CM, Snyderman CH, Gardner P, Prevedello D, Wheless S, Kassam AB, Carrau RL, Germanwala A, Zanation A. Nasoseptal "rescue" flap: a novel modification of the nasoseptal flap technique for pituitary surgery. Laryngoscope. 2011;121:990–3.
12. Zhang X, Wang EW, Wei H, Shi J, Snyderman CH, Gardner PA, Fernandez-Miranda JC. Anatomy of the posterior septal artery with surgical implications on the vascularized pedicled nasoseptal flap. Head Neck. 2015;37:1470–6.

Revision Sinus Surgery for Recalcitrant Chronic Frontal Rhinosinusitis: Draf IIA/Draf IIB

7

Amar Miglani and Devyani Lal

Key Points

- Recalcitrant frontal sinus disease is influenced by a combination of technical factors, patient-specific factors, and anatomic factors. Effective management requires a tailored approach, utilizing various surgical techniques that have demonstrated high success rates.
- For most refractory cases, the Draf IIa (frontal sinusotomy extending from medial orbital wall to vertical attachment of middle turbinate), Draf IIa with removal of the nasal beak, or a Draf IIb (partial middle turbinate resection with medial extension of frontal sinusotomy to septum) will be sufficient in restoring patency to the frontal outflow tract.
- Meticulous dissection with maximal mucosal preservation is necessary to optimize sinus patency and minimize the risk of restenosis.
- An individualized, patient-centered approach should consider disease severity, local anatomy, procedure risks, patient health, and patient preference to identify the most suitable frontal sinus approach.

Supplementary Information The online version contains supplementary material available at https://doi.org/10.1007/978-3-031-89191-5_7.

A. Miglani · D. Lal (✉)
Department of Otolaryngology-Head & Neck Surgery, Mayo Clinic Arizona, Phoenix, AZ, USA
e-mail: Miglani.amar@mayo.edu; Lal.Devyani@mayo.edu

J. T. Lee et al. (eds.), *Advances in Surgical and Medical Interventions for Recalcitrant Chronic Rhinosinusitis*,
https://doi.org/10.1007/978-3-031-89191-5_7

Background

Frontal sinus surgery has evolved significantly from its origins, which were dominated by extirpative procedures such as radical frontal sinus ablation and trephine-based obliteration [1]. Advances in our knowledge and technology have fueled the evolution of techniques. Contemporary frontal sinus surgery aims to restore physiological drainage of the frontal outflow tract through endoscopic endonasal approaches that emphasize mucosal preservation and wide osteotomies. The goals of frontal sinus surgery are threefold: (1) maintain ostial patency, (2) optimize the delivery of topical medications to the sinonasal mucosa, and (3) prevent obstruction of the drainage pathway, which may lead to mucocele formation.

Wolfgang Draf described varied approaches to frontal sinus surgery in the 1990s, categorizing them as type I, IIa, IIb, and III (Table 7.1) [2, 3]. The type I frontal sinusotomy refers to an anterior ethmoidectomy without manipulation of the frontal sinus outflow tract. Type IIa involves removal of ethmoidal cells extending into the frontal sinus, creating an opening between the middle turbinate medially and lamina papyracea laterally. Type IIb includes resection of the anterior middle turbinate superior attachment with subsequent removal of the frontal sinus floor between the nasal septum medially and the lamina papyracea laterally. Type 3 involves creation of a median drainage pathway with resection

Table 7.1 Approaches to frontal sinus surgery

<table>
<tr><th colspan="2">Draf approaches</th><th colspan="2">Classification of the extent of frontal sinus surgery (EFSS)</th></tr>
<tr><td></td><td></td><td>Grade 0</td><td>Balloon sinus dilation</td></tr>
<tr><td>Draf 1</td><td>Anterior ethmoidectomy without manipulation of the frontal sinus outflow tract/frontal ositum</td><td>Grade 1</td><td>Clearance of cells in frontal recess without surgery within ostium</td></tr>
<tr><td rowspan="3">Draf 2a</td><td rowspan="3">Removal of all anterior ethmoidal cells in the frontal recess with widening of the frontal ostium from the vertical attachment of the middle turbinate to the medial orbital wall</td><td>Grade 2</td><td>Clearance of cells obstructing frontal sinus ostium</td></tr>
<tr><td>Grade 3</td><td>Clearance of cells pneumatizing through frontal ostium to frontal sinus</td></tr>
<tr><td>Grade 4</td><td>Clearance of cells pneumatizing through frontal ostium with removal of bone of frontal beak</td></tr>
<tr><td>Draf 2b</td><td>Removal of the medial/anterior attachment of the middle turbinate with extension of the frontal ostium extending to the nasal septum</td><td>Grade 5</td><td>Enlargement of the frontal ostium from lamina papyracea to nasal septum</td></tr>
<tr><td>Draf 3</td><td>Removal of entire floor of frontal sinus, creating common ostium via septal window</td><td>Grade 6</td><td>Removal of entire floor of frontal sinus, creating common ostium via septal window</td></tr>
</table>

The Draf approaches and EFSS classification systems of frontal sinus surgery are outlined. Within the EFSS system, there is no analogous Draf approach to Grade 0 (Balloon sinus dilation). Grade 1, Grade 5, and Grade 6 are analogous to Draf 1, Draf 2b, and Draf 3, respectively. Grade 2, 3, and 4 are most similar to varying degrees of aggressiveness of a Draf 2a procedure.

of bilateral frontal sinus floors with resection of the superior septum. A more updated classification system discussing the extent of frontal sinus surgery (EFSS) was developed by Wormald, et al. and ranges from Grade 0 (Balloon sinus dilation) to Grade 6 (analogous to a Draf III) (Table 7.1) [4]. The focus herein will be to discuss Draf IIa and Draf IIb procedures in context of revision frontal sinus surgery.

Causes of Frontal Sinus Surgery Failures

Improvements in our understanding of the nuanced anatomy of the frontal sinus recess, along with advances in endoscopic instrumentation, image guidance, and adjuvant therapies, have led to more effective management of frontal sinus disease. A review of frontal sinus surgery outcomes over a 25-year period revealed that success rates increased in each subsequent decade, with Draf IIa surgery success ranging from 68% to 92% in the most recent 10 years [5]. Most studies demonstrate success rates in the mid-80% range, highlighting the real risk of surgical failure inherent in all surgical approaches of the frontal sinus and the possible need for revision frontal sinus surgery.

Surgical failure and the need for revision surgery can be attributed to technical factors, anatomic factors, and patient factors (Table 7.2) [6].

Table 7.2 Factors contributing to surgical failure

Patient factors
Non-compliance
Inadequate postoperative irrigations
Inadequate debridement
Aggressive biological subtype
Anatomic factors
Narrow A-P diameter
Complex frontoethmoidal pneumatization
Presence of suprabullar or frontal septal cells
Prominence of the anterior frontal beak
Small ostial size
Technical factors
Failure to remove cells narrowing the frontal drainage pathway
Circumferential removal of frontal recess mucosa leading to cicatricial scarring and new bone formation
Overly aggressive drilling resulting in exposed bone and excessive crusting, leading to subsequent scar and new bone formation
Recurrence/ progression of disease
Inadequate postoperative debridement
Middle turbinate lateralization
Incomplete removal of the uncinate process

Technical Factors

Technical factors include variables that may decrease the size of the drainage pathway such as incompletely removing cells (e.g., frontoethmoidal cells) or structures (e.g., retained uncinate process) that impinge on the drainage pathway. Other variables include mucosal stripping, which predisposes patients to cicatricial scarring and osteoneogenesis. A review of previous revisions of frontal sinusotomies in 149 cases, Otto et al. identified that most patients had multiple causes of frontal sinus surgical failure [7]. Common factors include ongoing mucosal edema, osteoneogenesis, and technical factors such as lateralized middle turbinates, scarring of the frontal recess, and retained ethmoid air cells (Fig. 7.1). Similar findings have been found in separate studies. Valdes et al. found that the presence of a residual agger nasi cell and mucosal edema were the most common causes of surgical failure [8]. Lateralization of both an intact and remnant middle turbinate can occur, leading to scarring across the frontal recess with impedance of sinus drainage and subsequent inflammation. Avoiding destabilization of middle turbinate's anterior and posterior attachments in addition to medialization techniques such as suture conchopexy (i.e., bolgerization) [9] and middle meatal packing may help minimize risk of lateralization, although long-term outcomes have not been reported.

Critical ostial size has also been investigated. In general, larger openings have higher likelihood of success, but the postoperative size is largely dependent on the patient's frontal recess anatomy and the thoroughness of frontal recess dissection. An important variable that should be assessed on preoperative imaging is the anteroposterior dimension of the frontal recess which provides a measure of how large a potential frontal ostium can be made. The risk of restenosis increases with narrower A-P dimension. Naidoo et al. investigated outcomes of Draf IIA sinusotomy and odds of persistent frontal patency. An ostial size of >4.8 mm and A-P dimension <3.7 mm was strongly associated with surgical success and neo-ostium stenosis,

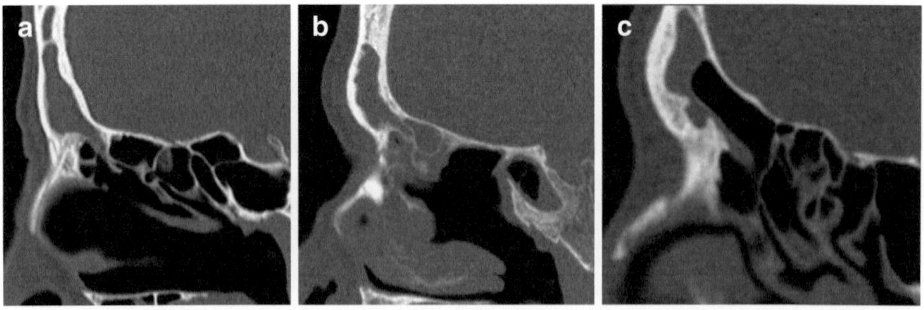

Fig. 7.1 Examples of persistent disease following ESS. Residual ethmoidal cells are present in all images (1**a**, 1**b**, 1**c**). Osteitic bone with ongoing mucosal disease is most pronounced in Fig. 1**b**. These examples highlight that frequently multiple factors may contribute to refractory frontal sinus disease (Property of Mayo Clinic Arizona)

respectively [10]. Hosemann et al. identified 5 mm as a critical ostial size, whereas a drop below 5 mm increased stenosis rate from 16% to 30% and a 2 mm ostium was associated with a 50% risk of surgical failure [11].

Patient Factors

Non-compliance with postoperative oral or topical medical management or inadequate debridement, including intolerance to debridement, is a patient-specific factor that may contribute to refractory frontal sinus disease [12]. Historically, certain chronic rhinosinusitis (CRS) subtypes, including chronic sinusitis with nasal polyps (CRSwNP), aspirin exacerbated respiratory disease (AERD), and CRS with asthma patients were described as refractory patients at risk for recurrent disease [13–16]. However, recent studies have demonstrated that there is no increased risk of ostial restenosis in patients with nasal polyps, eosinophilic mucin, asthma, allergy or elevated Lund-Mackay CT scores [10, 17]. A separate study found that revision sinus surgery rates in AERD, allergic fungal sinusitis (AFS), and CRSwNP cohorts were low measuring approximately 4% over a 30-month follow-up period [13]. Regarding postoperative debridement, when there is concern for a stenosing frontal outflow tract, close follow-up with early debridement can aid in maintaining frontal outflow patency.

Anatomic Factors

The frontal sinus drainage pathway is contained between the medial orbital wall (laterally), the cribriform (medially), the nasal beak (anteriorly), and ethmoid roof (posteriorly). A narrow baseline anteroposterior (AP) diameter has shown to increase risk of restenosis [10]. Within the international classification system of complexity of frontal sinus surgery, factors that increase difficulty (and possibly subsequent risk of failure) include a narrow A-P diameter and frontoethmoidal cells encroaching into the ostium or cells extending significantly into the frontal sinus (e.g., supragger frontal cells, suprabullar frontal cells, supraorbital ethmoid cells, and frontal septal cells) [4]. Careful preoperative review of imaging, use of image guidance, and mucosal preserving techniques are helpful in optimizing complete dissection and successful frontal sinus surgery outcomes.

Indications and Considerations for Draf IIa/IIb Frontal Sinus Surgery

The indications for the Draf IIa and Draf IIb [18] are detailed in Table 7.3. Generally, Draf IIa is suitable for most recalcitrant chronic frontal sinusitis cases. In cases with a narrow AP diameter, presence of osteoneogenesis, a need for wider exposure, or

Table 7.3 Indications for Draf IIa and Draf IIb

Procedure	Description	Indications for revision surgery
Draf IIA	Complete removal of all anterior ethmoidal cells in the frontal recess with widening of the frontal ostium from the medial orbital wall to the vertical attachment of the middle turbinate medially.	– Revision surgery for chronic sinusitis without nasal polyps (CRSsNP) and CRSwNP – Frontal mucoceles – Frontal mucopycoceles – Acute frontal sinusitis – Frontal barotrauma – Recurrent acute frontal sinusitis – Lateralized middle turbinate – Synechiae
Draf IIb	Removal of the medial/anterior attachment of the middle turbinate with extension of the frontal ostium extending from the medial orbital wall to the nasal septum.	– Revision surgery for CRSsNP and CRSwNP – Lateralized middle turbinate or turbinate remnant – Frontal mucocele – Frontal mucopycocele – Osteoneogenesis – Resection of benign of malignant neoplasm – Posterior table cerebrospinal fluid leak or encephalocele – Unilateral approach to cranial base of medial and superior orbit

other complicating factors, an extended Draf IIa with removal of the nasal beak or a Draf IIb procedure may be necessary.

Imaging Review

A decision to pursue revision frontal sinus surgery is often associated with the persistence or recurrence of CRS symptoms. Updated computed tomography (CT) imaging is indicated for revision surgery planning. Imaging review for revision frontal sinus surgery should determine the following features [19]:

- Nature and extent of previous surgery.
- Patency of the drainage pathway.
- If frontal outflow is occluded, determine if the occlusion is related to soft tissue, bone, or both.
- Presence of residual structures narrowing the frontal recess, with specific attention to a lateralized middle turbinate, residual frontoethmoidal cells, and remnant uncinate tissue.
- AP dimension of the frontal ostium.
- Integrity of the skull base or orbital roof and medial wall.
- Degree of opacification of the frontal sinus.
- Any expansile features to raise concern for underlying mucocele.

Magnetic resonance imaging may play a complementary role with its superior soft tissue characterization and should be employed in cases of suspected intracranial complications of rhinosinusitis or concern for neoplasm [19]. The radiographic features can help determine the most suitable approach and extent of revision surgery.

Determining Extent of Revision Surgery

The extent of surgery and choice of technique remain subjects of healthy debate within the rhinologic community. Decision-making involves determining what approach will provide an adequate neo-ostium size to facilitate delivery of topical medications while minimizing risks and convalescence for the patient.

The Draf IIa procedure may be considered for primary and revision frontal surgery for CRS, frontal mucoceles, acute frontal sinusitis, frontal barotrauma, and recurrent acute frontal sinusitis. Askar, et al. reviewed 48 patients undergoing revision Draf IIa frontal sinusotomy for CRS, finding a 92.4% ostial patency rate at 6 months, suggesting that most patients with refractory frontal sinus disease can be managed with such an approach [20]. An extended Draf IIa with removal of part of the nasal beak may also be considered as described by the EFSS classification. This allows for a wider ostium, more direct access using 0-degree scope to the frontal recess, improved ease of debridement, and improved ability to instrument high up within the frontal sinus.

The Draf IIb procedure is typically considered for revision surgery for CRS, particularly in setting of a lateralized middle turbinate or its remnant, mucocele, osteoneogenesis, frontal neoplasm, or for endoscopic repair of posterior table cerebrospinal fluid leak or meningoencephalocele. In a series of 18 patients undergoing Draf IIb, 13 were revision and long-term patency was achieved in 91% of patients [18]. In a separate series of 21 patients, all had patent neo-ostium at 15.7 months and no complications were noted except hyposmia that was reported in 14.3% of patients [21]. Comparing outcomes to the Draf III approach, similar patency and long-term symptom outcomes were noted, but Draf III patients were found to require more frequent office visits and debridement as well as antibiotics compared to Draf IIa patients.

There are trade-offs when comparing less aggressive to more aggressive approaches. A less aggressive approach such as a Draf IIa may minimize risks of complications but could also result in an inadequate opening to control frontal sinus disease. Conversely, a more aggressive approach such as the Draf IIB may provide a larger ostium, but may be associated with increased risk of complications (e.g., cerebrospinal fluid leak secondary to middle turbinate resection and hyposmia). Ultimately, an individualized approach with consideration of the severity of disease, local anatomy, procedure risks, patient health, and patient preference should be undertaken to identify a suitable approach.

Surgical Technique

Draf IIA

The approach to Draf IIA is dictated by the extent of prior surgery and remnant bony and soft tissue obstruction. A complete and thorough ethmoidectomy with removal of any remnant frontoethmoidal cells, lateralized middle turbinate tissue, or remnant uncinate tissue that may narrow the drainage pathway is crucial. Preservation of mucosa is paramount to minimize risk of cicatrization. The steps are as follows:

1. Perform a complete ethmoidectomy, delineating the medial orbital wall and the mid/posterior ethmoid skull base.
2. Identify the skull base just posterior to the frontal recess and frontoethmoidal cells (i.e., just behind bulla and suprabulla cells).
3. Probe and identify the natural drainage pathway if intact, resecting partitions including frontoethmoidal cells and any remnant uncinate process.
4. Using angled scopes and instrumentation, meticulously dissect any cells extending to and above the frontal ostium, including supra agger/supra agger frontal cells and suprabullar/suprabullar frontal cells.
5. Widen the frontal outflow tract from the nasal beak anteriorly to the ethmoid roof posteriorly, to the medial orbital wall laterally, and to the middle turbinate medially.

Extended Draf IIA with Removal of Nasal Beak (Video 7.1)

In settings of osteitis, narrow anatomy, or frontoethmoidal cells extending above the frontal ostium, and extended Draf IIa with removal of part of the nasal beak aids in achieving a wider frontal sinus access and visualization. This technique involves creating a mucosal flap, drilling the nasal beak between the middle turbinate attachment and medial orbital wall, and widening of the frontal sinusotomy. The steps are as follows:

1. Perform a Draf IIa as described above.
2. Create an inferiorly based lateral nasal wall mucosal flap with three mucosal incision (Video 7.1).
3. Elevate the mucosal flap and reflect it inferiorly.
4. Drill the bone overlying the frontal process of the maxilla, resecting the axilla and nasal beak while skeletonizing the periosteum overlying the medial orbital wall.
5. Continue dissection with a Kerrison, curette, or further drilling to widen the frontal outflow tract.

6. Redrape the inferiorly based flap to cover the lateral nasal wall and promote re-mucosalization.
7. Place a Merocel pack or other packing material in the middle meatus to stabilize the flap and stent the middle meatus, minimizing the risk of middle turbinate lateralization.

Draf IIB (Video 7.2)

The Draf IIB involves completion of the Draf IIa followed by resection of the anterior attachment of the middle turbinate with medial extension of the frontal sinusotomy to the nasal septum. The steps are as follows:

1. Perform a Draf IIa as described above.
2. Verify the anticipated location of the middle turbinate resection using CT navigation.
3. Conduct a targeted and controlled middle turbinate resection using through-cutting instruments, resecting the anterior portion of the middle turbinate to the level of the cribriform plate.
4. Extend the frontal sinusotomy medially to the nasal septum by resecting the frontal sinus floor anterior to the cribriform. Consider use a combination of rongeurs, through-cutting instruments, and a diamond burr as needed.

Postoperative nasal endoscopies for the three approaches can be visualized in Fig. 7.2.

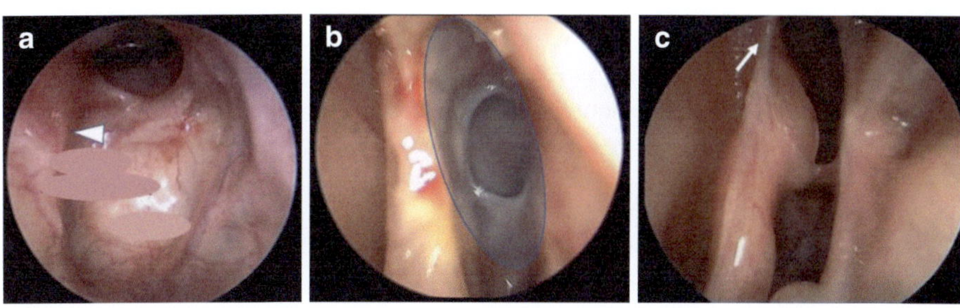

Fig. 7.2 Postoperative clinic nasal endoscopies reveal patency of frontal outflow tracts. Figure 2**a** represents a standard revision Draf 2**a** with intact middle turbinate (white arrowhead). Figure 2**b** demonstrates a Draf 2**a** with resection of nasal beak (blue shaded oval). Figure 2**c** demonstrates a postoperative Draf 2**b** with resection of the anterior attachment of the middle turbinate (white arrow) (Property of Mayo Clinic Arizona)

Adjunctive Techniques and Reported Outcomes

Trephine and external techniques: In the last century, endoscopic techniques have become standard of care for most frontal sinus procedures. Despite this shift in practice, open approaches still retain utility in appropriate clinical circumstances and may be considered as part of a sinus surgeon's armamentarium, particularly in revision frontal sinus operations.

Indications for external approaches include specific instances of frontal sinus trauma, CSF leaks, complicated rhinosinusitis, mucoceles with orbital involvement, and tumors. Perhaps the most commonly employed external frontal procedure is the trephine. The trephine's initial indication was treatment of acute complicated frontal sinusitis (i.e., Pott's puffy tumor). However, indications have expanded and it is commonly used as an adjunct to endoscopic frontal approaches to identify the frontal outflow tract or access regions high within the frontal sinus (e.g., cells extending high above the frontal ostium). In acutely inflamed, infected, or highly recalcitrant cases, placement of a small cannula may be performed to deliver topical medications directly to the sinus and outflow tract.

Most providers prefer to perform the trephination under general anesthesia with patient supine. Important anatomic landmarks to identify include the superior orbital rim and supraorbital notch as the trephine will always be medial to the notch. Incision location should be at the inferomedial quadrant at the apex of the frontal bossing anterior projection of the sinus. Computerized image guidance can assist in confirming appropriate incision placement. Once the incision is marked, local anesthetic is infiltrated in this region and an approximately 1.5 cm incision is made taking care to avoid injury to the supraorbital bundle. The soft tissue and periosteum is incised and a freer or similar elevator is used to elevate the periosteum circumferentially. Hemostasis can be achieved using cautery, dissolvable hemostatic agents, and pledgets as needed. Confirmation of the trephination site can be performed throughout the procedure as needed using image guidance. A high speed 3–4 mm drill can be used to drill away anterior table [22]. Before entering the mucosa (and encountering further bleeding), further surrounding bone can frequently be removed with a Kerrison as needed. Lastly, the mucosa is incised and entered completing the trephination.

Outcomes within the published literature are favorable. Crozier used trephines for repair of frontal sinus CSF leak and found no recurrences with follow-up period of 37 months [23, 24]. A separate study found excellent frontal outflow patency in 86% of patients with 16 months of follow-up who underwent a combined above and below approach for complex frontal sinus indications [25].

Other external techniques include frontal sinusotomy with osteoplastic flap, external frontoethmoidectomy, frontal sinus obliteration, and cranialization. While endoscopic approaches have become the mainstay for most frontal sinus procedures, external techniques including the trephine retain a crucial role despite the higher burden of immediate and long-term postoperative complications and sequela. External procedures may be considered for frontal sinus neoplasms, fractures, cerebrospinal fluid leaks, or in cases of recalcitrant inflammatory sinus disease that are not adequately addressed by prior endoscopic procedures or where disease is far lateral and inaccessible through endoscopic approach.

Stents: Early literature regarding stenting focused on non-dissolvable materials such as silastic sheeting/tubing. More recent innovation has introduced dissolvable drug eluting stents. A recent review evaluating steroid-eluting implants analyzed six prospective randomized clinical trials and demonstrated that the implants can improve postoperative results following ESS with reduction in recurrence of nasal polyp and decrease the need for additional surgery. These results suggest that implants could be used as a substitute for the beneficial effect of systemic steroid use. A limitation is the long-term results and impact of steroid eluting stents. Additionally, there is concern whether these interventions are cost effective [26]. While these interventions hold promise, further high-level studies with longer follow-up are needed.

Tips and Pearls

- Detailed review of preoperative imaging will help inform the appropriate frontal sinus procedure.
- An individualized, patient-centered approach with consideration of the severity of disease, local anatomy, procedure risks, patient health, and patient preference should be undertaken to identify the most suitable frontal sinus approach.
- Meticulous and thorough dissection to maximize frontal recess dimensions while preserving mucosa within the frontal recess is important in optimizing patency and minimizing risk of restenosis.
- Use of angled scopes and angled instrumentation can improve visualization and access of cells pneumatizing high within the frontal sinus.
- Draf IIa is suitable for most recalcitrant chronic frontal sinusitis cases. Extended Draf IIa with removal of the nasal beak and Draf IIb may improve access through a wider frontal drainage pathway and should be considered in appropriate clinical circumstances.
- Ideally, the postoperative ostia size should measure 4.5–5 mm to maintain long-term patency.
- Treatment adjuncts, including frontal trephination, use of dissolvable drug-eluting stents, and postoperative debridement, can aid in maintaining frontal outflow patency.

References

1. McLaughlin RBJ. History of surgical approaches to the frontal sinus. Otolaryngol Clin N Am. 2001;34(1):49–58.
2. Draf W. Endonasal micro-endoscopic frontal sinus surgery: The fulda concept. Oper Tech Otolaryngol Neck Surg [Internet]. 1991;2(4):234–40. https://www.sciencedirect.com/science/article/pii/S1043181010800879.

3. Draf W. In: Kountakis SE, Senior BA, Draf W, editors. Endonasal frontal sinus drainage type I–III according to Draf BT—The Frontal Sinus. Berlin: Springer; 2005. p. 219–32. https://doi.org/10.1007/3-540-27607-6_24.
4. Wormald P-J, Hoseman W, Callejas C, Weber RK, Kennedy DW, Citardi MJ, et al. The international frontal sinus anatomy classification (IFAC) and classification of the extent of endoscopic frontal sinus surgery (EFSS). Int Forum Allergy Rhinol. 2016;6(7):677–96.
5. DeConde AS, Smith TL. Outcomes after frontal sinus surgery: an evidence-based review. Otolaryngol Clin N Am. 2016;49(4):1019–33.
6. Schuman TA, Senior BA. In: Lal D, Hwang PH, editors. Identifying and addressing causes of failure in frontal sinus surgery BT—frontal sinus surgery: a systematic approach. Cham: Springer International Publishing; 2019. p. 199–209. https://doi.org/10.1007/978-3-319-97022-6_12.
7. Otto KJ, DelGaudio JM. Operative findings in the frontal recess at time of revision surgery. Am J Otolaryngol. 2010;31(3):175–80.
8. Valdes CJ, Bogado M, Samaha M. Causes of failure in endoscopic frontal sinus surgery in chronic rhinosinusitis patients. Int Forum Allergy Rhinol. 2014;4(6):502–6.
9. Bolger WE, Kuhn FA, Kennedy DW. Middle turbinate stabilization after functional endoscopic sinus surgery: the controlled synechiae technique. Laryngoscope. 1999;109(11):1852–3.
10. Naidoo Y, Wen D, Bassiouni A, Keen M, Wormald PJ. Long-term results after primary frontal sinus surgery. Int Forum Allergy Rhinol. 2012;2(3):185–90.
11. Hosemann W, Kühnel T, Held P, Wagner W, Felderhoff A. Endonasal frontal sinusotomy in surgical management of chronic sinusitis: a critical evaluation. Am J Rhinol. 1997;11(1):1–9.
12. Shen SA, Jafari A, Qualliotine JR, DeConde AS. Follow-up adherence is associated with outcomes after endoscopic sinus surgery. Ann Otol Rhinol Laryngol. 2020;129(7):707–14.
13. Miglani A, Divekar RD, Azar A, Rank MA, Lal D. Revision endoscopic sinus surgery rates by chronic rhinosinusitis subtype. Int Forum Allergy Rhinol. 2018;8(9):1047–51.
14. Wu AW, Ting JY, Platt MP, Tierney HT, Metson R. Factors affecting time to revision sinus surgery for nasal polyps: a 25-year experience. Laryngoscope. 2014;124(1):29–33.
15. Mendelsohn D, Jeremic G, Wright ED, Rotenberg BW. Revision rates after endoscopic sinus surgery: a recurrence analysis. Ann Otol Rhinol Laryngol. 2011;120(3):162–6.
16. Hopkins C, Slack R, Lund V, Brown P, Copley L, Browne J. Long-term outcomes from the English national comparative audit of surgery for nasal polyposis and chronic rhinosinusitis. Laryngoscope. 2009;119(12):2459–65.
17. Chandra RK, Palmer JN, Tangsujarittham T, Kennedy DW. Factors associated with failure of frontal sinusotomy in the early follow-up period. Otolaryngol Neck Surg. 2004;131(4):514–8.
18. Turner JH, Vaezeafshar R, Hwang PH. Indications and outcomes for Draf IIB frontal sinus surgery. Am J Rhinol Allergy. 2016;30(1):70–3.
19. Hoxworth JM, Lal D. In: Lal D, Hwang PH, editors. Radiologic review for frontal sinus surgery BT - frontal sinus surgery: a systematic approach. Cham: Springer International Publishing; 2019. p. 27–53. https://doi.org/10.1007/978-3-319-97022-6_3.
20. Askar MH, Gamea A, Tomoum MO, Elsherif HS, Ebert C, Senior BA. Endoscopic Management of Chronic Frontal Sinusitis: prospective quality of life analysis. Ann Otol Rhinol Laryngol. 2015;124(8):638–48.
21. Patel VS, Choby G, Shih L-C, Patel ZM, Nayak JV, Hwang PH. Equivalence in outcomes between Draf 2B vs Draf 3 frontal sinusotomy for refractory chronic frontal rhinosinusitis. Int Forum Allergy Rhinol. 2018;8(1):25–31.
22. Choby GW, Nayak JV. In: Lal D, Hwang PH, editors. Frontal trephination: indications, anatomy, techniques, and outcomes BT—frontal sinus surgery: a systematic approach. Cham: Springer International Publishing; 2019. p. 137–42. https://doi.org/10.1007/978-3-319-97022-6_8.

23. Patel AB, Cain RB, Lal D. Contemporary applications of frontal sinus trephination: a systematic review of the literature. Laryngoscope. 2015;125(9):2046–53.
24. Crozier DL, Hwang PH, Goyal P. The endoscopic-assisted trephination approach for repair of frontal sinus cerebrospinal fluid leaks. Laryngoscope. 2013;123(2):321–5.
25. Batra PS, Citardi MJ, Lanza DC. Combined endoscopic trephination and endoscopic frontal sinusotomy for management of complex frontal sinus pathology. Am J Rhinol. 2005;19(5):435–41.
26. Gadkaree SK, Rathi VK, Scangas GA, Naunheim MR, Metson R. Use of corticosteroid-eluting sinus stents between 2012 and 2017. JAMA Otolaryngol Neck Surg. 2019;145(1):90–1. https://doi.org/10.1001/jamaoto.2018.2944.

Modified Mini/Hemi/Subtotal/Central Lothrop for Recalcitrant Chronic Frontal Sinusitis

8

Michael S. Hegazin, Christina H. Fang, Prayag S. Patel, Jordon G. Grube, and Jean Anderson Eloy

Key Points

- The Draf I-III can provide adequate access to the frontal sinuses, but modifications can be made to accommodate the surgical needs of the individual patient.
- The modified hemi-Lothrop procedure (**Eloy IIC**) involves an ipsilateral Draf IIB and an anterosuperior septectomy window for access to the lateral recess of the ipsilateral frontal sinus via the contralateral nasal cavity.
- The modified mini-Lothrop procedure (**Eloy IID**) involves a contralateral Draf IIB and a frontal intersinus septectomy. This allows drainage of an ipsilaterally obstructed frontal sinus through the intersinus septectomy window and eventually through the contralateral frontal sinus floor opening.
- The modified subtotal-Lothrop procedure (**Eloy IIE**) involves an ipsilateral Draf IIB with a superior septectomy and frontal intersinus septectomy. The contralateral frontal sinus recess is preserved in this technique.

Supplementary Information The online version contains supplementary material available at https://doi.org/10.1007/978-3-031-89191-5_8.

M. S. Hegazin
Department of Otolaryngology—Head and Neck Surgery, Rutgers New Jersey Medical School, Newark, NJ, USA

C. H. Fang
Department of Otorhinolaryngology—Head and Neck Surgery, Montefiore Medical Center, The University Hospital of Albert Einstein College of Medicine, Bronx, NY, USA

P. S. Patel
Department of Otolaryngology—Head & Neck Surgery, Maimonides Medical Center, Brooklyn, NY, USA

J. G. Grube
Department of Otolaryngology—Albany Medical College, Albany Medical Center, Albany, NY, USA

J. T. Lee et al. (eds.), *Advances in Surgical and Medical Interventions for Recalcitrant Chronic Rhinosinusitis*,
https://doi.org/10.1007/978-3-031-89191-5_8

- The modified central-Lothrop procedure (**Eloy IIF**) involves resection of the frontal sinus floor bilaterally, with a superior septectomy and frontal intersinus septectomy, while preserving both frontal sinus recesses.
- These alterations represent expansion on the current Draf or nasofrontal classification systems and approaches.

Background

The frontal sinus has proven to be anatomically challenging, both with respect to surgical access and management of chronic and recurrent disease. There exist numerous anatomic variations between patients and even between sides in the same patient [1]. Treatments for frontal sinus disease range from conservative medical management to more aggressive open surgical procedures. Advances in frontal sinus surgery have allowed for movement away from the more invasive and potentially disfiguring open approaches to less aggressive, endonasal endoscopic approaches.

The Lothrop procedure, first described in 1914, consisted of an intranasal ethmoidectomy followed by an external Lynch-type approach with resection of the medial frontal sinus floor, superior nasal septum, and intersinus septum, which created a large frontonasal communication. The micro-endoscopic and endoscopic modifications to Lothrop's original technique have been described in the literature, notably by Draf [2], Gross, et al. [3], and Close, et al. [4] These authors have detailed an endonasal approach similar in concept to Lothrop that also involves creating a large common drainage pathway between the paired frontal sinuses. In the last decade, further modifications to the procedure have been developed to reduce invasiveness and preserve the natural architecture of the frontal sinus. This has led to the description of the modified hemi-Lothrop procedure [5–8], the modified mini-Lothrop procedure [9, 10], and the modified subtotal-Lothrop procedure by the senior author [11, 12].

Current and common methods of classification for endonasal frontal sinus drainage techniques include the Draf and nasofrontal approaches [13]. In the last decade, modifications of endonasal frontal sinus techniques have been developed, but are

J. A. Eloy (✉)
Department of Otolaryngology—Head and Neck Surgery, Rutgers New Jersey Medical School, Newark, NJ, USA

Department of Otolaryngology—Facial Plastic Surgery, Cooperman Barnabas Medical Center, Robert Wood Johnson Barnabas Health, Livingston, NJ, USA

Center for Skull Base and Pituitary Surgery, Neurological Institute of New Jersey, Rutgers New Jersey Medical School, Newark, NJ, USA

Department of Neurological Surgery, Rutgers New Jersey Medical School, Newark, NJ, USA

Department of Ophthalmology and Visual Science, Rutgers New Jersey Medical School, Newark, NJ, USA not included within these classification systems. For this reason, a new classification system consolidating the two previous methods and allowing for inclusion of the four more recently published modifications has been designed (Table 8.1). Here we discuss these modifications in the context of the new classification scheme.

Table 8.1 Classification schemes of endoscopic approaches to the frontal sinus

Draf	Nasofrontal approach	Eloy's proposed modifications	Description
I	I	I	Anterior ethmoidectomy with drainage of the frontal sinus recess without touching the frontal sinus outflow pathway
IIA	II	IIA	Removal of the anterior ethmoidal cells and frontal cells protruding into the frontal sinus outflow pathway creating an opening between the middle turbinate medially and the lamina papyracea laterally
IIB	III	IIB	Removal of the frontal sinus floor between the nasal septum medially and the lamina papyracea laterally
		IIC	Ipsilateral removal of the frontal sinus floor between the nasal septum medially and the lamina papyracea laterally; superior septectomy for access from the contralateral side and enhanced access to the lateral supraorbital frontal sinus and supraorbital ethmoid regions. This also provides bi-nostril, bimanual manipulation; previously described as a modified hemi-Lothrop procedure
		IID	Contralateral removal of the frontal sinus floor between the nasal septum medially and the lamina papyracea laterally with addition of an intersinus septectomy for drainage of the diseased frontal sinus to the contralateral recess; previously described as a modified mini-Lothrop procedure
		IIE	Ipsilateral removal of the frontal sinus floor between the nasal septum medially and the lamina papyracea laterally; superior septectomy for access from the contralateral side and enhanced access to the lateral supraorbital frontal sinus and supraorbital ethmoid regions; intersinus septectomy for access to the entire posterior wall of the frontal sinus; preservation of the contralateral frontal sinus recess; previously described as a modified subtotal-Lothrop procedure
		IIF	Central resection of the frontal sinus floor bilaterally, with a superior septectomy and frontal intersinus septectomy, while preserving both frontal sinus recesses; also termed a modified central-Lothrop procedure
III	IV	III	Bilateral removal of the floor of the frontal sinus anterior to the middle turbinates from one lamina papyracea to the next with superior septectomy and intersinus septectomy; also termed a modified Lothrop procedure

Surgical Techniques

Standard Frontal Sinus Approaches

Draf I (Nasofrontal approach I or Eloy I): This procedure consists of an anterior ethmoidectomy for drainage of the frontal sinus recess without dissection of the frontal sinus outflow pathway (Fig. 8.1a). This involves removal of obstructing disease inferior to the frontal sinus recess. In this technique, the anterosuperior ethmoidal cells (including the agger nasi) are resected without disrupting the frontal sinus outflow pathway.

Draf IIA (Nasofrontal approach II or Eloy IIA): This procedure entails the removal of the anterior ethmoidal cells and frontal cells protruding into the frontal sinus outflow pathway, creating an opening between the middle turbinate medially and the lamina papyracea laterally (Fig. 8.1b). This in turn leads to enlargement of the frontal sinus outflow pathway.

Draf IIB (Nasofrontal approach III or Eloy IIB): This procedure also enlarges the frontal sinus outflow pathway and consists of the removal of the frontal sinus floor between the nasal septum medially and the lamina papyracea laterally (Fig. 8.1c).

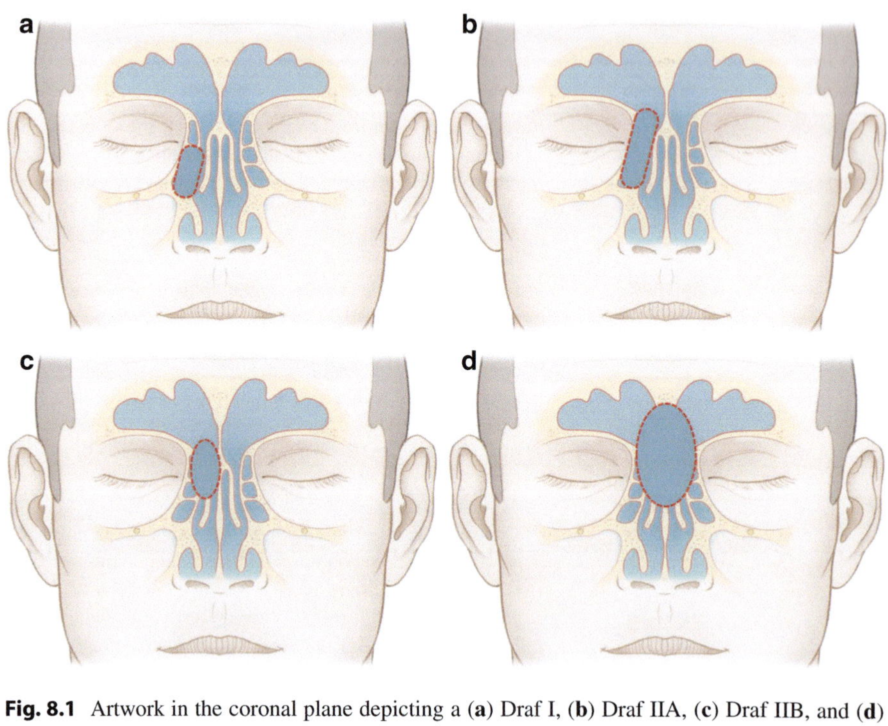

Fig. 8.1 Artwork in the coronal plane depicting a (**a**) Draf I, (**b**) Draf IIA, (**c**) Draf IIB, and (**d**) Draf III procedure. Area containing the resected structures is depicted with the red outline. © 2015 Chris Gralapp

The goal of this procedure is to achieve maximal opening of the frontal sinus outflow pathway on one side.

Draf III (Nasofrontal approach IV or Eloy III): In this procedure, bilateral removal of the floor of the frontal sinus anterior to the middle turbinates from one lamina papyracea to the next is performed, with a superior septectomy and intersinus septectomy; this is also termed a modified Lothrop procedure (Fig. 8.1d). With this procedure, a contiguous bilateral enlargement of the frontal sinus drainage pathway is achieved.

Common Surgical Techniques and the Draf 3

After intubation, the operating room table is rotated 90 degrees with the patient's left side facing towards the ventilator and anesthesia team, the patient's right arm is tucked, and the head of bed is elevated to 30 degrees. The patient's nasal hairs are trimmed, and the nasal cavities decongested using adrenaline (1:1000) soaked cottonoid pledgets that have been marked with fluorescein. One percent lidocaine with 1:100,000 epinephrine is used to perform a sphenopalatine block, as well as injected into the middle turbinate axilla and lateral nasal wall. Depending on the disease process, the appropriate sinuses are opened widely in the standard fashion using both hand and powered instruments and the bilateral frontal sinus ostia are identified when possible.

Depending on the extent of surgical resection that is planned, a superior septectomy is performed beginning at the level of the head of the middle turbinate and carried anteriorly and superiorly up to the level of the axilla of the middle turbinate. Superior septal mucosa can be harvested and used later as a graft or can be sacrificed. Using the inside-out technique, the bilateral frontal sinusotomies are widened using powered instrumentation (combination of cutting and diamond burrs) anteriorly and then connected in the midline, staying anterior to the first olfactory fiber. The nasofrontal beak is drilled down to the periosteum anterolaterally. Drilling is continued, with the help of curettes where necessary, to create the largest common cavity feasible. A free mucosal graft, either from the septectomy or harvested from the nasal floor, can be placed over the exposed bone on the anterior table. This may be utilized in select cases to minimize post-operative stenosis. Silastic sheeting, or a steroid eluting stent, is used to secure the graft.

Modifications to Draf Techniques

Modified Hemi-Lothrop Procedure (Eloy IIC)

The modified hemi-Lothrop procedure (Eloy IIC) has previously been described as a technique used to improve access to the lateral recess (supraorbital extension) of an affected frontal sinus or supraorbital ethmoid cell (Fig. 8.2a–d) [5–7]. The procedure combines an ipsilateral Draf IIB (removal of the frontal sinus floor from the nasal septum medially to the lamina papyracea laterally) and a superior septectomy.

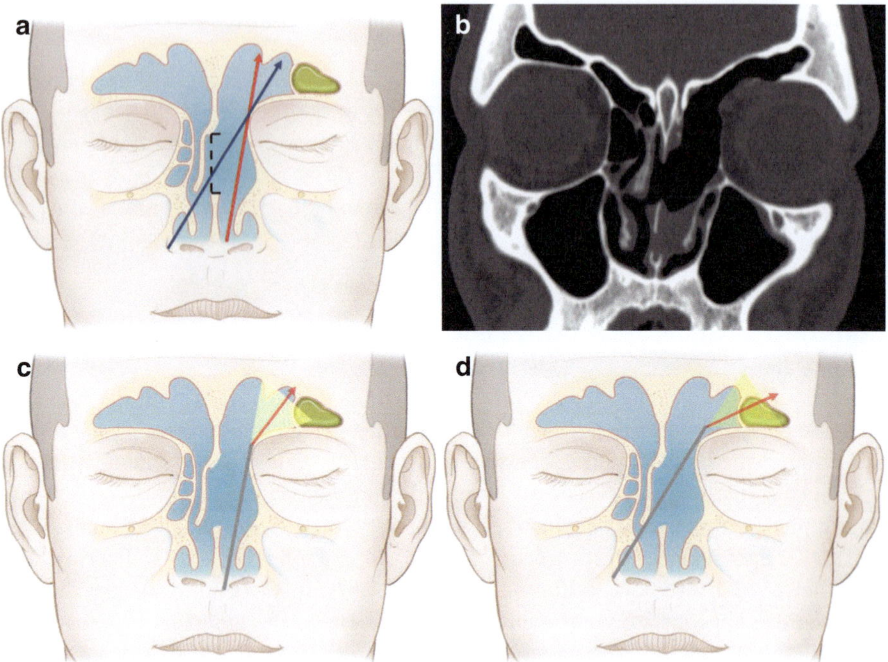

Fig. 8.2 (**a**) Artwork in the coronal plane showing the approach to the contralateral frontal sinus with Eloy IIC procedure, also known as the modified hemi-Lothrop procedure. (**b**) Coronal computed tomography scan in patient post procedure. (**c**, **d**) This technique allows for bi-nostril bimanual instrumentation. © 2011 Chris Gralapp

The superior septectomy window allows insertion of an endoscope and instruments via the contralateral side, thus providing greater access and visualization of the lateral frontal sinus recess of the affected ipsilateral frontal sinus or supraorbital ethmoid. This technique also provides bi-nostril and bimanual instrumentation (Fig. 8.3a, b). The ability to perform bi-nostril and bimanual dissection is of particular importance in cases of soft tissue tumors of the lateral frontal sinus recess or supraorbital ethmoid.

Modified Mini-Lothrop Procedure (Eloy IID)

The modified mini-Lothrop procedure (Eloy IID) is a procedure intended to treat frontal sinus disease when ipsilateral access to the frontal sinus recess is not possible [9, 10]. Ipsilateral access to the frontal sinus recess can be hindered by one of many circumstances, including scarring, outflow tract osteogenesis, or orbital fat prolapse from previous medial orbital wall decompression or trauma (Fig. 8.4a–d). The procedure combines the removal of the contralateral frontal sinus floor (Draf IIB) and an endoscopic frontal intersinus septectomy (Fig. 8.5a, b). While the modified Lothrop procedure as originally described did not require a complete intersinus septectomy, it is desirable to perform a total intersinus septectomy in the modified

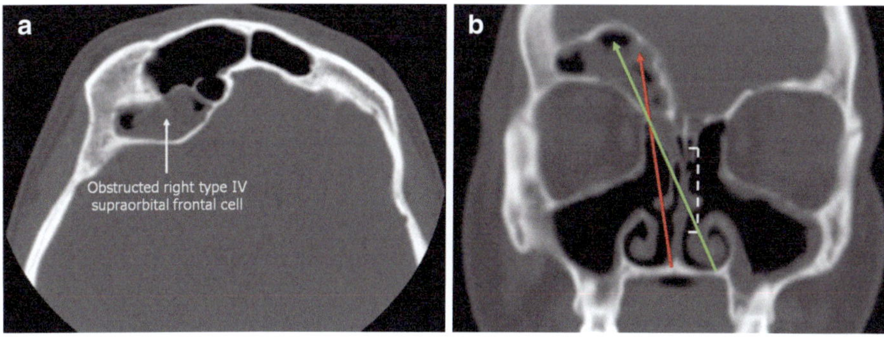

Fig. 8.3 Axial (**a**) and coronal (**b**) computed tomography scan of a patient with an obstructed right frontal sinus. There is improved access with Eloy IIC (green arrow with white bracket showing the septectomy window) compared to standard ipsilateral approach (red arrow). © 2013 American Academy of Otolaryngology—Head and Neck Surgery Foundation

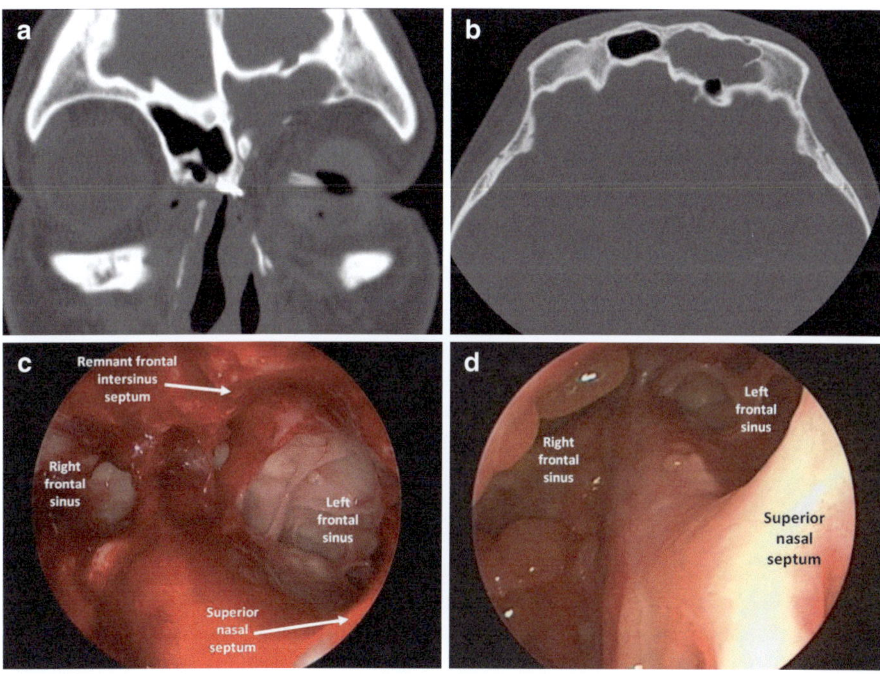

Fig. 8.4 Coronal (**a**) and axial (**b**) computed tomography scan in a patient with orbital fat prolapse. (**c**) Intraoperative view of nasal cavity and sinus immediately after Eloy IID or modified mini-Lothrop procedure. (**d**) Eight-month postoperative nasal endoscopic view of the sinonasal cavity after the Eloy IID procedure. © 2012 American Rhinological Society—American Academy of Otolaryngologic Allergy, LLC

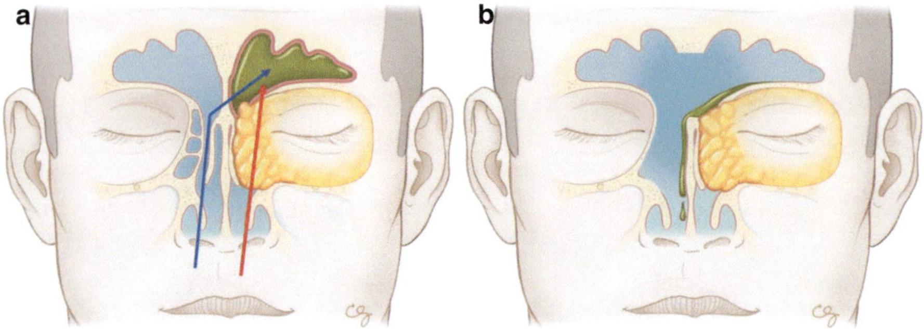

Fig. 8.5 (**a**) Artwork in the coronal-plane demonstrating Eloy IID (green arrow) in a patient with fat prolapse preventing an ipsilateral frontal sinusotomy (red arrow). (**b**) Depiction of drainage via the contralateral nasal cavity after the Eloy IID procedure. © 2011 Chris Gralapp

mini-Lothrop procedure (Eloy IID) since this window is designed to be the contralateral diseased frontal sinus only drainage pathway.

Modified Subtotal-Lothrop Procedure (Eloy IIE)

The modified subtotal-Lothrop procedure (Eloy IIE) is designed for the treatment of recalcitrant bilateral frontal sinus disease and ipsilateral anterior skull base lesion resection, with an emphasis on preserving as much of the normal sinonasal architecture as possible (Fig. 8.6a–d) [11, 12]. This procedure can be used for large posterior frontal sinus encephaloceles, in which access to the bilateral posterior frontal sinus table and bimanual manipulation are desired. This technique is also appropriate for unilateral sinonasal tumor resection in which the contralateral frontal sinus recess is uninvolved (Figs. 8.7a-f and 8.8a-d). The procedure involves the removal of the frontal sinus floor unilaterally (Draf IIB) with the addition of a superior septectomy and an intersinus septectomy. This allows for access and visualization of the ipsilateral and contralateral frontal sinus and bi-nostril and bimanual instrumentation (Video 8.1). The contralateral frontal sinus recess and contralateral middle turbinate are left undisturbed.

Modified Central-Lothrop Procedure (Eloy IIF)

The modified central-Lothrop procedure (Eloy IIF) has not been previously described in the literature. In this procedure, emphasis is on preserving as much of the normal sinonasal architecture as feasible (Figs. 8.9a–d and 8.10a–f). The procedure involves the removal of the medial frontal sinus floor bilaterally with the addition of a superior septectomy and an intersinus septectomy. This allows for access and visualization of both frontal sinuses and affords bi-nostril and bimanual instrumentation. This procedure can be used for frontal sinus disease located near the midline. It can result in scarring and subsequent obstruction of the created central opening. However, preservation of both frontal sinus recesses lateral to the midline opening, and resection of the frontal intersinus septum should allow ample

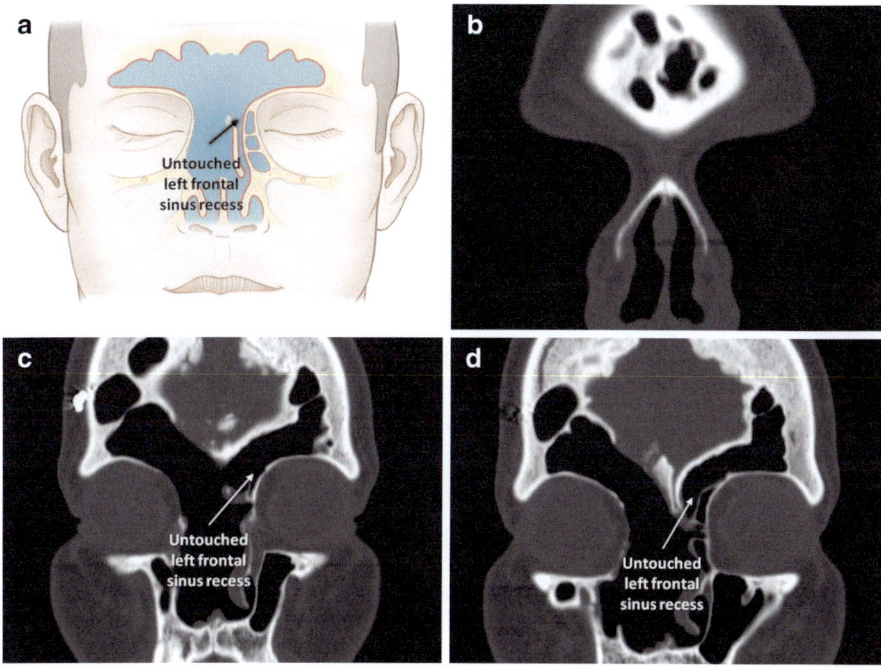

Fig. 8.6 (**a**) Artwork in the coronal plane showing bilateral frontal sinus access with Eloy IIE (modified subtotal-Lothrop procedure) with preservation of the contralateral frontal sinus recess. (**b–d**) Coronal computed tomography scans of patient postoperatively after tumor resection utilizing Eloy IIE. Intact anterior septum (**b**), access to both frontal sinuses (**c**), and intact contralateral frontal sinus recess (**d**) are seen. © 2014 Chris Gralapp

communication between the two sides with an exit pathway in either of the untouched frontal sinus recess.

Tips and Pearls

- Choosing the appropriate approach to the frontal sinus depends on the patient's individual anatomy and surgical needs.
- The modified hemi-Lothrop procedure (Eloy IIC) is a good option for those patients in which lateral recess access is required.
- The modified mini-Lothrop (Eloy IID) can be used to access the bilateral frontal sinuses in situations where access to one frontal sinus is impossible.
- The modified subtotal-Lothrop procedure (Eloy IIE) is useful in situations where an anterior skull base resection has been performed to preserve normal sinonasal architecture as much as possible.
- The modified central-Lothrop procedure (Eloy IIF), a newer technique, can be useful for midline frontal sinus disease with preservation of both frontal sinus recesses.

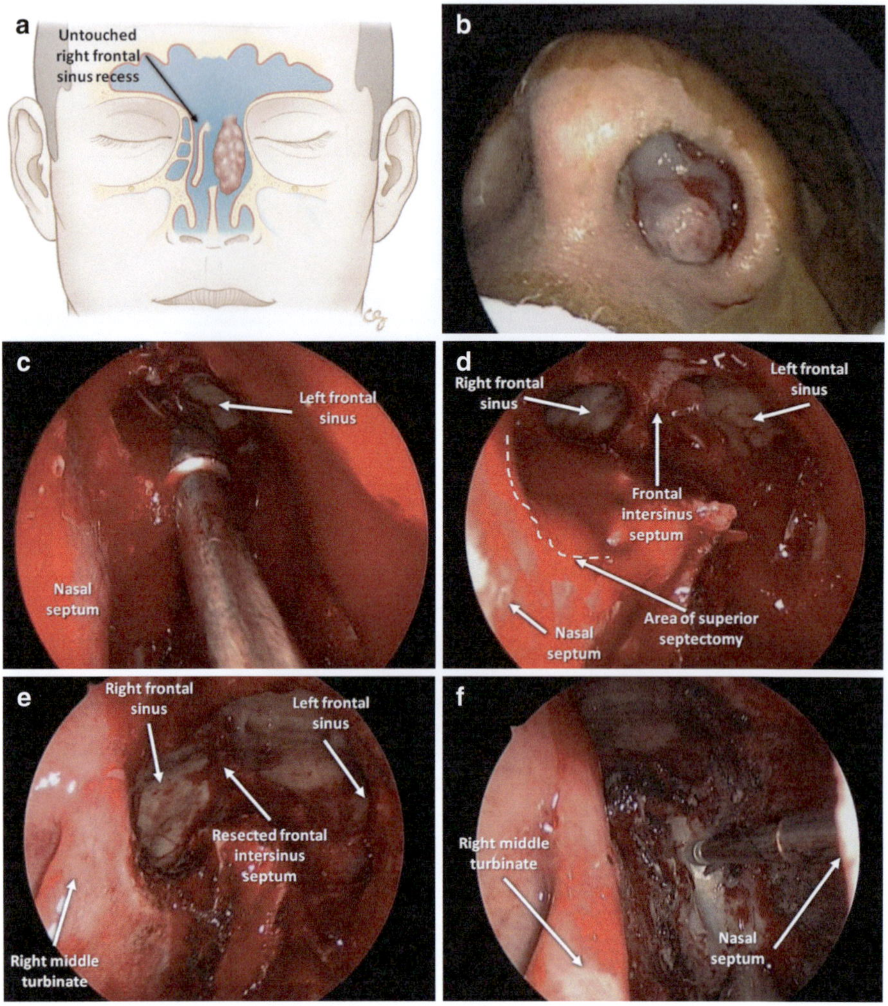

Fig. 8.7 (**a**) Artwork in the coronal plane showing bilateral frontal sinus access with a left Eloy IIE (modified subtotal-Lothrop procedure) with preservation of contralateral frontal recess. Endonasal view of intraoperative modified subtotal-Lothrop procedure in a patient with an olfactory neuroblastoma: (**b**) Initial intraoperative view of the lesion. (**c**) Using a 30-degree rigid endoscope, a left Draf IIB is performed. (**d**) A superior septectomy is performed and the medial contralateral frontal sinus floor is resected. (**e**) The intersinus septectomy is subsequently performed. The right (contralateral) frontal sinus recess as well as the right middle turbinate are preserved. (**f**) View from the contralateral (right) nasal cavity after completion of left Draf IIB, superior septectomy, and intersinus septectomy. © 2014 American Rhinological Society—American Academy of Otolaryngologic Allergy, LLC

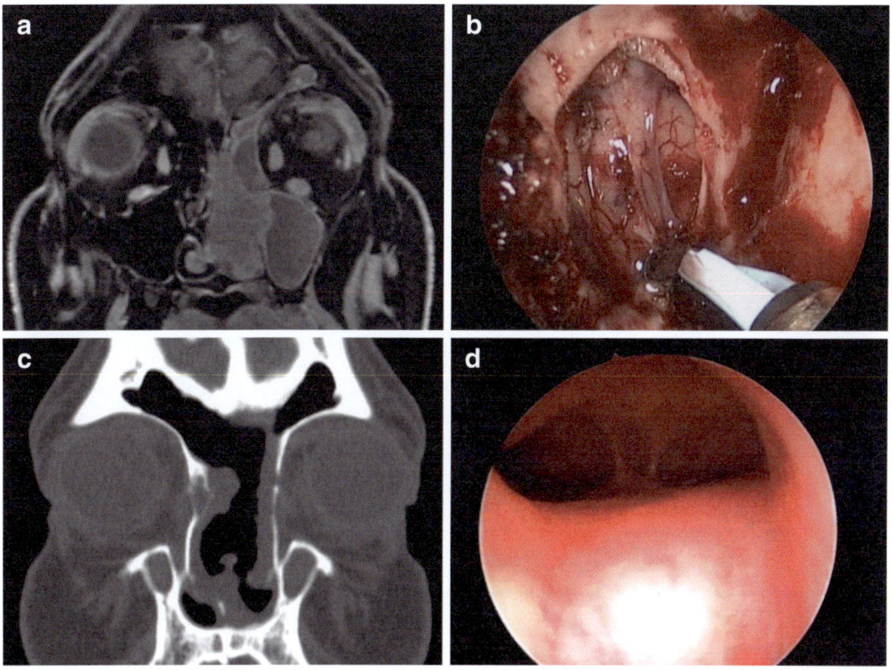

Fig. 8.8 (**a**) Preoperative coronal T1-weighted gadolinium enhanced paranasal sinus MRI of a patient with a left sinonasal olfactory neuroblastoma. (**b**) Intraoperative endoscopic view of the anterior skull base defect after tumor resection. (**c**) Coronal postoperative CT scan of the same patient showing a patent modified subtotal-Lothrop procedure (Eloy IIE). (**d**) Six-month postoperative endoscopic image of the patent frontal sinus cavity. © 2014 American Rhinological Society—American Academy of Otolaryngologic Allergy, LLC

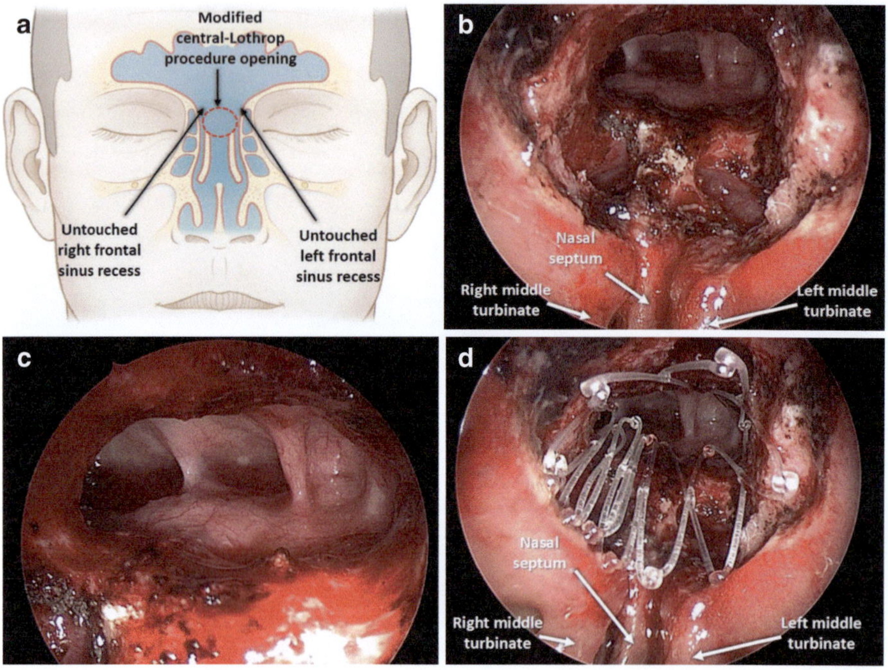

Fig. 8.9 (**a**) Artwork in the coronal plane showing bilateral frontal sinus access with Eloy IIF (modified central-Lothrop procedure) with preservation of the bilateral frontal sinus recesses © 2015 Chris Gralapp. (**b**) Intraoperative 30-gegree endoscopic view of the modified central-Lothrop procedure (Eloy IIF). (**c**) Close up view of the central opening. (**d**) Endoscopic view of steroid eluting stent placement

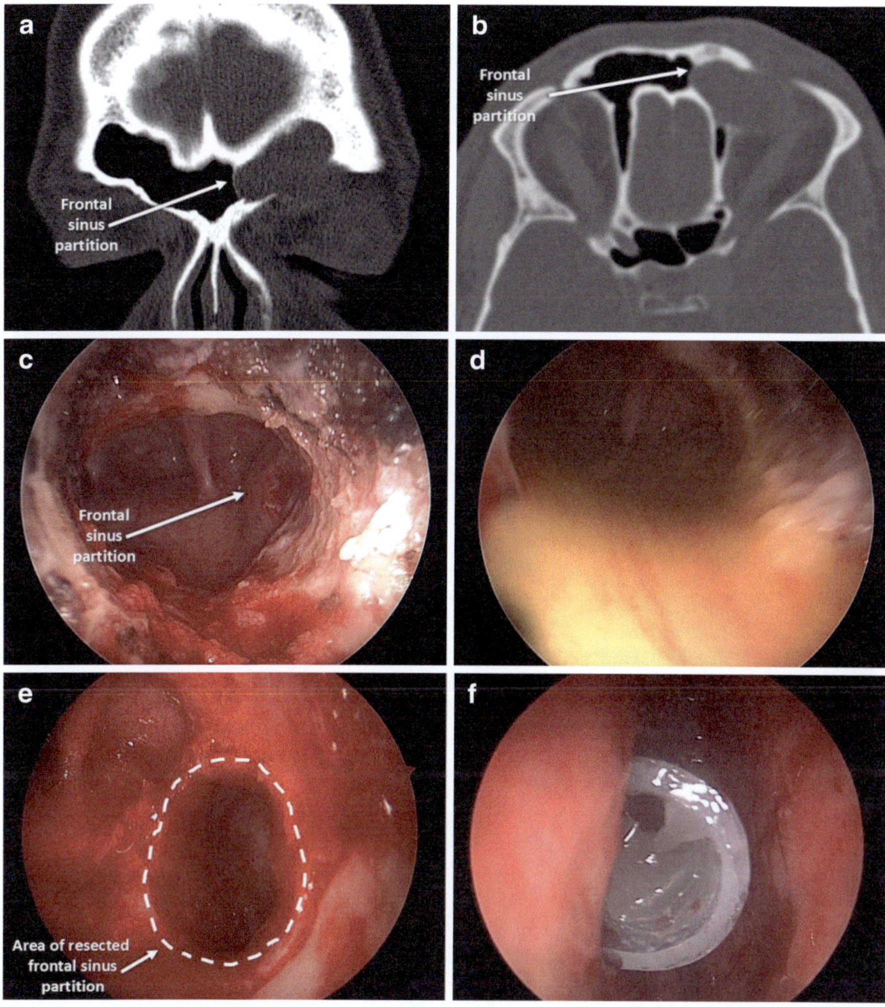

Fig. 8.10 Preoperative coronal (**a**) and axial (**b**) CT scan of a patient with proptosis and a right fronto-orbital mucopyocele causing destruction of the superomedial orbital wall. Note the partition separating the mucopyocele and the frontal sinus. This lesion was approached via a modified central-Lothrop procedure (Eloy IIF). (**c**) Intraoperative endoscopic view of the modified central-Lothrop procedure (Eloy IIF) prior to the resection of the dividing partition. (**d**) Copious mucopurulent extravasation is noted after resection of the partition. (**e**) Depiction of the opening after resection of the partition. (**f**) A silastic splint is used to stent the created opening after adequate drainage of the mucopyocele

Financial Disclosures None.

Conflicts of Interest None.

References

1. Javer AR, Alandejani T. Prevention and management of complications in frontal sinus surgery. Otolaryngol Clin N Am. 2010;43:827–38.
2. Draf W. Endonasal micro-endoscopic frontal sinus surgery: the Fulda concept. Op Tech Otolaryngol Head Neck Surg. 1991;2:234–40.
3. Gross WE, Gross CW, Becker D, Moore D, Phillips D. Modified transnasal endoscopic Lothrop procedure as an alternative to frontal sinus obliteration. Otolaryngol Head Neck Surg. 1995;113:427–34.
4. Close LG, Lee NK, Leach JL, Manning SC. Endoscopic resection of the intranasal frontal sinus floor. Ann Otol Rhinol Laryngol. 1994;103:952–8.
5. Eloy JA, Friedel ME, Murray KP, Liu JK. Modified hemi-Lothrop procedure for supraorbital frontal sinus access: a cadaveric feasibility study. Otolaryngol Head Neck Surg. 2011;145:489–93.
6. Eloy JA, Kuperan AB, Friedel ME, Choudhry OJ, Liu JK. Modified hemi-lothrop procedure for supraorbital frontal sinus access: a case series. Otolaryngol Head Neck Surg. 2012;147:167–9.
7. Friedel ME, Li S, Langer PD, Liu JK, Eloy JA. Modified hemi-lothrop procedure for supraorbital ethmoid lesion access. Laryngoscope. 2012;122:442–4.
8. Liu JK, Mendelson ZS, Dubal PM, Mirani N, Eloy JA. The modified hemi-Lothrop procedure: a variation of the endoscopic endonasal approach for resection of a supraorbital psammomatoid ossifying fibroma. J Clin Neurosci. 2014;21:2233–8.
9. Eloy JA, Friedel ME, Kuperan AB, Govindaraj S, Folbe AJ, Liu JK. Modified mini-lothrop/extended draf IIb procedure for contralateral frontal sinus disease: a cadaveric feasibility study. Otolaryngol Head Neck Surg. 2012;146:165–8.
10. Eloy JA, Friedel ME, Kuperan AB, Govindaraj S, Folbe AJ, Liu JK. Modified mini-lothrop/extended draf IIB procedure for contralateral frontal sinus disease: a case series. Int Forum Allergy Rhinol. 2012;2:321–4.
11. Eloy JA, Liu JK, Choudhry OJ, et al. Modified subtotal lothrop procedure for extended frontal sinus and anterior skull base access: a cadaveric feasibility study with clinical correlates. J Neurol Surg B Skull Base. 2013;74:130–5.
12. Eloy JA, Mady LJ, Kanumuri VV, Svider PF, Liu JK. Modified subtotal-Lothrop procedure for extended frontal sinus and anterior skull-base access: a case series. Int Forum Allergy Rhinol. 2014;4:517–22.
13. Weber R, Draf W, Kratzsch B, Hosemann W, Schaefer SD. Modern concepts of frontal sinus surgery. Laryngoscope. 2001;111:137–46.

Draf III: Overall Concepts and the Mucosal Graft and Laterally Based Flap Techniques

9

Shilpa M. Rao and Bradford A. Woodworth

Key Points

- The Draf 3 (or Draf III) technique, also known as the modified endoscopic Lothrop or the frontal sinus drill-out procedure, has emerged as a vital tool in the endoscopic era to treat recalcitrant frontal sinus disease.
- This technique is also useful in the treatment of lateral mucoceles, skull base tumors, anterior/posterior table fractures, and CSF leaks of the frontal sinus.
- The Draf 3 has also decreased the need for aggressive open approaches like osteoplastic flap with obliteration and frontal sinus cranialization.
- Mucosal grafts and laterally based flaps have shown short-term and long-term efficacy in preventing stenosis and closure of the neo-ostium.

Background

Surgical management of frontal sinus disease is one of the most challenging areas in sinus surgery because of narrow frontal sinus ostia, anatomical variability, proximity to skull-base and orbital structures, and difficult visualization. A gradual

Supplementary Information The online version contains supplementary material available at https://doi.org/10.1007/978-3-031-89191-5_9.

S. M. Rao
Department of Otolaryngology-Head and Neck Surgery, University of Alabama in Birmingham, Birmingham, AL, USA

B. A. Woodworth (✉)
Department of Otolaryngology-Head and Neck Surgery, University of Alabama in Birmingham, Birmingham, AL, USA

Gregory Fleming James Cystic Fibrosis Research Center, Birmingham, AL, USA
e-mail: bwoodwo@uab.edu

J. T. Lee et al. (eds.), *Advances in Surgical and Medical Interventions for Recalcitrant Chronic Rhinosinusitis*,
https://doi.org/10.1007/978-3-031-89191-5_9

stepwise approach is often suggested for the management of frontal sinus pathology, with endoscopic frontal sinusotomy as the preferred initial surgical intervention in patients that do not respond favorably to medical treatment [1]. Aggressive open approaches like osteoplastic flap with frontal sinus obliteration are reserved for severe cases. However, this procedure is associated with a 20% rate of intraoperative complications including, but not limited to, exposure of orbital fat, unintentional fracture of the anterior table, and dural injury, as well as a 10% risk of long-term complications like mucocele and dissatisfied esthetic appearance [2].

Surgical techniques have evolved in the endoscopic era to prioritize functional frontal sinus drainage and minimize complications. Open techniques like the Lothrop procedure, external Lynch incision, and osteoplastic flap have given way to extended endoscopic approaches that markedly increase the pathway for frontal sinus drainage [3]. A minimally invasive technique called the Draf 3 procedure, also known as the endoscopic modified Lothrop or frontal drill-out procedure, has gained wide acceptance as the primary alternative to frontal sinus obliteration [4]. The Draf 3 method, initially described by Wolfgang Draf [5] in 1991 and Becker, et al. [4] in 1995, involves surgical resection of the superior nasal septum, inter-frontal sinus septum, and the floor of the frontal sinus to create a single common frontal sinus drainage pathway [5]. Wolfgang Draf employed an operating microscope to perform the surgery, but it is now adapted to use of an endoscope. While complications from the Draf 3 are lower than open approaches, the primary issue in a meta-analysis of the procedure is a 19% rate of neo-ostium stenosis and closure rate of 4%. Osteogenesis due to the exposed drilled bone of the anterior neo-ostium is often the culprit and can lead to narrowing and recurrence of symptoms [6, 7]. The other causes of Draf 3 stenosis include postoperative adhesions, scarring, and inflammation of bare bone causing mucosal edema and hypertrophy [6, 8]. In an effort to improve stenosis and closure rates, the senior author (BAW) developed the Draf 3 mucosal graft technique with laterally based flaps and first described the technique with the results of a prospective study in 2012 [6]. This study demonstrated marked improvement over pooled analyses of Draf 3 results in the literature.

Indications for the Draf 3 Procedure

The Draf 3 procedure is traditionally recommended for patients with chronic frontal sinusitis who have not experienced successful outcomes with initial conservative surgical management techniques like endoscopic enlargement of frontal sinus ostia or Draf 2 or Draf 2b procedure. These techniques are discussed in Chap. 7. The Draf 3 procedure should be considered before choosing aggressive open approaches like frontal sinus obliteration, because of its minimally invasive nature and decreased morbidity. The primary intent is to create a common frontal sinus drainage pathway for maintaining functional mucociliary clearance and adequate ventilation [9]. Anderson and Sindwani [10] reported chronic frontal sinusitis and mucocele as the most common indications for the Draf 3 in their systematic review and meta-analysis of 18 studies. The technique is usually suggested for patients with chronic rhinosinusitis associated with high risk features like severe sinonasal polyposis, aspirin intolerance, narrow frontal ostium, and ciliary dysmotility [11]. The Draf 3 is also considered for approaches to benign (i.e., osteoma and inverted papilloma) and malignant neoplasms involving the frontal sinus or the frontal sinus ostium. In conjunction with periorbital suspension techniques, access to tumors in the far lateral frontal sinus or narrow supraorbital recess is now possible [12]. It is frequently used as an approach during endoscopic skull base surgery to mark the anterior limits of surgical resection and prevent iatrogenic postoperative frontal sinus disease [13–15]. The approach can also be used to manage frontal sinus trauma and cerebrospinal fluid leaks [16–24]. Fractures involving the frontal sinus have been treated in the past with open approaches such as sinus obliteration or cranialization, with the objective of preventing complications such as mucoceles and cerebrospinal fluid leak from the posterior table [25]. Recently, clinical management has shifted towards endoscopic approaches using a Draf 3 (or Draf 2b) for access to reduce anterior table fractures and repair posterior table fractures and CSF leaks with successful outcomes [26–28]. Other less frequently reported indications include frontal sinus osteomyelitis and frontal cholesterol granuloma [29–31]. Overall, the Draf 3 allows for better postoperative monitoring, prevents frontal bossing and external scar, improves cosmetic appearance, and lessens overall morbidity compared to open approaches [32].

Surgical Techniques

The patient is prepped and draped under general anesthesia. Image guided surgical navigation may be used to confirm landmarks during surgery. The nasal cavity is decongested with 1:1000 epinephrine-soaked cotton pledgets and inspected with a 0-degree endoscope for the presence of diseased mucosa. The extent of sinus surgery overall is based on the purpose of the procedure. Patients with isolated frontal sinus mucoceles or other pathology and no other mucosal disease rarely need more than maxillary antrostomies and anterior +/− posterior ethmoidectomy to identify the skull base as a landmark for the surgery. However, CRS patients with diffuse patchy mucosal inflammation or polyps require "full house" endoscopic sinus surgery with wide maxillary antrostomies, and complete sphenoethmoidectomy [33].

The Draf 3 procedure may be carried out in two ways, viz., the "inside-out" and "outside-in" techniques which were based originally on the diameter of the frontal recess, as reported by Noller, et al. [11] According to their group, the inside-out technique was considered when the antero-posterior diameter of the frontal recess was >4 mm, which provides adequate space for instrumentation. The outside-in technique was performed when the diameter was <4 mm, because the restriction impeded the ability to pass frontal instruments. The other facet of the outside-in approach was the ability to use a 0 degree endoscope for the entire procedure. The outside-in method is generally performed in the reverse order in comparison to the inside-out technique and involves the removal of nasofrontal beak followed by the frontal recess progressing towards the intersinus septum.

Modifications

Our surgical technique has evolved in the last 15 years from using an exclusively inside-out technique to incorporating various aspects of both procedures. The ability to use the 0 degree endoscope with the outside-in increases operative speed, but can also be incorporated into an inside-out approach, especially when the frontal sinus has already been opened with a Draf 2a bilaterally. We also describe our original technique using mucosal grafts from the upper septum (Video 9.1, Figs. 9.1, 9.2 and 9.3)

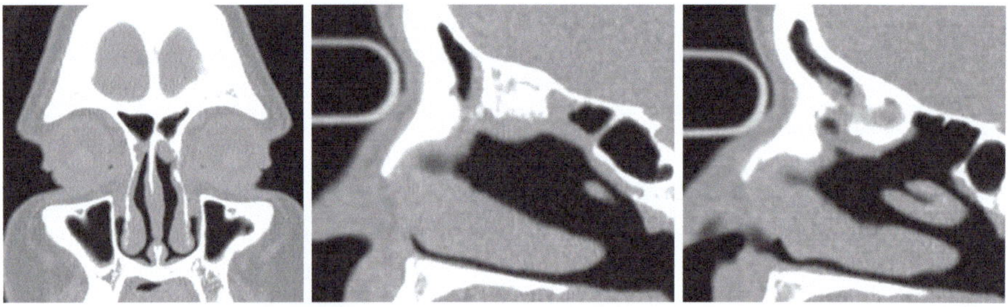

Fig. 9.1 Coronal (**a**) and sagittal HRCT (**b**, **c**) imaging of paranasal sinuses showing small stenotic frontal sinus ostia with a poor A/P diameter

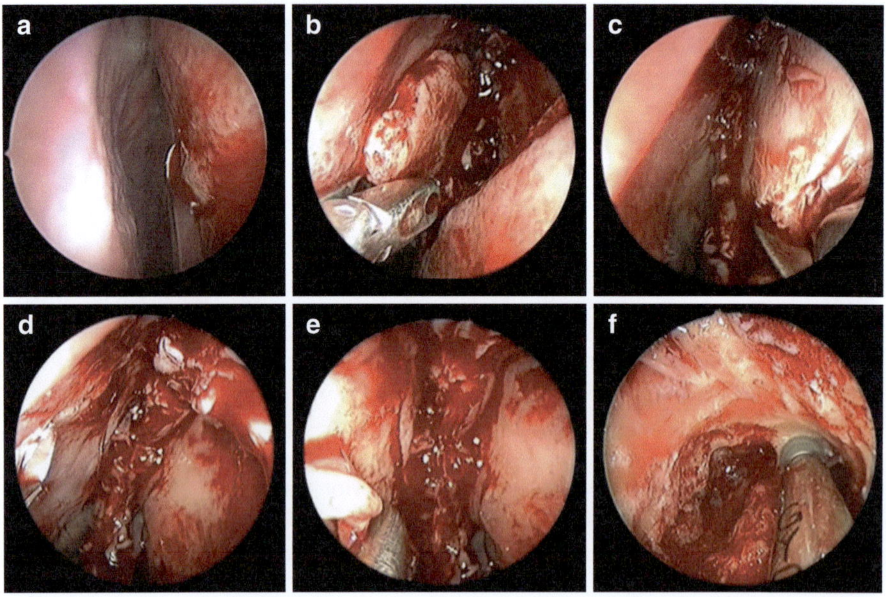

Fig. 9.2 Intraoperative images of Draf 3 mucosal graft and laterally based flap technique for the patient in Fig. 9.1. The upper septectomy is outlined with a beaver blade (**a**) and the right upper septal mucosal graft removed (**b**). A scissor is used to complete the incisions and harvest the left upper septal mucosal graft. Laterally based flaps ending at the nasal vault are incised with a beaver blade (**d**) and displaced inferiorly with an elevator (**e**) to the level of the inferior turbinate head so that they are out of the way for drilling the Draf 3 (**f**)

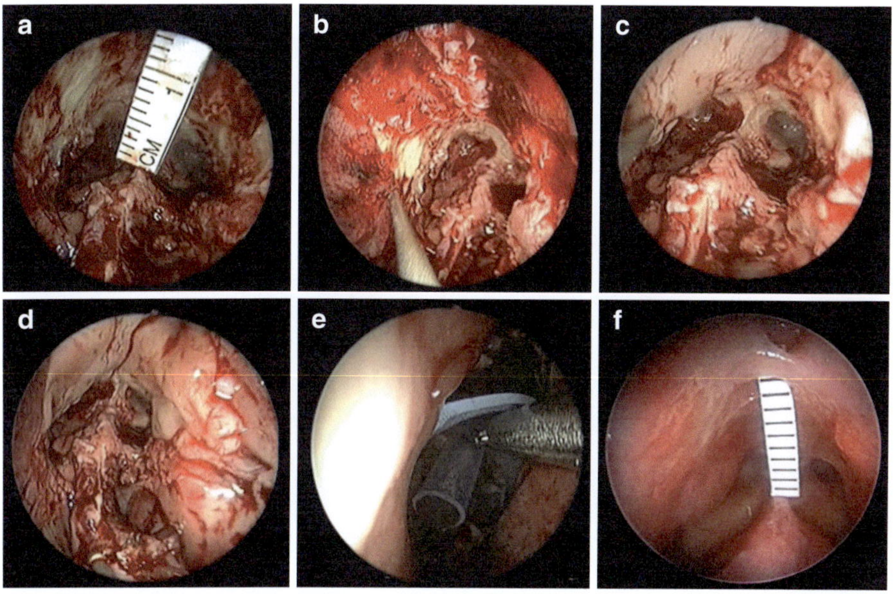

Fig. 9.3 Intra-operative views of the completed Draf 3 with measurement of the A/P diameter (**a**). The laterally based flaps are placed back into position over the bone that was drilled laterally (**b**) and the first mucosal graft placed over the drilled frontal beak (**c**). 70 degree endoscopic view of both mucosal grafts over all the drilled bone and the lateral flaps covering the lateral bone (**d**). Rolled silastic sheets are placed to cover the grafts (**e**) and postoperative healing and diameter show similar diameter at 3 months (**f**)

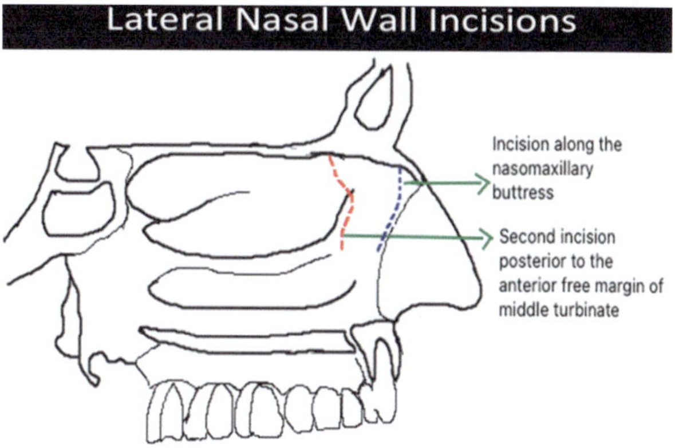

Fig. 9.4 Incisions along the lateral nasal wall—anterior (in blue) and posterior incision (in red), in preparation for the Draf III procedure

as well as a newer modification of the technique that incorporates the upper septal mucosa with our laterally based flaps (Video 9.2, Figs. 9.4, 9.5, 9.6 and 9.7).

Starting with a 0 degree scope, the upper septectomy is outlined with an angled Beaver blade or, more recently, with an extended needle-tip bovie cautery. The mucosal grafts are harvested, placed on the back table, the perichondrium and submucosa thinned, and placed in saline for later in the case. Alternatively, the posterior aspect of one or both inferior turbinates can be harvested and thinned out for use if

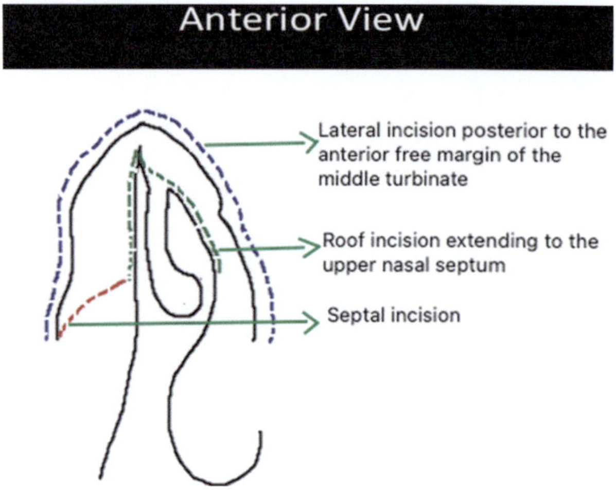

Fig. 9.5 Incisions depicted in the anterior nasal view—anterior incision (in blue), posterior incision (in green) and inferior septal incision (in red)

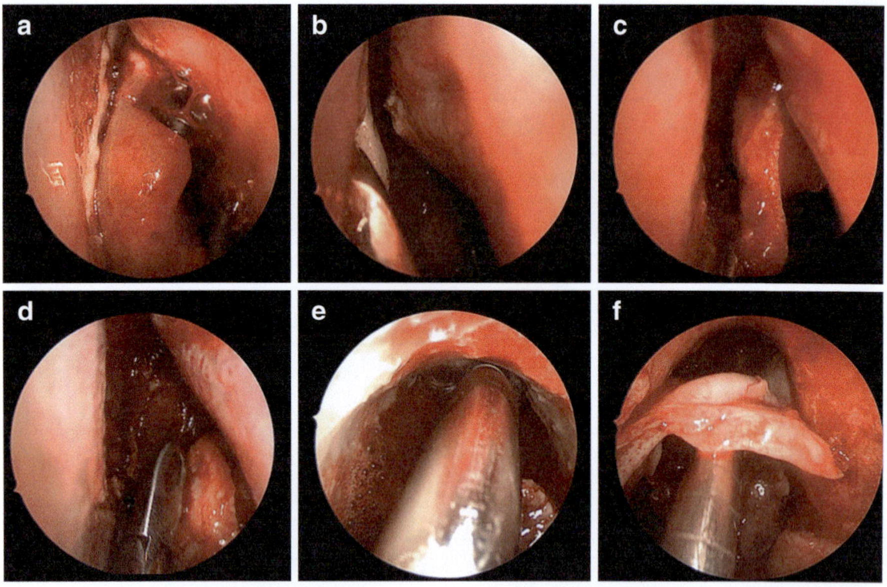

Fig. 9.6 A lateral nasal wall incision for a complete flap technique (**a**) is demonstrated using a needle tip bovie cautery followed by elevation of the upper septal mucosa connected to the lateral flap (**b–d**). The Draf 3 is performed (**e**) and the right flap is placed into the frontal sinus over the beak (**f**)

the mucosa is unusable (i.e., polypoid change, already perforated). Next, laterally based mucoperiosteal flaps based on the front portion of the inferior turbinate are elevated following a lateral incision posterior to the anterior free margin of the middle turbinate extended to the upper nasal septum approximately a half centimeter posterior to the anterior most middle turbinate attachment. Another lateral incision

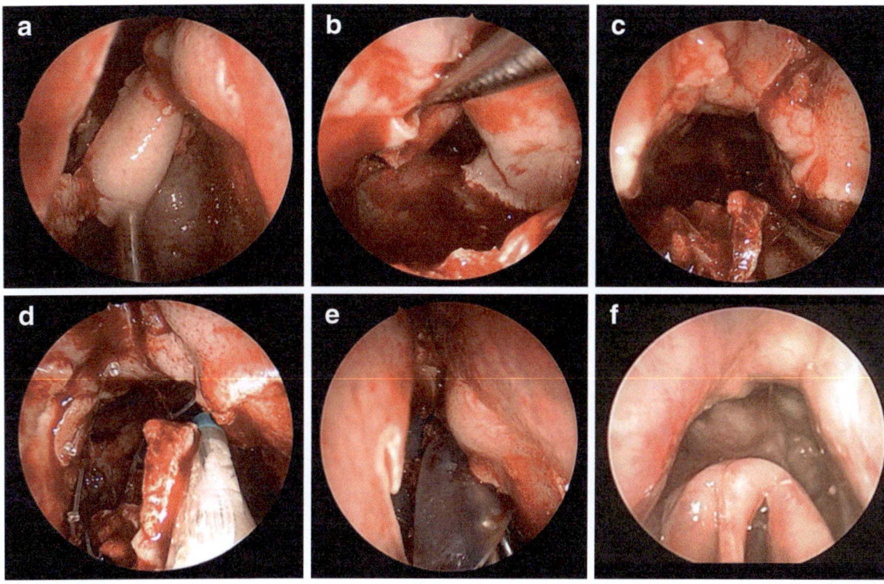

Fig. 9.7 The left flap is then placed into the frontal sinus (**a**) and both flaps positioned over the exposed bone of the sinus (**b**). Endoscopic view of the flaps in position (**c**). Mometasone eluting stents are placed over the flaps to tack them down (**d**) and additional silastic sheets are placed to cover the flaps (**e**). Endoscopic view at 3 months reveals a stable diameter with well healed flaps (**f**)

along the nasomaxillary buttress just posterior to the cartilaginous nose is made superiorly to the nasal vault under the nasal bones but posterior to the cartilaginous attachments to avoid exposure of the anterior cartilage. The flap is elevated in the subperiosteal plane and preserved for later in the procedure. Recently, we have transitioned the majority of the time to elevating one continuous flap on each side that incorporates the laterally based flap with the upper septal mucosa. This is a difficult technique to master due to the thin, friable nature of the mucosa that spans the upper nasal vault. The flaps are placed out of the way of the instruments and endoscope on the nasal floor.

The septal mucosa of the posterior aspect of the septectomy is elevated to identify the first olfactory filia on both sides. The procedure then continues using 15-degree cutting and diamond burrs to thin the nasolacrimal area and lateral bone to improve width. While we may proceed with a classic outside-in approach depending on the circumstances (i.e., osteoma filling the frontal sinus recess), more commonly we use the 0 degree view and 15-degree bur to drill anteriorly from the Draf 2a, removing the frontal sinus floor/nasofrontal beak on both sides and crossing over to create a common cavity. Once the basic cavity is sculpted, we switch to a 70-degree endoscope and 70-degree diamond burr to polish the corners of the neo-ostium, as well as remove the remainder of the intersinus septum and any lateral partitions within the frontal sinus to achieve maximal diameter.

Next, the laterally based flaps are transferred to the lateral and inferior aspect of the neo-ostium and, if raised attached to the upper septal mucosa, the additional length covers the anterior aspect of the ipsilateral portion of the Draf 3. Otherwise, the upper septal or inferior turbinate mucosal grafts harvested earlier are placed onto the anterior aspect of the neo-ostium and rolled 0.5 mm silastic sheeting cut to fit are placed into the frontal sinus to cover the mucosal grafts or flaps. Frontal Propel steroid-eluting stents can also be used to help provide pressure and tack the grafts or flaps down. Nasopore® or other bioabsorbable material can also be placed into the Draf 3 to provide additional pressure.

Reported Outcomes

Numerous studies describe the benefits of the Draf 3 procedure and validate it as the preferred procedure over an osteoplastic flap. However, it should be noted that closure or stenosis is the most common reason for revision and the most common complication. Shih, et al. [34] reviewed 29 articles that described the Draf 3 in 1205 patients, and identified symptom improvement with an overall rate of 85.6% and an overall patency rate of 90.7%. This was compared to results of an earlier meta-analysis that had an overall patency rate of 86.1%, but the stenosis rate of the earlier cohort was 15% with an additional 4% with complete closure [10]. Several groups, including our own, use the mucosal graft technique which may have contributed to the improved patency rate in the later cohort [6, 8, 32, 35, 36]. Ting, et al. [37], in their retrospective study of 204 patients, saw a recurrence rate of 30% due to frontal sinus restenosis after 10 years of follow-up. Eloy, et al. [38], in their retrospective multi-institutional study of 120 patients who underwent Draf 3 procedure, noticed stenosis of the neo-ostium in 16 patients (13%) and a complete closure in 15 patients (12.5%). There was an increased risk of restenosis in patients with aspirin sensitivity, asthma, and cystic fibrosis [7, 38]. Several studies have shown that the success rates remain unchanged with short- and long-term follow-up whereas the rates of revision surgery gradually increase with time [34, 38].

The senior author (BAW) developed the Draf 3 mucosal grafting technique with laterally based flaps in 2008 due to frustration with the prolonged healing time of the bare bone of the frontal beak and the subsequent decrease in neo-ostial size/diameter that was observed in the first 3 months postoperatively. We hypothesized that covering the bare bone with mucosal grafts or flaps would minimize postoperative osteoneogenesis, decrease stenosis, and avoid revision surgery. A prospective study to evaluate the technique was performed with measurement of the intraoperative antero-posterior diameter with a trimmed paper ruler inserted into the Draf 3 cavity at the level of the drilled nasofrontal beak to the anterior aspect of the central cribriform plate. A ruler was also inserted into the neo-ostium at their clinical follow-up visits and the results recorded. Patients followed up to 3 months were included in the study where we observed excellent results with an average neo-ostium diameter of 10.8 mm at 3 months compared to 11.7 mm pre-operatively. Importantly, no patients developed stenosis (<50% original diameter) and there was a 100% success rate (no closure >50% and no revisions) [6]. While overall follow-up was an average of 16 months (3–30), we subsequently published our 1 year follow-up study in 2016 which enrolled 67 patients with a year or more follow-up (average 34 m, R 12–85) with measurements of 11.0 mm+/−1.9 AP diameter preoperatively and 9.9 mm+/−2.2 at last clinical follow-up. There were two failures by definition with stenosis (97% success rate) but they had an effective outcome since they did not require revision. In fact, there were no revisions of the Draf 3 in the entire cohort [8].

In a later study, Hildenbrand et al. [36] reported a high success rate of 94% using a similar technique. More recently, Wang et al. [7] performed a controlled trial of subjects receiving a Draf 3 that were randomized to mucosal grafting or controls. He used calipers to measure the neo-ostium and found that subjects receiving mucosal grafts and pedicled flaps had significantly greater lateral and A-P dimensions at all time-points postoperatively up to 1 year. Another described technique to cover the exposed bone with a vascularized septal mucosal flap based on the anterior ethmoidal artery and nasoseptal artery was reported and noted to have patent neo-ostiums in the post-operative period [39, 40]. However, these studies lacked adequate patient sampling (n δ 4) and require further investigation. Studies using a superior lateral anterior pedicled flap to cover the exposed bone in Draf 2 and 3 procedures have reported 100% success rate in 25 patients [41, 42]. While further evaluation with larger numbers of specifically Draf 3 subjects is required to evaluate superiority over mucosal grafting techniques, these studies add further support to the overwhelming evidence that the drilled bone should be covered in a Draf 3 to improve clinical outcomes.

Tips and Pearls

- Adequate care to preserve the posterior table mucosa.
- Cover the bare bone with mucosal grafts or pedicled flaps to help prevent re-stenosis.
- Start with the 0 degree scope to raise the flaps and harvest mucosal grafts.
- Prolonged follow-up is necessary for early identification of complications and timely intervention.

Disclosures Bradford A. Woodworth serves as a consultant for Cook Medical.

References

1. Metson R, Sindwani R. Endoscopic surgery for frontal sinusitis--a graduated approach. Otolaryngol Clin N Am. 2004;37(2):411–22.
2. Weber R, Draf W, Keerl R, et al. Osteoplastic frontal sinus surgery with fat obliteration: technique and long-term results using magnetic resonance imaging in 82 operations. Laryngoscope. 2000;110(6):1037–44.
3. Eloy JA, Vázquez A, Liu JK, Baredes S. Endoscopic approaches to the frontal sinus: modifications of the existing techniques and proposed classification. Otolaryngol Clin N Am. 2016;49(4):1007–18.

4. Becker DG, Moore D, Lindsey WH, Gross WE, Gross CW. Modified transnasal endoscopic Lothrop procedure: further considerations. Laryngoscope. 1995;105(11):1161–6.
5. Draf W. Endonasal micro-endoscopic frontal sinus surgery: the Fulda concept. Oper Tech Otolaryngol Head Neck Surg. 1991;2:234–40.
6. Conger BT Jr, Riley K, Woodworth BA. The Draf III mucosal grafting technique: a prospective study. Otolaryngol Head Neck Surg. 2012;146(4):664–8.
7. Wang YP, Shen PH, Hsieh LC, Wormald PJ. Free mucosal grafts and anterior pedicled flaps to prevent ostium restenosis after endoscopic modified Lothrop (frontal drillout) procedure: a randomized, controlled study. Int Forum Allergy Rhinol. 2019;9(11):1387–94.
8. Illing EA, Cho Do Y, Riley KO, Woodworth BA. Draf III mucosal graft technique: long-term results. Int Forum Allergy Rhinol. 2016;6(5):514–7.
9. Wormald PJ. Salvage frontal sinus surgery: the endoscopic modified Lothrop procedure. Laryngoscope. 2003;113(2):276–83.
10. Anderson P, Sindwani R. Safety and efficacy of the endoscopic modified Lothrop procedure: a systematic review and meta-analysis. Laryngoscope. 2009;119(9):1828–33.
11. Noller M, Fischer JL, Gudis DA, Riley CA. The Draf III procedure: a review of indications and techniques. World J Otorhinolaryngol Head Neck Surg. 2022;8(1):1–7.
12. Tilak A, Purvis J, Pena-Garcia A, et al. Above and beyond: periorbital suspension for endoscopic access to difficult frontal sinus pathology. Laryngoscope. 2022;132(3):538–44.
13. Grayson JW, Khichi SS, Cho DY, Riley KO, Woodworth BA. Management strategies for skull base inverted papilloma. Otolaryngol Head Neck Surg. 2016;155(1):179–83.
14. Illing E, Chaaban MR, Riley KO, Woodworth BA. Porcine small intestine submucosal graft for endoscopic skull base reconstruction. Int Forum Allergy Rhinol. 2013;3(11):928–32.
15. Blount A, Riley K, Cure J, Woodworth BA. Cerebrospinal fluid volume replacement following large endoscopic anterior cranial base resection. Int Forum Allergy Rhinol. 2012;2(3):217–21.
16. Banks C, Grayson J, Cho DY, Woodworth BA. Frontal sinus fractures and cerebrospinal fluid leaks: a change in surgical paradigm. Curr Opin Otolaryngol Head Neck Surg. 2020;28(1):52–60.
17. Illing EA, Woodworth BA. Management of Frontal Sinus Cerebrospinal Fluid Leaks and Encephaloceles. Otolaryngol Clin N Am. 2016;49(4):1035–50.
18. Chaaban MR, Woodworth BA. Complications of skull base reconstruction. Adv Otorhinolaryngol. 2013;74:148–62.
19. Jones V, Virgin F, Riley K, Woodworth BA. Changing paradigms in frontal sinus cerebrospinal fluid leak repair. Int Forum Allergy Rhinol. 2012;2(3):227–32.
20. Chaaban MR, Conger B, Riley KO, Woodworth BA. Transnasal endoscopic repair of posterior table fractures. Otolaryngol Head Neck Surg. 2012;147(6):1142–7.
21. Virgin F, Baranano CF, Riley K, Woodworth BA. Frontal sinus skull base defect repair using the pedicled nasoseptal flap. Otolaryngology—Head Neck Surg. 2011;145(2):338–40.
22. Virgin FW, Bleier BS, Woodworth BA. Evolving materials and techniques for endoscopic sinus surgery. Otolaryngol Clin N Am. 2010;43(3):653–72. xi
23. Purkey MT, Woodworth BA, Hahn S, Palmer JN, Chiu AG. Endoscopic repair of supraorbital ethmoid cerebrospinal fluid leaks. ORL J Oto-rhino-laryngol Relat Spec. 2009;71(2):93–8.
24. Woodworth BA, Schlosser RJ, Palmer JN. Endoscopic repair of frontal sinus cerebrospinal fluid leaks. J Laryngol Otol. 2005;119(9):709–13.
25. Woodworth BA, Harvey RJ, Neal JG, Palmer JN, Schlosser RJ. Endoscopic management of frontal sinus mucoeceles with anterior table erosion. Rhinology. 2008;46(3):231–7.
26. Grayson JW, Jeyarajan H, Illing EA, Cho DY, Riley KO, Woodworth BA. Changing the surgical dogma in frontal sinus trauma: transnasal endoscopic repair. Int Forum Allergy Rhinol. 2017;7(5):441–9.
27. Song X, Wang D, Sun X, et al. Endoscopic repairs of Sinonasal cerebrospinal leaks: outcome and prognostic factors. J Craniofac Surg. 2018;29(1):182–7.
28. Derise N, Vandiver B, McCormick J, et al. Transnasal endoscopic management of frontal sinus anterior table fractures improves cosmetic quality-of-life outcomes. Int Forum Allergy Rhinol. 2022.

29. Thompson HM, Tilak AM, Miller PL, Grayson JW, Cho DY, Woodworth BA. Treatment of frontal sinus osteomyelitis in the age of endoscopy. Am J Rhinol Allergy. 2021;35(3):368–74.
30. Yokoi H, Yamanaka H, Matsumoto Y, et al. Modified Lothrop (Draf III) procedure for the treatment of a recurrent orbitofrontal cholesterol granuloma: a case report. SAGE Open Med Case Rep. 2020;8:2050313x20907809.
31. Deep NL, Chaaban MR, Chaudhry AL, Woodworth BA. Frontal sinus cholesterol granuloma: case report. Allergy Rhinol. 2014;5(1):36–8.
32. Conger BT Jr, Illing E, Bush B, Woodworth BA. Management of lateral frontal sinus pathology in the endoscopic era. Otolaryngol Head Neck Surg. 2014;151(1):159–63.
33. McCormick JP, Thompson HM, Cho DY, Woodworth BA, Grayson JW. Phenotypes in chronic rhinosinusitis. Curr Allergy Asthma Rep. 2020;20(7):20.
34. Shih LC, Patel VS, Choby GW, Nakayama T, Hwang PH. Evolution of the endoscopic modified Lothrop procedure: a systematic review and meta-analysis. Laryngoscope. 2018;128(2):317–26.
35. Naidoo Y, Bassiouni A, Keen M, Wormald PJ. Long-term outcomes for the endoscopic modified Lothrop/Draf III procedure: a 10-year review. Laryngoscope. 2014;124(1):43–9.
36. Hildenbrand T, Wormald PJ, Weber RK. Endoscopic frontal sinus drainage Draf type III with mucosal transplants. Am J Rhinol Allergy. 2012;26(2):148–51.
37. Ting JY, Wu A, Metson R. Frontal sinus drillout (modified Lothrop procedure): long-term results in 204 patients. Laryngoscope. 2014;124(5):1066–70.
38. Eloy P, Vlaminck S, Jorissen M, et al. Type III frontal sinusotomy: surgical technique, indications, outcomes, a multi-university retrospective study of 120 cases. B-ENT. 2011;7(Suppl 17):3–13.
39. Seyedhadi S, Mojtaba MA, Shahin B, Hoseinali K. The Draf III septal flap technique: a preliminary report. Am J Otolaryngol. 2013;34(5):399–402.
40. Erdur O, Ozturk K, Erkan K. Feasibility of a septal mucosal flap for preventing re-stenosis following the Draf III procedure. J Laryngol Otol. 2018;132(1):79–82.
41. Omura K, Nomura K, Aoki S, et al. Effect of a superior lateral anterior pedicle flap for Draf procedures. J Craniofac Surg. 2019;30(4):e350–2.
42. Omura K, Nomura K, Aoki S, Katori Y, Tanaka Y, Otori N. Lacrimal sac exposure and a superior lateral anterior pedicle flap to improve outcomes of Draf type II and III procedures. Int Forum Allergy Rhinol. 2018.

The Superior Lateral Anterior Pedicled Flap (SLAP) for the Draf III Procedure

10

Kazuhiro Omura and Nobuyoshi Otori

Key Points

- Stenosis and bony regrowth can result in failures of frontal sinus patency even after endoscopic frontal sinus drainage via a Draf II or III procedure.
- The Superior Lateral Anterior Pedicle (SLAP) flap is a good option for preventing restenosis of the frontal cavity and promotes mucosal epithelization over the bare bone of the nasal beak.
- This is a simple, efficient, and effective technique that can be used in the majority of patients without added morbidity.

Background

Surgical management of the frontal sinus is difficult for several reasons. First, access to the frontal sinus through complicated and varied frontal recesses requires anatomical knowledge and operative skill. Second, not all of the mucosa of the frontal sinus is accessible with curved surgical instruments. Third, once fenestrated, a frontal drainage pathway has a high likelihood of stenosis during the follow-up period. Draf II and III procedures were introduced in 1991 [1], and since then, have been widely used for frontal sinus diseases.

Supplementary Information The online version contains supplementary material available at https://doi.org/10.1007/978-3-031-89191-5_10.

K. Omura (✉) · N. Otori
Department of Otorhinolaryngology, The Jikei University School of Medicine, Tokyo, Japan
e-mail: kazuhiro.omura@jikei.ac.jp; otori@jikei.ac.jp

J. T. Lee et al. (eds.), *Advances in Surgical and Medical Interventions for Recalcitrant Chronic Rhinosinusitis*,
https://doi.org/10.1007/978-3-031-89191-5_10

The goals of the Draf procedures are to increase patency of the frontal sinuses to allow drainage of secretions and aid in administration of nasal irrigations and topical medications to the mucosa of the frontal sinus. The Draf III procedure seeks to address these problems by maximizing the size of the frontal outflow tract, but there are still some limitations [2–5]. Postoperative stenosis after the Draf III procedure remains a limiting factor and tends to occur in cases in which a small-sized frontal ostium is created intraoperatively. Thus, creating the largest possible frontal neo-ostium at the time of the operation is recommended [3]. On the other hand, exposed bone tends to cause osteitis and results in scar formation and osteoneogenesis which can further narrow the sinus cavity [4]. To prevent osteitis, the mucosa can be used to cover exposed bone. Recently, several techniques applying a mucosal flap to Draf III procedures were reported [5–10]. The types of mucosal flaps varied from free flaps to anterior and posterior pedicled flaps. A free flap is easy to manipulate but is lacking in viability. The author and Kosuke Tochigi with senior author (N.O.) examined mucosal flap techniques in rabbits and demonstrated that the pedicled flap demonstrated improved mucosalization of the frontal beak with less inflammation than free mucosal flaps [11].

This chapter will discuss the superior lateral anterior pedicle (SLAP) flap for use in the Draf II and III procedures. A SLAP flap is easy to manipulate and avoids the limitations of other pedicled flaps that may impair visibility in the operative field [12, 13]. Additionally, harvest of this flap fully exposes the lacrimal sac during the Draf procedure to reduce the amount of bone surface area exposed for quicker re-mucosalization.

Surgical Technique

The patient is induced under general anesthesia and prepped and draped in the usual fashion for sinus surgery. Intraoperative navigation may be used to verify anatomic landmarks. Sinus surgery is carried out in the usual fashion to include uncinectomy and total ethmoidectomy. A modified Killian incision is first made along the nasal septum, extending to the nasal floor. Extension to the nasal floor aids in access for future steps. The underlying septal cartilage can be removed, taking care to ensure preservation of an L-strut for nasal support (Fig. 10.1a–e). Once this is completed, a vertical incision is made along the axilla at the same depth as the septal incision and extending superiorly and across the nasal cavity roof, joining the septal mucosal incision (Fig. 10.1f). The mucosa along the superior nasal cavity is very thin and we recommend sharp dissection along this plane to minimize the risk of tearing. Then a parallel vertical incision of the lateral wall of the nasal cavity is made 10–15 mm anterior to the incision at the agger or just behind the line of piriform aperture (Fig. 10.2a, b). A slit knife for orbital surgery or #15c blade is suitable for this anterior incision. The superior end of the flap should be preserved and is supplied by branches of the facial artery. Take care to avoid extending this incision along the anterior aspect of the inferior turbinate to preserve the mucosa of the head of the turbinate. This aids in minimizing crust formation in this area. An inferior

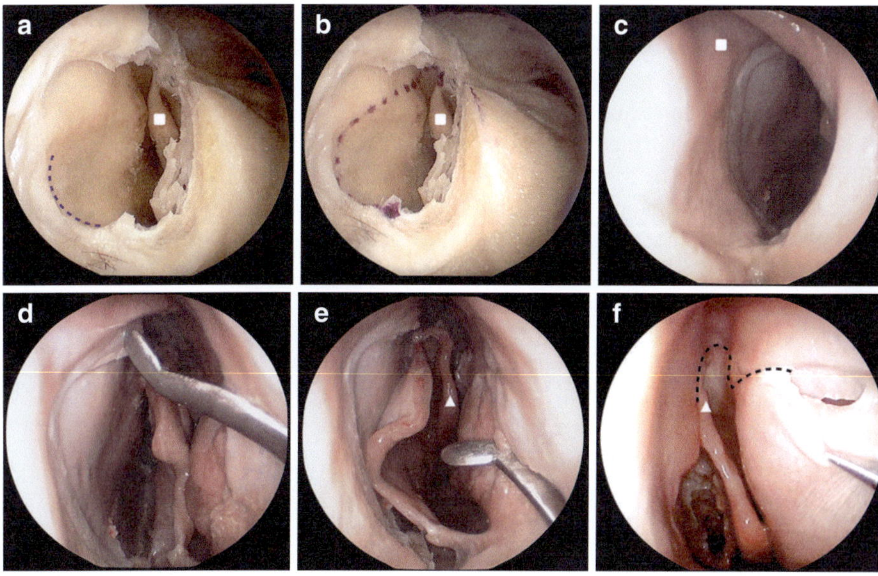

Fig. 10.1 Incision line on the septum . Figure 10.1. Zero-degree endoscopic view of the left nasal cavity of cadaveric specimen. (**a**) The septum and middle turbinate (white square) are seen with left septal deviation. (**b**) Anticipated incision line marked in purple along the anticipated L-strut of the septal cartilage. (**c**) Septal mucosal cut with preservation of the L-strut (white square). (**d**) The tip of the golf shaped elevator indicates the cartilage of the L-strut. (**e**) The entire incision line from the base of the nasal floor to middle turbinate (white triangle). (**f**) View of right nasal cavity depicting the superior horizontal incision that will connect the septal mucosal incision to the middle turbinate (black dotted line)

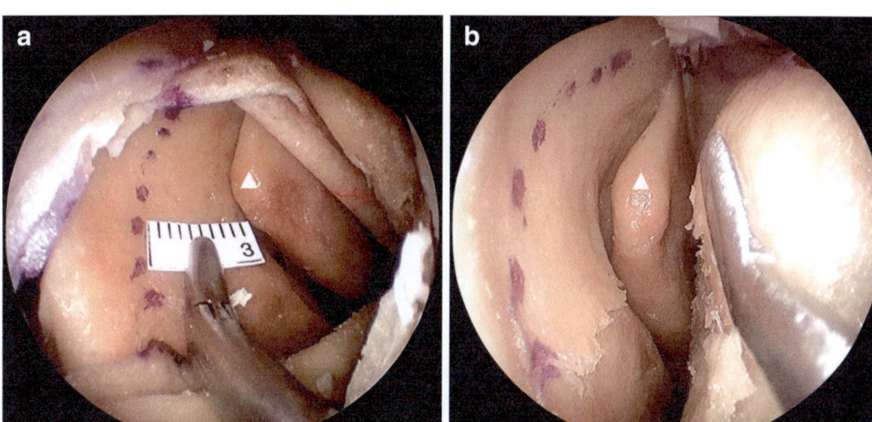

Fig. 10.2 Incision line on the lateral wall. (**a**) Zero-degree endoscopic view of the right nasal cavity of the cadaver specimen. Purple dotted line is the incision marked 1 cm anterior from the tip of the middle turbinate. (**b**) Second view of the planned incision line. Placement of the incision too anteriorly can result in disruption of nasal support and nasal saddling

horizontal incision across the flap will free it inferiorly, just above the inferior turbinate. This releases the flap such that it can be rotated and stored in the anterior-superior corner of the nasal cavity during dissection. **Surgical** Video 10.1 demonstrates the technique for harvest of this flap.

To minimize the surface area of the exposed bone, the lacrimal sac and duct are fully exposed. The authors generally recommend avoiding drilling directly over the nasolacrimal sac to avoid damage and potential postoperative epiphora. Insead, once the periosteum of the nasolacrimal duct is encountered, Kerrison punches can often efficiently remove the overlying bone (Fig. 10.3a, b). Once this is

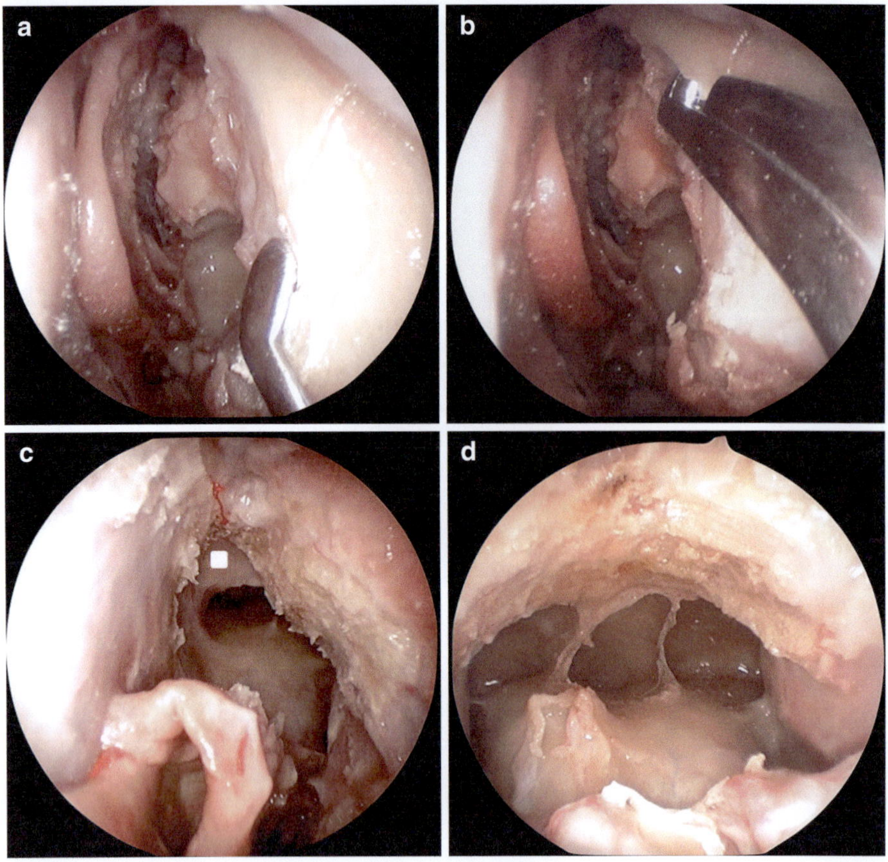

Fig. 10.3 Drilling and exposing the bone over the nasolacrimal duct . Zero-degree endoscopic view of a left nasal cavity of the cadaver specimen. (**a**) Drilling should start from the inferior aspect of the lateral nasal wall as indicated by the instrument tip. (**b**) Once periosteal membrane of the nasolacrimal duct was detected, a Kerrison punch can remove the lacrimal bone without tearing the lacrimal duct. (**c**) After Draf IIb. The bone of the nasal beak should be drilled until the anterior wall of the frontal sinus (white square) is seen by 0 degree endoscopy. (**d**) After Draf III. The bone of the nasal beak should be drilled until the anterior wall of the frontal sinus is seen by 0 degree endoscopy. The membrane of the posterior wall of the frontal sinus should be preserved as much as possible

accomplished, drilling of the nasal beak can be performed. The authors seek to be able to visualize the anterior wall of the frontal sinus with a zero-degree endoscope (Fig. 10.3c, d).

After the Draf procedure is completed, the SLAP flap is positioned to cover the exposed bone over the anterior surface of the frontal beak. Once the lacrimal bone is removed as high as the superior end of a lacrimal sac, the edge of the SLAP flap can also cover the periosteum of a lacrimal duct. This minimizes the exposed bony surface along the neo-ostium of the frontal sinus and aids in preventing restenosis during recovery. At the end of the procedure, packing should be placed to hold the flap in place (Fig. 10.4a–d).

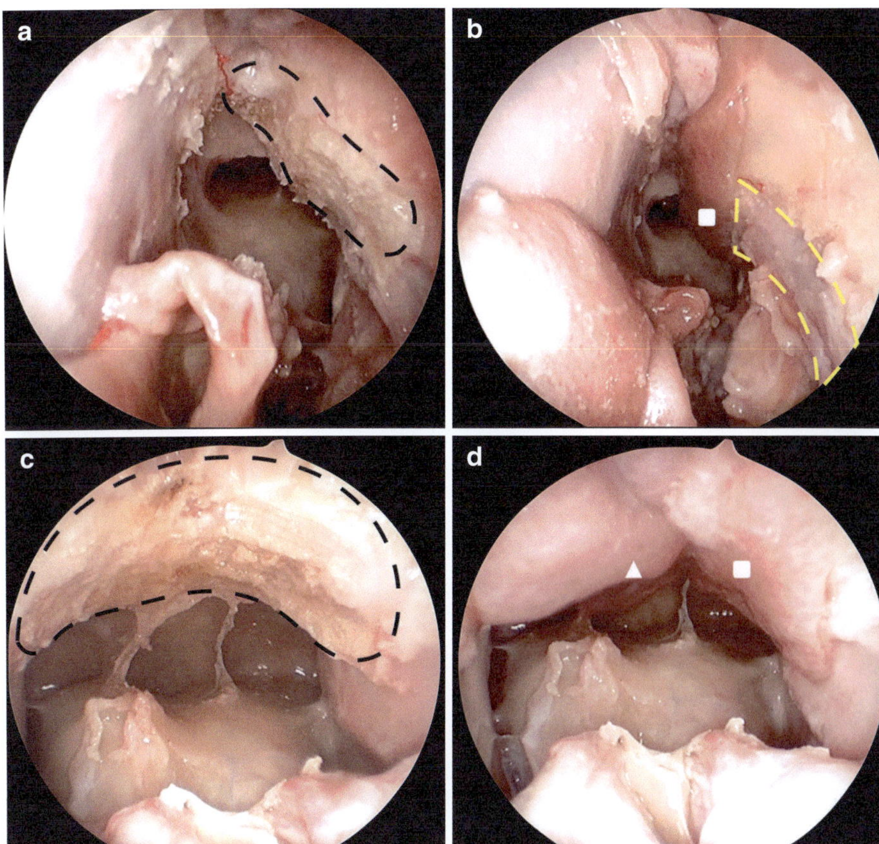

Fig. 10.4 Superior Lateral Anterior Pedicled (SLAP) Flap after Draf procedure. (**a**) 0 degree endoscopic view of a left nasal cavity of the cadaver specimen after Draf type IIb. Exposed bone demarcated by black dotted line. (**b**) View after placement of SLAP flap (white square) over bony exposure. The bony exposure is fully covered with the SLAP flap. The periosteum of a nasolacrimal duct demarcated by the yellow dotted line. (**c**) Endoscopic view of a left nasal cavity of the cadaver specimen after Draf III. Exposed bone demarcated by black dotted line. (**b**) View after placement of left SLAP flap (white square) and right SLAP flap (white triangle) over the exposed frontal bone. Note that the exposed bone is fully covered by SLAP flaps

Tips and Pearls

- An assistant can elevate the tip of the nose with a suction or elevator to aid in identification of the pyriform aperture (Fig. 10.5a).
- Make the posterior vertical incision prior to flap elevation. Once the flap is elevated, it becomes substantially more difficult to elevate the flap, particularly high in the nasal cavity where the mucosa is most delicate (Fig. 10.5b).
- Branches of the facial artery may be encountered inferiorly along the lateral nasal wall during flap elevation. These can be controlled with electrocautery or bipolar (Fig. 10.5c).

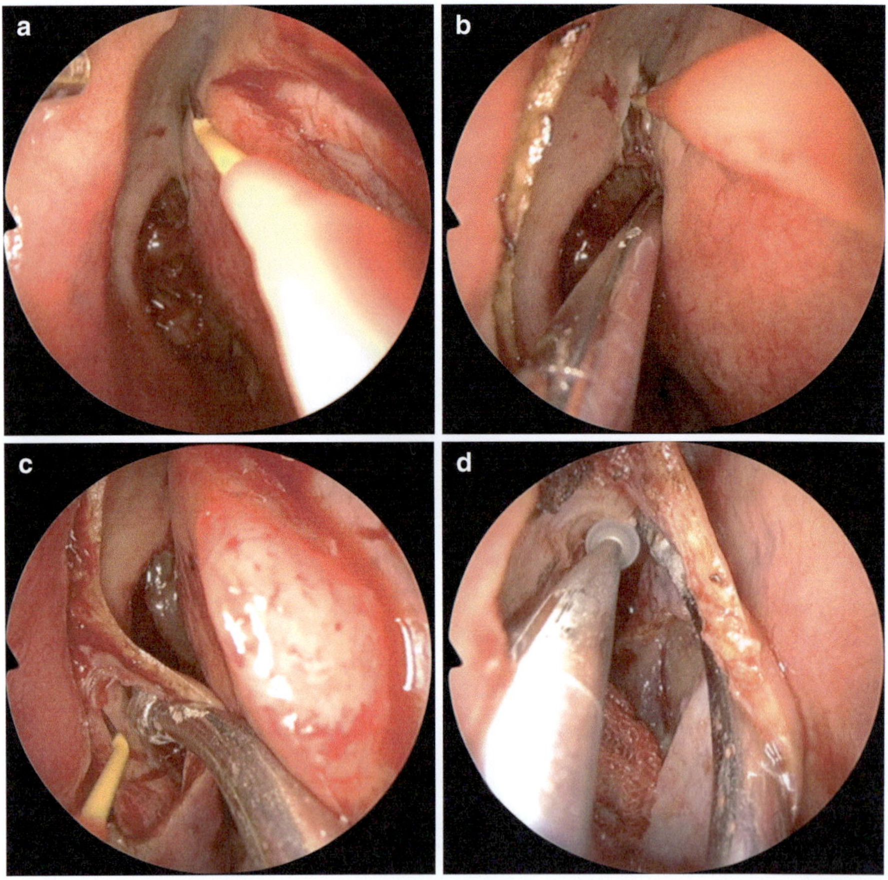

Fig. 10.5 Four-handed, two-surgeon techniques to aid in surgical exposure . 0 degree endoscopic view of a right nasal cavity. (**a**) Assistant using suction tip (upper left quarter) to elevate the nasal tip and cartilages and help identify the edge of the piriform aperture. (**b**) Assistant using suction tip (ethmoid sinus) to medialize the middle turbinate and improve working space and visualization. (**c**) Curved suction elevating the mucosal flap to demonstrate bleeding points from lateral nasal wall from branches of the facial artery. (**b**) Curved suction medializing slap flap during drilling to prevent injury

- Drilling can be performed without performing the inferior cut along the SLAP flap, but the flap may need to be held with an elevator to avoid damage (Fig. 10.5d).

References

1. Draf W. Endonasal micro-endoscopic frontal sinus surgery, the Fulda concept. Oper Tech Otolaryngol Head Neck Surg. 1991;2:234–40.
2. Li C, Sun X, Zhao M, Shen Y, Huang Q, Zhang X, Huang Z, Cui S, Zhou B. Comparison of airflow characteristics after Draf III frontal sinus surgery and normal person by numerical simulation. Math Biosci Eng. 2019;16(4):1750–60.
3. Shih L-C, Patel VS, Choby GW, Nakayama T, Hwang PH. Evolution of the endoscopic modified Lothrop procedure: a systematic review and meta-analysis. Laryngoscope. 2018;128(2):317–26.
4. Barham HP, Hall CA, Hernandez SC, Zylicz HE, Stevenson MM, Zito BA, Harvey RJ. Impact of Draf I, Draf IIb, and Draf IIa frontal sinus surgery on nasal irrigation distribution. Int Forum Allergy Rhinol. 2020;10(1):49–52.
5. Anderson P, Sindwani R. Safety and efficacy of the endoscopic modified Lothrop procedure: a systematic review and meta-analysis. Laryngoscope. 2009;119:1828–33.
6. Tran KN, Beule AG, Singal D, Wormald PJ. Frontal ostium restenosis after the endoscopic modified Lothrop procedure. Laryngoscope. 2007;117:1457–62.
7. Bhandarkar ND, Sautter NB, Kennedy DW, Smith TL. Osteitis in chronic rhinosinusitis: a review of the literature. Int Forum Allergy Rhinol. 2013;3:355–63.
8. Conger BT Jr, Riley K, Woodworth BA. The Draf III mucosal grafting technique: a prospective study. Otolaryngol Head Neck Surg. 2012;146:664–8.
9. Fiorini FR, Nogueira C, Verillaud B, et al. Value of septoturbinal flap in the frontal sinus drill-out type IIb according to Draf. Laryngoscope. 2016;126:2428–32.
10. Wang Y-P, Shen P-H, Hsieh L-C, Wormald P-J. Free mucosal grafts and anterior pedicled flaps to prevent ostium restenosis after endoscopic modified Lothrop (frontal drillout) procedure: a randomized, controlled study. Int Forum Allergy Rhinol. 2019;9(11):1387–94.
11. Tochigi K, Omura K, Miyashita K, Aoki S, Otori N, Tanaka Y. Pathological Features of Free Graft and Pedicled Flap in the Nasal Cavity: an animal study. Laryngoscope. 2021;131(2):E428–33.
12. Omura K, Nomura K, Aoki S, Tochigi K, Miyashita K, Tanaka Y, Otori N, Kojima H. Effect of a superior lateral anterior pedicle flap for Draf procedures. J Craniofac Surg. 2019;30(4):e350–2.
13. Omura K, Nomura K, Aoki S, Katori Y, Tanaka Y, Otori N. Lacrimal sac exposure and a superior lateral anterior pedicle flap to improve outcomes of Draf type II and III procedures. Int Forum Allergy Rhinol. 2018.

The Outside-in Draf III Procedure

11

Peta-Lee Sacks, Kachorn Seresirikachorn,
and Richard J. Harvey

Key Points

- The Draf III procedure is an important technique for accessing the frontal sinus and can be useful in some situations as a primary surgery and in recalcitrant frontal sinusitis.
- The outside-in approach is a method to approach the frontal sinus that relies on landmarks and uses near-straight instrumentation to avoid entry into the frontal sinus until the end of the procedure.
- The outside-in technique may be particularly useful in situations where frontal recess anatomy is complex or there is a substantial disease or tumor burden.

Supplementary Information The online version contains supplementary material available at https://doi.org/10.1007/978-3-031-89191-5_11.

P.-L. Sacks (✉)
Department of Otolaryngology, Macquarie University Hospital, Sydney, NSW, Australia

K. Seresirikachorn
Department of Otolaryngology, Faculty of Medicine, Chulalongkorn University, Bangkok, Thailand

R. J. Harvey
Rhinology and Skull Base, Applied Medical Research Centre, St Vincent's Hospital, Darlinghurst, NSW, Australia

Department of Otolaryngology, UNSW and Macquarie University, Sydney, NSW, Australia
e-mail: richard@richardharvey.com.au

J. T. Lee et al. (eds.), *Advances in Surgical and Medical Interventions for Recalcitrant Chronic Rhinosinusitis*,
https://doi.org/10.1007/978-3-031-89191-5_11

Background

The modified endoscopic Lothrop was initially performed for salvage surgery but over the past two to three decades, with the advancement of endoscopic endonasal surgery, it has become a commonly performed operation both for access in neoplastic and inflammatory disease as well as in anterior skull base reconstruction. Draf III procedures are important techniques for accessing the frontal sinus, the purpose of which depends on the pathology or anatomy involved. Classically, the Draf III was an operation that typically took a prolonged period of time and required multiple angled instruments, angled endoscopy, and curved powered instrumentation. The evolution of anterior skull base surgery created the need for the Draf III procedure to be just a small part of the surgery and therefore needed to be performed more efficiently and with a lower risk of complications.

The traditional approach to the Draf III focused on the identification and dissection of the frontal recess using angle endoscopes and early entry into the frontal sinus cavity in order to complete the bone removal. This is often referred to as the "inside-out" approach and the technique has been well defined by Wormald, et al. [1], who is often credited as bringing the original "lothrop" into the modern endoscopic era.

The outside-in approach does not require navigation of complex and variable frontal recess anatomy. Rather, it relies on anatomic landmarks, of the nasofrontal beak and anterior cranial fossa, that serve as boundaries for creating a common cavity. The limits of the endoscopic Lothrop cavity are well recognized. Laterally, these are the orbital plates of the frontal bone and periosteum of the skin over the frontal process of the maxilla laterally. Posteriorly, the first olfactory neuron on each side demarcates the forward projection of the olfactory bulb. Anteriorly, the dissection is taken to the plane of the anterior table of the frontal sinus [2].

This approach both utilizes a straight or zero-degree endoscope and near-straight instrumentation and avoids entry into the frontal sinus where mucosa is often inflamed and risk of intraoperative bleeding is higher, until very near the end of the procedure. It also successfully avoids the need for dissection of the frontal recess, until the end of the procedure, and this is particularly useful where frontal recess anatomy is complex and significant disease or tumor burden is present. The technique allows a significantly quicker operative time with bone drilling usually less than 30 min [2]. The evolution of the modified endoscopic Lothrop procedure to an Outside-In approach has allowed for a frontal recess-independent orientation, safer and more efficient Draf III common sinusotomy of frontal sinus to be performed. Indications for the outside-in Draf III are listed in Table 11.1.

Table 11.1 Surgical indications for the Outside-In Draf-III

–	Alternative to external access to frontal sinus
–	Frontal sinus intraoperative access where:
	Drilling in the frontal sinus is required
	Access to anterior skull base
	Lateral access within the frontal sinus
	Bimanual dissection in the frontal sinus
–	Frontal sinus post surgery access for:
	Access for topical therapies
	Prevent mucus plugging
	Overcome mucostasis—From disease or treatment (e.g., radiotherapy)
	Disease surveillance
	Rarely utilized for simple frontal sinus ventilation which is adequately achieved with Draf IIa or IIb for all but very complex anatomy

Surgical Technique

Patient Positioning and Preparation

The patient is positioned with the head extended using an under-shoulder support cushion. The surgical bed is placed at 20 degrees reverse Trendelenburg. The endotracheal tube is placed towards the right side. Nasal preparation is adrenaline based. The authors' preference is to use topical 1% ropivacaine and 1:2000 adrenaline on neurosurgical cottonoids. The surgical field is infiltrated with 10 mL comprised of 8 mL 1% ropivacaine, 1 ml adrenaline 1:10,000 adrenaline and 1 mL of 100 mg/mL of tranexamic acid which is infiltrated locally into the septum, lateral nasal wall down to the inferior turbinate and anterior to the piriform, and middle turbinate. The patient should be given a bradycardic (HR < 70 pbm) anesthetic with the use of either total intravenous anaesthesia or the use of a beta-blocker and clonidine.

Surgical Steps

Often a complete sphenoethmoidectomy will be performed; however this is not always essential and would be dictated by the indication for the Draf III procedure. At a minimum, the osteomeatal complex is dissected in order to define the medial orbital wall.

Large inferior based lateral wall flaps are created that commence at about the root of the middle turbinate, superiorly in the apex of the nasal cavity and then down the piriform bone edge. The incision on the lateral wall begins high above the axilla at the nasal roof by needle-point diathermy, setting 12 (0016 AM Megadynne, NJ, USA).

The posterior incision, at a depth of the middle turbinate insertion, is carried vertically down to the middle turbinate. The superior incision is carried at the very apex of the nasal cavity forward to the pyriform aperture and then vertically down, just behind the pyriform aperture, to a level approximating the midpoint of the middle meatus. These incisions are to the bone, and the inferior-based lateral wall mucosal flap is elevated subperiosteally, with the flap retracted down and exposing the axilla and lateral wall bone (Fig. 11.1). The septal window mucosa is often removed anterior enough to allow a direct approach to the anterior aspect of the nasofrontal beak or frontal sinus. This septal window can be extended to include any superior septal deviation but is usually less than one third the height of the septum. The mucosa on the septum is folded back to the olfactory cleft. A small emissary vein is usually seen prior to the first olfactory neuron running in a lateral direction. The first olfactory neuron is more adherent to the skull base and defines the posterior limit of dissection. It is only in the midline where inadvertent entry into the anterior cranial fossa can potentially occur and so it is vital that the surgeon expose the first olfactory neuron to prevent posterior dissection.

Once the olfactory neuron is identified, a superior septectomy is performed with a 2 mm 40 degree Kerrison rongeur. A full thickness incision is made in the antero-inferior location. The rongeur is placed in the anteroinferior opening and taken to the

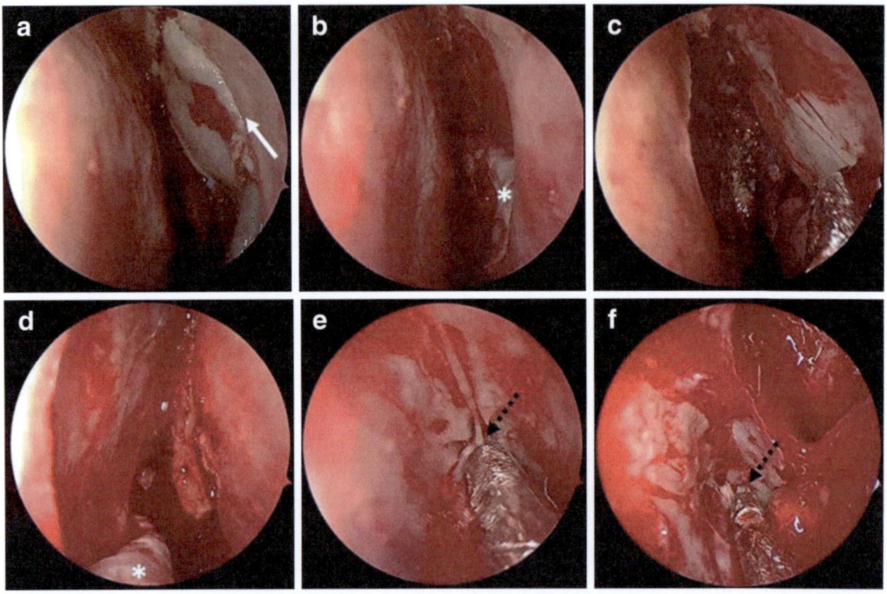

Fig. 11.1 Large inferior-based lateral wall flaps, septal window creation, and first olfactory neuron identification. (**a**) The posterior incision of left lateral wall flaps is carried vertically down to the middle turbinate. The superior incision is carried at the very apex of the nasal cavity forward to the pyriform aperture (white arrow) and then vertically down, just behind the pyriform aperture, to a level approximating the midpoint of the middle meatus. (**b**) The inferior-based lateral wall mucosal flap is elevated subperiosteally, with the flap (asterisk) retracted down and exposing the axilla and lateral wall bone. (**c**) The septal window mucosa is folded back to the olfactory cleft. (**d**) Right inferior-based lateral wall flaps (asterisk) (**e**) The right first olfactory neuron is defined as the posterior limit of dissection. (**f**) The left first olfactory neuron is defined

anterior limit on the floor of the frontal sinus. The septum is then resected up to the skull base as drilling will start at the septal attachment to the floor of the frontal sinus. A 4 or 5 mm 15 degree high speed rough diamond bur is used to remove the bone.

Drilling proceeds with a zero-degree endoscope and 4-mm 15° diamond burr, at 30,000 revolutions-per-minute (Straightshot M5 Micordebrider, Medtronic, FL, USA), removing the entire axilla-agger nasi-maxillary-frontal process complex. The bone is removed laterally to define the periosteum overlying the maxillary process of the frontal bone. The lateral limits are the periosteum and nasolacrimal sac at the level of the frontal process of the maxilla. Identification of these landmarks allows for maximal widening of the surgical field. Drilling then proceeds to remove the entire axilla lateral to the middle turbinate insertion. This defines the lateral boundary of resection. As the lateral boundary is approached, there is a transition in color from the yellow hue of bone to the white of the periostium. The bone lateral to the middle turbinate, anterior to the frontal recess, and medial to the periosteum is referred to as "Ritter's triangle" and needs to be removed until the mucosa of the frontal recess is "blue lined" before the nasofrontal beak is removed (Fig. 11.2).

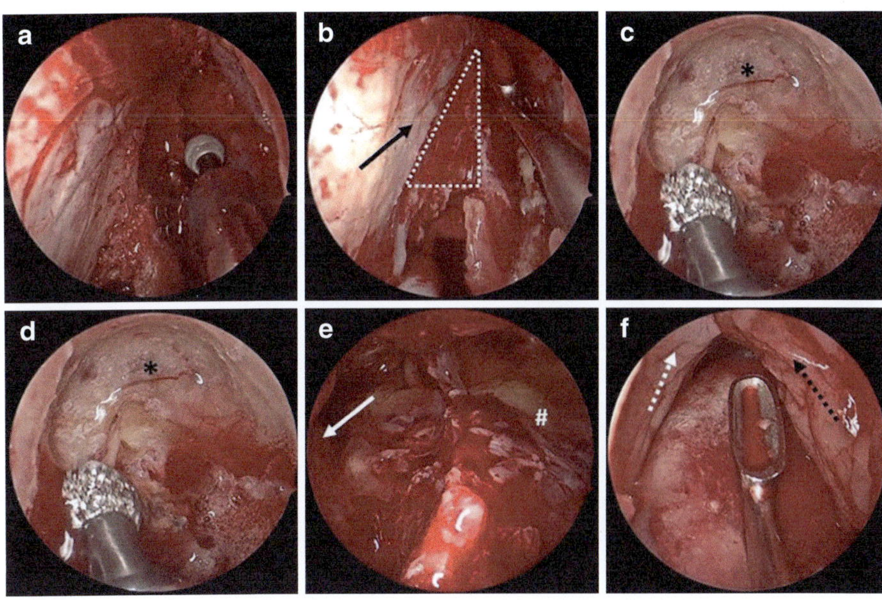

Fig. 11.2 Drilling and flap and free graft replacement steps. (**a**) Drilling removes the septal bone attachment to the floor of the frontal sinus. (**b**) Drilling removes the entire axilla-agger nasi-maxillary-frontal process complex. The lateral limits at the level of the frontal process of the maxilla bone are the periosteum (black arrow) and nasolacrimal sac. Then, drilling proceeds to remove the entire axilla, lateral to the middle turbinate insertion. The bone lateral to the middle turbinate, anterior to the frontal recess, and medial to the periosteum is referred to as "Ritter's triangle (dash line triangle)." (**c**) The nasofrontal beak bone centrally is drilled away. (**d, e**) Complete resection of the bone anteriorly to the level of the anterior table of the frontal sinus and laterally to remove bone in order to "square off" the common frontal sinusotomy and be able to visualize the orbital roof (white arrow). (**f**) The right (white dash arrow) and left (black dash arrow) thin free mucosal grafts are placed to cover exposed bone. Posterior table of left frontal sinus (number sign)

Once both the posterior (first olfactory neuron and frontal recess mucosa) and lateral limits (periosteum) have been defined, all the bone centrally is drilled away. It is preferable to avoid entering the frontal sinus itself until late in the dissection in order to prevent any mucosal bleeding due to mucosal inflammation in the cavity. The bone being drilled is the bone of the frontal beak. The frontal recess and the frontal sinus itself lies between the anterior nasal beak and thus protects against entry into the anterior cranial fossa as long as the surgeon remains anterior to the first olfactory neuron.

Complete resection of the bone anteriorly to the level of the anterior table of the frontal sinus and laterally to remove bone in order to "square off" the common frontal sinusotomy and visualize the orbital roof.

Once the bone between the surgical cavity and the frontal recess is thinned, the remaining thin bone is removed with a 2 mm 40 degree Kerrison rongeur, either from above down or from below up. The frontal recess partitions are removed with the 2.5-mm 45° cutting forceps and 4.3 m quadcut straight microdebrider (Straightshot M5 Microdebrider, Medtronic, FL, USA). The 5-mm 70° Hosemann frontal sinus punch can complete the removal of bone edges.

The use of both inferiorly based lateral wall flaps and free mucosal grafts can aid in remucosalization of the exposed frontal bone at the anterior aspect of the dissection cavity and minimize osteoneogenesis. The free mucosal grafts are best harvested from the soft tissue posterior ends of the inferior turbinates. It is important to ensure that the submucosa of the graft is excised to create a thin graft (Fig. 11.3). Multiple techniques for vascularized flaps have been described [3].

Once all grafting materials are placed, the Draf III cavity is packed. The authors prefer to use a silastic sheet template that is fashioned (0.51 mm Medtronic, Jacksonville, FL) into the frontal sinus cavity. This is then supported in situ by either carboxycellulose foam (nasopore, stryker, MI) with or without hyaluronic acid gel (Bioregen, Changzhou, China). Alternatives include drug-eluting frontal stents or finger-in-glove Merocel packs (Video 11.1).

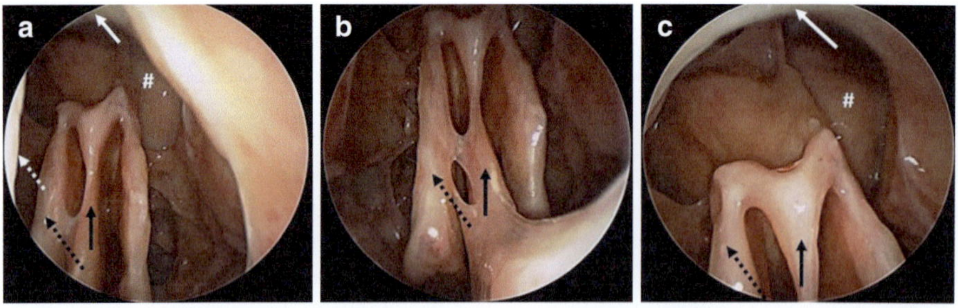

Fig. 11.3 Postoperative view of outside in Lothrop cavity. (**a**) Postoperative view from the left nasal cavity. (**b**, **c**) Postoperative view from the right nasal cavity. Anterior nasal beak that covers with free mucosal graft (white arrow), anterior edge of the septal window (white dash arrow), right middle turbinate (black dash arrow), posterior edge of the septal window (black arrow), posterior table of the left frontal sinus (number sign)

Post-Operative Management

Patients are often discharged on the day of surgery. Amoxicillin/ clavulanic acid is given for 10 days, and prednisone was given at 25 mg maximum daily for 7–21 days to reduce edema/congestion and varies on pathology. Nasal saline irrigations commence day 1 postoperatively and are performed twice daily. The silastic template and any residual packing is removed after 3–4 weeks post-operatively (Video 11.2).

Reported Outcomes

Patient Reporting Outcome Measures

Disease-specific quality of life scores (SNOT-22 and nasal symptom score) and global nasal function have been shown to have significant improvement following the Outside-In Draf III in a retrospective study [4]. Similarly, olfactory function has been shown to have improved significantly following surgery [4]. The olfactory neuroepithelium of the septum and superior turbinate is protected throughout the procedure and hence may explain these outcomes.

Operative Time

The Outside-In approach to Draf III procedure has been demonstrated to be an efficient technique for finding the frontal sinus regardless of pathology. Chin et al. demonstrated a mean time to frontal sinus floor discovery of 7.82+/− 6.79 min and to completion of cavity of 26.92+/−11.20 min. For endoscopic skull base surgery and chronic rhinosinusitis without nasal polyposis, the mean time to completion was 18.45 and 24.66 min respectively and was significantly faster then when it was performed for chronic rhinosinusitis with nasal polyposis with a measured mean time of 33.32 min ($p = 0.02$) [2].

Complications

Potential complications include CSF leak, orbital or intracranial complications, bleeding, infection, and stenosis. Serious complications are rare. Chin et al. found one patient with early post-operative skin edema which settled over 1 week without intervention but no other complications recorded [2]. Takeda reported a single case of inadvertent CSF leakage where the first olfactory neuron was defined intraoperatively but the anatomy of the anterior cranial fossa was aberrant and the point is made that a pre-operative CT scan in a sagittal view is important to ensure the validity of the first olfactory neuron as a landmark to the posterior table of the frontal sinus [5].

Failure of Draf III procedures includes neoosteogenesis and stenosis. This can be dramatically reduced by the use of free mucosal grafting and vascularised flaps with success being reported as high as 97% [6]. If hypertrophic soft tissue is present at the anterior limit of the common sinusotomy at 3 months post-op, then 0.2–0.4 mL of triamcinolone (40 mg/mL) is injected with 1 mL syringe and long (1.5 inch) 25G needle.

Tips and Pearls

- The septal window can be variable but is rarely much more anterior than the bone-cartilage junction.
- The septal window should incorporate any high septal deflections and the septal swell body.
- Trim the middle turbinate root back to just posterior to the posterior septal window and both of these are just anterior to the first olfactory neuron exit point.
- Remove all of Ritter's triangle and see the "blue" of the frontal recess before continuing the superior bone removal.
- When removing the bone, do so on a broad front and avoid tunneling.
- Square off the opening to ensure that the orbital roof can be visualized.
- Very large and broad inferior based lateral wall flaps provide better access and healing.
- Soft tissue of the interior turbinate tail is a low morbidity option to harvest for free mucosal grafting. Stay outside the bone/inferior turbinate artery when harvesting.
- Leave silastic sheeting or other packing in for at least 3–4 weeks postoperatively.

References

1. Wormald PJ. Salvage frontal sinus surgery: the endoscopic modified Lothrop procedure. Laryngoscope. 2003;113(2):276–83.
2. Chin D, Snidvongs K, Kalish L, Sacks R, Harvey RJ. The outside-in approach to the modified endoscopic Lothrop procedure. Laryngoscope. 2012;122(8):1661–9.
3. Oostra A, Koutsarnakis C, Georgalas C. Advances in vascularized flaps for skull base reconstruction. Curr Opin Otolaryngol Head Neck Surg. 2021;29(1):36–43.
4. Wong EH, Do TQ, Harvey RJ, Orgain CA, Sacks R, Kalish L. Patient-reported olfaction improves following outside-in Draf III frontal sinus surgery for chronic rhinosinusitis. Laryngoscope. 2019;129(1):25–30.
5. Takeda T, Omura K, Torng H, Ebihara T, Aoki S, Tochigi K, et al. Frontal sinus "hump": an anatomical risk factor for anterior Skull Base injury in the endoscopic modified Lothrop approach (outside-in frontal drill-out). Case Rep Otolaryngol. 2021;2021:3402496.
6. Illing EA, do Cho Y, Riley KO, Woodworth BA. Draf III mucosal graft technique: long-term results. Int Forum Allergy Rhinol. 2016;6(5):514–7.

Part III

In-Office Procedures for Recalcitrant Chronic Sinusitis, Chronic Rhinitis, and Chronic Nasal Obstruction

Balloon Sinuplasty

12

Angela M. Donaldson

Key Points

- Chronic rhinosinusitis is a common condition impacting 28 million adults.
- Most patients may successfully treat symptoms with medical therapy. However, despite appropriate medical therapy, some patients have persistent or progressive disease requiring surgical intervention.
- Balloon sinuplasty is a treatment option for patients with limited chronic rhinosinusitis without nasal polyps and those with recurrent acute rhinosinusitis.
- This technique was a rapidly accepted procedure based on its short procedure time, recovery time, and flexibility to perform the procedure in the office.

Background

Chronic rhinosinusitis has an estimated prevalence of 2.1–13.8% in the United States. While medical therapy is successful in most cases, approximately 320,000 endoscopic sinus surgeries (ESS) are performed each year [1]. Balloon sinuplasty (BSP) is a minimally invasive technique in which the device microfractures and thus dilates the natural ostium of the maxillary, frontal, and/or sphenoid sinuses. The major benefit of this technique is that bone and soft tissue are displaced without

Supplementary Information The online version contains supplementary material available at https://doi.org/10.1007/978-3-031-89191-5_12.

A. M. Donaldson (✉)
Department of Otolaryngology Head and Neck Surgery, Mayo Clinic Florida, Jacksonville, FL, USA
e-mail: Donaldson.angela@mayo.edu

J. T. Lee et al. (eds.), *Advances in Surgical and Medical Interventions for Recalcitrant Chronic Rhinosinusitis*,
https://doi.org/10.1007/978-3-031-89191-5_12

disrupting native mucosa. This allows for shorter recovery time and less risk of intraoperative bleeding compared to traditional sinus surgery. This procedure may also be more desirable to patients because it can be performed in both the office and operative setting.

The FDA approved the use of balloon sinus dilation in 2005. Currently, there are four FDA approved devices each with multiple iterations. In addition, image guidance technology now includes balloon dilation instrumentation which may help to prevent inadvertent creation of false passages [2]. The utilization of this device has increased exponentially, with the Medicare database reporting that between 2011 and 2017, there has been a 468% increase in the use of balloon sinuplasty [3].

Indications for Balloon Sinuplasty

Indications for balloon sinuplasty include recurrent acute rhinosinusitis (RARS), chronic rhinosinusitis without nasal polyps (CRSsNP), and acute rhinosinusitis with complications in patients who are unable to undergo ESS [4]. Balloon sinuplasty can also be used as a hybrid procedure with ESS in those with CRSsNP or after previous sinus surgery. Hathorn, et al. performed a randomized controlled trial (RCT) on patients with CRS who underwent frontal sinusotomy using a traditional Draf 2a technique on one side and a hybrid technique using balloon dilation on the other frontal sinus. They found that the hybrid side had less blood loss and a shorter operative time. Additionally, there was no statistically significant difference in sinus patency at 5 weeks and 3 months between the two groups [5]. Use of BSP in the setting of frontal bullar and suprabullar cells has been suggested, as it may be easier to advance through a narrowed frontal sinus outflow tract. This suggestion should be considered with caution as complex frontal sinus anatomy has a higher risk of false passage or skull base injury. BSP can be utilized in complex revision surgery to identify and dilate the natural drainage pathway with subsequent enlargement of the sinus ostium using ESS instrumentation [6, 7].

There is a paucity of literature on the extent of sinus disease best treated with BSP alone. In 2018, a clinical consensus statement (CCS) on balloon sinus dilation was published based on expert opinion and available evidence-based literature. Clear indications for the use of BSP were limited by the lack of consistent descriptions of limited/mild disease in the literature. For example, there was "no consensus" on the use of BSP as a standalone procedure in patients with CRS without polyps. This result was primarily based on enrollment limited to disease involving isolated maxillary +/− anterior ethmoid disease in early industry sponsored RCTs. The CCS did identify patient populations that do not meet criteria for the use of BSP. These patients include those without sinonasal symptoms and positive findings on CT scan, those with sinus headache or sleep apnea not meeting criteria for CRS or RARS, and those with sinonasal symptoms but CT imaging shows no evidence of sinus disease [8]. Diagnoses such as allergic fungal sinusitis, cystic fibrosis, and malignancies are also contraindications to this procedure. Additionally, relative exclusion criteria for BSP include presence of osteoneogenesis, skull base dehiscences, and nasal polyps. Special consideration should also be made to those on anticoagulation medication, as this has been associated with increased risk of bleeding during the procedure [1].

Reported Outcomes

While most patients can be successfully managed with medical therapy, a large portion will need surgical intervention. Outcomes after BSP have consistently shown positive results in symptom improvement and other quality of life measures. The ORIOS study was a multi institutional, prospective, nonrandomized trial of patients undergoing in-office BSP. Follow-up at 24 weeks showed improvement in SNOT-20 and Lund MacKay scores [9]. In the MERLOT study, 198 patients with CRS self-selected between medical therapy and BSP followed by medical therapy. Patients undergoing surgery were allowed to have adjuvant procedures including septoplasty, inferior turbinate reduction, ethmoidectomy, and polypectomy. At 24 weeks SNOT-20 and other quality of life (QOL) metrics had more improvement in the BSP group compared to medical therapy and these results were sustained at 1 year [10, 11]. The lack of a standardized protocol for medical therapy, allowance of various procedures in addition to the BSP, and uneven distribution of patients in each group did limit the impact of this study. Sikand et al. randomized RARS patients to BSP and medical therapy versus medical therapy alone and were followed for 48 weeks. In contrast to the previous publication, patients requiring additional procedures were excluded. Their outcomes were similar, however, with the BSP and medical therapy group reporting better outcome scores compared to medical therapy alone, including number of post operative sinus infections and severity of sinus symptoms [12]. There are two RCTs comparing outcomes of BSP to endoscopic sinus surgery. All patients had maxillary disease +/− anterior ethmoid disease with a diagnosis of CRS or RARS. At 6 months, the mean change in SNOT-20 was similar between groups. However, secondary outcomes including number of debridements, post operative pain, and timing to return to work favored BSP over ESS [13–15]. Several cadaveric studies have evaluated irrigation penetration after balloon sinuplasty. Gantz, et al. found no difference in irrigation penetration to the frontal sinus when comparing ESS and balloon sinuplasty techniques. In contrast, the maxillary sinus penetration was better after ESS compared to BSP [16]. This is consistent with findings that partial uncinectomy improves maxillary sinus penetration after BSP [17].

Revision rates after balloon sinuplasty vary within the literature from 7% to 15% [18]. However, these values are associated with a wide range of follow up periods. The risk of revision ESS after balloon sinuplasty was assessed by Jang, et al. They evaluated a total of 146 patients undergoing revision ESS. Of those revision cases 16 patients had a history of previous BSP. Factors such as history of ESS prior to BSP, presence of nasal polyps, and positive skin prick testing were associated with need for revision ESS [19]. In another study, a large claim-based database was used to identify the frequency of balloon sinuplasty in revision sinus procedures. Patients with a 2 year follow-up history were included. Revision rates were similar between those who underwent endoscopic sinus surgery and those who had a balloon sinuplasty procedure 10.99% and 10.89%, respectively. In this study, they found that revision rates were significantly higher in frontal sinus disease initially treated with ESS vs BSP, 4.2% versus 3.7% [18]. Jang, et al. found that only 11% of patients had revision surgery performed using the BSP approach. However, approximately 40% of those patients had had a previous BSP [18]. Currently, there is no evidence or consensus over the use of balloon sinuplasty procedure after a previous balloon sinuplasty.

While there are relatively few serious complications from balloon sinuplasty, the risk of this procedure does deserve mention. Risk of severe bleeding, orbital complication, CSF leak, and synechiae formation have been documented. An open FDA database study looking at reported complications from 2015 to 2018 found a total of 78 reported adverse events, with the most common being skull base injury. Skull base injury with CSF leak was more common after dilation of the frontal or maxillary sinuses. Maxillary sinus dilation has also been associated with injury to the orbit including fracture of the orbital wall, pre and post septal cellulitis. Epistaxis during and after the procedure was more commonly associated with the sphenoid and frontal sinuses in this database. Device malfunction has also been reported. Rupture of the balloon during inflation is the most common device failure and is more common during frontal sinus balloon dilation [19]. Less serious complications such as scarring and persistent disease should also be noted. One of the causes of persistent disease may be dilation of a false passage. Jensen, et al. published a study on intraoperative accuracy of maxillary sinus balloon dilation in living patients. They found that BSP was unsuccessful in 31% of patients, which is a lower accuracy than previously reported in cadaveric studies [20].

Surgical Technique

The patient is brought into the procedure room and placed in a recumbent chair. A complete set of vitals are performed, and informed consent is obtained prior to commencing with topical anesthesia. Continuous blood pressure and heart rate monitoring are performed throughout the procedure. Prior to starting the procedure, a detailed nasal endoscopy is performed. Specific anatomic variants are noted including visualization of a posterior fontanelle, septal spur or deviation, concha bullosa, inferior turbinate hypertrophy.

Local Anesthesia Protocol

Oxymetazoline hydrochloride 0.05% and 4% Lidocaine topical mixture is placed on 4 cottonoid pledgets, 2 on each side. After 5 minutes these pledgets are removed and 2% topical tetracaine pledgets are placed in the middle meatus and sphenoethmoid recess under direct endoscopic visualization. A freer is used to ensure proper placement of pledgets. Pledgets are kept in place for 10 min and then removed. 1%

lidocaine with 1:100,000 epinephrine is then injected into the roof of the middle turbinate, uncinate, and sphenopalatine foramen using a 27 g spinal needle. The needle is aspirated prior to injection to avoid intravascular injection and subsequent tachycardia.

For patients with a concern for anxiety and excessive discomfort, the patient is pre-prescribed one Xanax 0.5 mg and encouraged to take acetaminophen 500 mg prior to the procedure. In certain cases, 2 tablets of acetaminophen/hydrocodone are prescribed.

Procedure: Maxillary Sinus Balloon Dilation

A 30-degree nasal endoscope is used. A maxillary double probe seeker is used to outfracture the uncinate. The seeker is advanced into the maxillary ostium inferiorly and gently slid superiorly to complete the outfracturing. The balloon dilation device is then advanced into the nasal cavity. The fiber optic illuminated transducer is carefully advanced into maxillary ostium. Transillumination of the maxillary sinus is noted and visual confirmation that the device is not in a posterior fontanelle is made. The balloon device is then advanced into the maxillary sinus and dilated to 12 mmHg and held in place for 5–10 s. The balloon is then deflated, and the transducer and balloon device are removed.

Procedure: Frontal Sinus Balloon Dilation

A 30-degree endoscope is used for this procedure. A freer is used to medialize the middle turbinate. Based on the vertical attachment of the middle turbinate, the balloon device is advanced into the nasal cavity, hugging the lateral aspect of the middle turbinate. This allows for more mobility and angulation of the tip of the balloon device without causing mucosal trauma. Once the ostium of the duct is noted the tip of the device is angled and the transducer is advanced into the outflow duct. Transillumination of the frontal sinus is evaluated. The balloon device is then advanced over the transducer and used to dilate the outflow duct. The balloon is then deflated, and the transducer and balloon device are removed.

Procedure: Sphenoid Sinus Balloon Dilation

A 0-degree endoscope is used for this procedure. A freer is used to gently push the middle and superior turbinate laterally. This should allow for better visualization of the sphenoid ostium. Once the ostium is visualized, the transducer is advanced into the ostium and the balloon device is advanced over it. The balloon device is then dilated to 12 mmHg and held in place for 5–10 s. The balloon is then deflated, and the transducer and balloon device are removed. Once this is complete, the freer is used to gently place the middle turbinate in a medialized position.

Tips and Pearls

- Additional topical anesthesia can be injected in areas which may be contacted during an in-office balloon sinuplasty procedure such as a small septal spur or the midportion of the vertical aspect of the middle turbinate.
- If the sphenoethmoid recess is edematous injecting additional 1% lidocaine with 1:100,000 epinephrine at the posterior aspect of the nasal septum may reduce bleeding during dilation.
- Study the CT scan prior to the procedure to identify the complexity of frontal sinus anatomy, determine the pathway of the frontal sinus outflow duct, check for presence of an Onodi cell.
- If an Onodi cell is present, try to place the fiber optic-illuminated transducer and balloon inferior and medial in the sphenoid ostium in order to prevent dilation of the Onodi cell.
- Repeat dilation of the sinus ostium may be necessary to get the desired size of dilation.
- For patients who need additional irrigation of the maxillary sinus, partial uncinectomy can be performed.

References

1. Orlandi RR, Kingdom TT, Smith TL, Bleier B, DeConde A, Luong AU, et al. International consensus statement on allergy and rhinology: rhinosinusitis 2021. Int Forum Allergy Rhinol. 2021;11(3):213–739.
2. Lopez EM, Farzal Z, Norris M, Canfarotta MW, Pappa AK, et al. Radiologic analysis of balloon Sinuplasty in a human cadaver model: observed effects on Sinonasal anatomy. Am J Rhinol Allergy. 2021;35(1):107–13. https://doi.org/10.1177/1945892420939430. Epub 2020 Jul 7. PMID: 32635741; PMCID: PMC7874344.
3. Kasle DA, Torabi SJ, Narwani V, Manes RP. Medicare reimbursement for balloon catheter dilations among surgeons performing high volumes of the procedures to treat chronic rhinosinusitis. JAMA Otolaryngol Head Neck Surg. 2020;146(3):264–9.
4. Cingi C, Bayar Muluk N, Lee JT. Current indications for balloon sinuplasty. Curr Opin Otolaryngol Head Neck Surg. 2019;27(1):7–13. https://doi.org/10.1097/MOO.0000000000000506.
5. Hathorn IF, Pace-Asciak P, Habib AR, Sunkaraneni V, Javer AR. Randomized controlled trial: hybrid technique using balloon dilation of the frontal sinus drainage pathway. Int Forum Allergy Rhinol. 2015;5(2):167–73. https://doi.org/10.1002/alr.21432. Epub 2014 Oct 31.
6. Eloy JA, Friedel ME, Eloy JD, Govindaraj S, Folbe AJ. In-office balloon dilation of the failed frontal sinusotomy. Otolaryngol Head Neck Surg. 2012;146(2):320–2. https://doi.org/10.1177/0194599811425885. Epub 2011 Oct 13.
7. Fleischman GM, Miller JD, Kim GG, Zanation AM, Ebert CS. Treatment of chronic frontal sinusitis with difficult anatomy: a hybrid balloon technique in four cases. Allergy Rhinol (Providence). 2014;5(3):120–4. https://doi.org/10.2500/ar.2014.5.0096. PMID: 25565046; PMCID: PMC4275456.
8. Piccirillo JF, Payne SC, Rosenfeld RM, Baroody FM, Batra PS, DelGaudio JM, Edelstein DR, Lane AP, Luong AU, Manes RP, McCoul ED, Platt MP, Reh DD, Corrigan MD. Clinical consensus statement: balloon dilation of the sinuses. Otolaryngol Head Neck Surg. 2018;158(2):203–14. https://doi.org/10.1177/0194599817750086.

9. Karanfilov B, Silvers S, Pasha R, et al. Office-based balloon sinus dilation: a prospective, multicenter study of 203 patients. Int Forum Allergy Rhinol. 2013;3(5):404–11.
10. Payne SC, Stolovitzky P, Mehendale N, et al. Medical therapy versus sinus surgery by using balloon sinus dilation technology: a prospective multicenter study. Am J Rhinol Allergy. 2016;30(4):279–86.
11. Stolovitzky JP, Mehendale N, Matheny KE, et al. Medical therapy versus balloon sinus dilation in adults with chronic rhinosinusitis (MERLOT): 12-month follow-up. Am J Rhinol Allergy. 2018;32(4):294–302.
12. Chandra RK, Kern RC, Cutler JL, Welch KC, Russell PT. REMODEL larger cohort with long-term outcomes and meta-analysis of standalone balloon dilation studies. Laryngoscope. 2016;126(1):44–50. https://doi.org/10.1002/lary.25507. Epub 2015 Jul 30. PMID: 26228589; PMCID: PMC5132108.
13. Cutler J, Bikhazi N, Light J, Truitt T, Schwartz M, Investigators RS. Standalone balloon dilation versus sinus surgery for chronic rhinosinusitis: a prospective, multicenter, randomized, controlled trial. Am J Rhinol Allergy. 2013;27(5):416–22.
14. Bikhazi N, Light J, Truitt T, Schwartz M, Cutler J. Standalone balloon dilation versus sinus surgery for chronic rhinosinusitis: a prospective, multicenter, randomized, controlled trial with 1-year follow-up. Am J Rhinol Allergy. 2014;28(4):323–9.
15. Gantz O, Danielian A, Yu A, Ference EH, Kuan EC, Wrobel B. Sinus irrigation penetration after balloon sinuplasty vs functional endoscopic sinus surgery in a cadaveric model. Int Forum Allergy Rhinol. 2019;9(9):953–7. https://doi.org/10.1002/alr.22386. Epub 2019 Jul 23.
16. Martinez-Paredes JF, Karatayli-Ozgursoy S, Gonzalez V, Olomu O, Donaldson AM. Effect of partial Uncinectomy after balloon Sinuplasty on maxillary sinus irrigant penetration: a cadaveric study. OTO Open. 2021;5(1):2473974X21989583. https://doi.org/10.1177/2473974X21989583. PMID: 33598598; PMCID: PMC7863165.
17. Jang DW, Cyr DD, Schulz K, Scher R, Ryan P, Abi Hachem R, Witsell DL. The use of balloon dilation in revision sinus surgery. Int Forum Allergy Rhinol. 2020;10(10):1158–64. https://doi.org/10.1002/alr.22571. Epub 2020 May 29.
18. Cooper M, Cheng T, Truong T, Kuchibhatla M, Hachem RA, Jang DW. Factors associated with revision surgery after balloon sinuplasty. Otolaryngol Head Neck Surg. 2019;160(4):734–9. https://doi.org/10.1177/0194599818813044. Epub 2018 Nov 20.
19. Wright AE, Davis ED, Khan M, Chaaban MR. Exploring balloon sinuplasty adverse events with the innovative OpenFDA database. Am J Rhinol Allergy. 2020;34(5):626–31. https://doi.org/10.1177/1945892420920505. Epub 2020 Apr 22.
20. Jensen BT, Holbrook EH, Chen PG, Luong AU, Marino MJ, Yao WC. The intraoperative accuracy of maxillary balloon dilation: a blinded trial. Int Forum Allergy Rhinol. 2019;9(5):452–7. https://doi.org/10.1002/alr.22286. Epub 2019 Jan 10.

In-Office Endoscopic Sinus Surgery for Recalcitrant Chronic Rhinosinusitis

13

Daniel B. Spielman and John M. DelGaudio

Key Points

- Patients with recalcitrant chronic rhinosinusitis require lifelong treatment, often requiring multiple revision surgeries under general anesthesia.
- In-office endoscopic procedures, in the appropriate patient, can lead to significant improvements in disease control and quality of life while avoiding the need for a general anesthetic.
- The use of in-office endoscopic sinus procedures can lead to decreased costs while being more convenient for patients, with comparable outcomes in some scenarios to procedures performed in the operating room.
- Proper patient selection, local anesthetic, and realistic expectations are essential to successful intervention with good outcomes.

Background

The management of CRS requires intensive medical and often surgical intervention. While endoscopic sinus surgery (ESS) is regarded to be a highly effective intervention, in itself is frequently not curative, and many patients experience residual or recurrent symptoms. Up to 15.9% of patients will require revision surgery for their CRS [1]. Individuals with atopy or with comorbidities such as aspirin exacerbated

Supplementary Information The online version contains supplementary material available at https://doi.org/10.1007/978-3-031-89191-5_13.

D. B. Spielman · J. M. DelGaudio (✉)
Department of Otolaryngology, Emory University, Atlanta, GA, USA
e-mail: jdelgau@emory.edu

J. T. Lee et al. (eds.), *Advances in Surgical and Medical Interventions for Recalcitrant Chronic Rhinosinusitis*,
https://doi.org/10.1007/978-3-031-89191-5_13

respiratory disease (AERD), allergic fungal rhinosinusitis (AFRS), or cystic fibrosis (CF) are at higher risk of requiring revision surgical intervention. For patients with advanced polyp burden, the risk of polyp recurrence postoperatively is 60% with 27% of patients ultimately undergoing revision ESS [2] and up to 29% of patients with CF will require revision ESS [3].

In-office rhinologic procedures have become increasingly common. Nearly all rhinologists perform office-based procedures with 77% of rhinologists reporting that they perform in-office polypectomy [4]. There is also noted to be a significant cost savings to the patient and insurers without a substantial impact on physician reimbursement [5]. Office-based procedures result in higher patient satisfaction due to decreased wait times and avoidance of general anesthesia. The objective of this chapter is to outline appropriate indications and techniques to perform in-office ESS.

Indications and Patient Selection

Careful patient selection is essential in conducting office-based rhinologic procedures. The surgical indication must be appropriate with reasonable outcome expectations by both the surgeon and the patient. Patients with severe comorbid anxiety, low pain tolerance, or inability to tolerate nasal endoscopy in the office are inappropriate candidates. Surgical indications and extent of disease must also be carefully considered. Patients with osteitic bone or those who require extensive bony work are not the best candidates for office-based ESS, as bony work is more challenging for patients to tolerate while awake.

For patients with CRS who are symptomatic despite appropriate medical therapy, primary or revision office-based endoscopic surgical procedures may be considered. The goals of surgery are often two-fold: to directly decrease the disease burden and to allow access for the delivery of topical irrigations and medications.

In the absence of other comorbidities, patients who require a primary full-house ESS are often better suited to surgical intervention in the operating room. However, an office-based procedure may be appropriate for patients with isolated disease, pregnant individuals, or for patients with comorbidities that make general anesthesia a higher risk. For those who have already had a complete primary ESS, but develop recurrent mucosal disease or polyps, an office-based procedure is ideal. Mucoceles may also be addressed in the office setting when present in an accessible area. Maxillary sinus ostium stenosis and recirculation sinusitis are noted to account for 42% of surgical failures, while frontal sinus outflow tract stenosis is responsible for 25% of surgical failures [6]. Many of these issues can be addressed in the office, avoiding a return trip to the operating room.

Severe burden of disease does not necessarily indicate that an office-based procedure cannot be performed safely and comfortably. Patients who have undergone a prior full-house ESS with removal of all bony septations are optimal candidates for in-office surgery. This concept has been demonstrated in the CF patient population [7]. For patients with significant medical comorbidities, especially pulmonary disease, the potential to avoid the risks associated with general anesthesia and mechanical ventilation is particularly palatable.

When performing an office-based procedure, the informed consent process should not differ from the standard consent discussion for procedures performed in the operating room. It is important that patients understand that despite the procedure being done in-office, it does not change the rare, but important risk of complications, including potential orbital or skull-base injury.

Setup and Local Anesthesia Technique

In order to successfully perform office-based procedures, adequate equipment, often similar to that used in the operating room, is necessary to ensure success. A reclining chair with adjustable height is needed. Patients are kept in a seated position. An endoscopic tower with recording ability as well as 0-degree and angled rigid endoscopes with adequate sinonasal instrumentation, including frontal sinus instruments if applicable, are necessary. Pediatric rigid endoscopes are a useful adjunct because their smaller size may be better tolerated by patients and they can allow for more posterior nasal cavity access. The microdebrider is very useful when addressing primary or recurrent polyp disease. Epistaxis management supplies must be on hand in the event that significant bleeding is encountered. This includes electrocautery, decongestant-soaked pledgets, thrombin-based surgical foam, and/or nasal packing. One should confirm that a patient's anticoagulation and antiplatelet therapy is discontinued several days prior. If unable to pause a patient's anticoagulation, it is safer to perform the procedure in the operating room.

A surgical time-out is performed to verify the patient, procedure, allergies, and any safety precautions. The type and extent of anesthetic agent used depends on the procedure type and location, along with surgeon preference and comfort. Topical anesthetic is used for all patients, and a combination of topical and injected anesthetic is used for some patients, especially when bony work is performed or posterior pathology is encountered. Although this is not our practice routinely, one can consider prescribing a one-time dose of a sedative to be taken immediately before the start of the procedure. Topical anesthetic (lidocaine 4%) mixed with a vasoconstrictor (oxymetazoline or phenylephrine) is sprayed initially to minimize discomfort for the remainder of the process. Next, pledgets or cotton balls soaked in oxymetazoline and lidocaine 4% are placed at the mucosal surfaces of the proposed site of surgery.

Under endoscopic visualization, lidocaine 1% with epinephrine 1:100,000 is injected into the axilla of the middle turbinate and the lateral nasal wall, as well as any other location that requires instrumentation. Allowing adequate time for anesthetic agents to take effect is important. The patient's sensitivity is tested by touching the area with an instrument before beginning the procedure. Additional directed injections of local anesthetic are given for persistent sensitivity and/or discomfort. Additional anesthetic, topical and/or injectable, may need to be applied throughout the course of the procedure if the patient does experience discomfort at any point.

Infraorbital and greater palatine nerve blocks can be considered for more involved procedures. The infraorbital nerve can be palpated exiting into the lower lid in a bony depression, just at or below the inferior orbital rim. Lidocaine 1% with epinephrine 1:100,000 is injected in the vicinity of the nerve, but not directly into the foramen. The greater palatine nerve can also be addressed by injecting in the vicinity of the foramen in the hard palate medial to the second or third molars [8]. A greater palatine block is specifically performed when working posteriorly within the nasal cavity or in the sphenoid sinus. Maximum lidocaine dose should be calculated to ensure lidocaine toxicity is not induced.

Surgical Technique

Nasal Polypectomy

For patients who have had primary ESS, but develop recurrent symptoms and nasal polyps, in-office polypectomy reduces disease burden and restores access for topical irrigations and steroids. Typically, these are patients with recalcitrant CRSwNP, such as those with AERD, CF, or AFRS, who have already had a complete primary ESS in the operating room with removal of all ethmoid partitions and opening of all sinus ostia. Nasal polypectomy in the office can also be considered for patients who have not previously had surgery, but who have a contraindication to full ESS in the operating room..

With appropriate local anesthesia, a microdebrider is used to remove polypoid disease, beginning anteriorly and inferiorly and progressing posteriorly and superiorly (Fig. 13.1; surgical video, Video 13.1). The inferior turbinate can be outfractured and the middle turbinate medialized to optimize access. Through-cutting instruments can also be used for polyp removal, but are less efficient and result in more bleeding and poorer visualization.

The middle turbinate often develops polypoid mucosa, especially in Central Compartment Atopic Disease (CCAD) and AFRS, and can be trimmed and sculpted to relieve obstruction while maintaining its form and function. When addressing disease adjacent to the orbit or skull base, the use of in-office surgical navigation with an updated CT scan is advantageous, as revision cases typically have fewer landmarks, although the authors have not utilized this technology in the office.

Maxillary Sinus Disease

The anterior location and distance of the maxillary sinus from the skull base makes it the safest sinus to address in the office. Indications for maxillary sinusotomy include odontogenic sinusitis, AFRS, postoperative stenosis of the maxillary antrostomy, maxillary recirculation, recurrent polyps, or mucocele formation. Maxillary sinus recirculation is a cause of postoperative recurrent disease in approximately

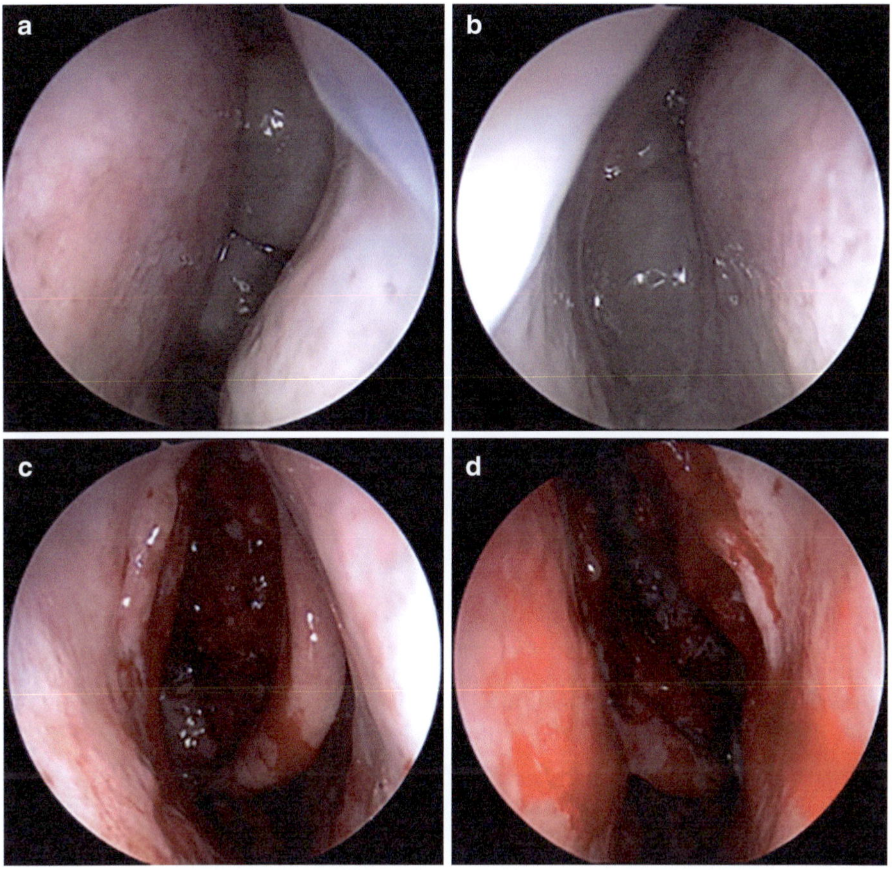

Fig. 13.1 (**a**, **b**) Preoperative endoscopy of R and L nasal cavity polyps in the middle meatus. (**c**, **d**) Postoperative endoscopy after in-office nasal polypectomy

15% of surgical failures. This occurs when there is an abnormal circular flow of sinonasal secretions between the natural ostium and a secondary surgically created opening [6, 9]. This can readily be addressed with an office-based procedure by removing any residual uncinate process and connecting the two ostia to create one large maxillary antrostomy [10]. If the previously placed antrostomy is inferior, it may be necessary to create a mega antrostomy, extending the sinusotomy through the inferior turbinate. Through-cutting instruments are used to remove the strut of bone and mucosa separating the natural and secondary ostia (Fig. 13.2).

When stenosis of the antrostomy exists, a ball tip probe can be used to identify the ostium and enlarge it using through-cutting and back-biting instruments. A microdebrider can be used to remove any residual inflammatory or polypoid disease. Care should be taken to avoid injury to the lacrimal duct and orbit. After completion, the ostium should be shaped in the form of a teardrop or pear. An angled

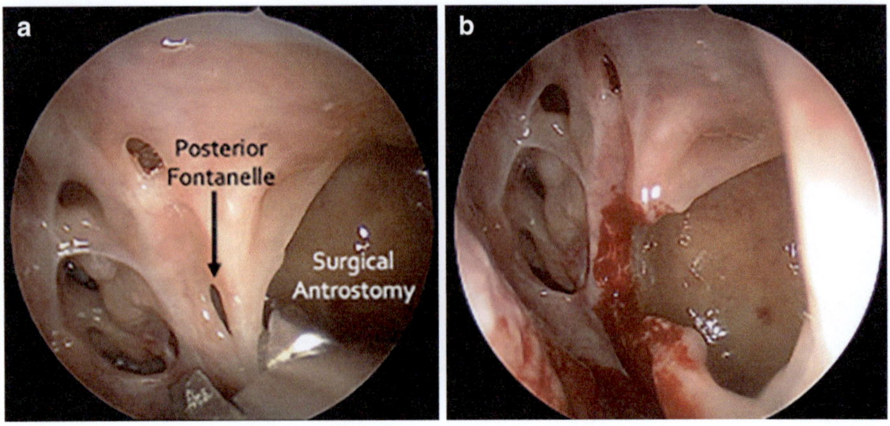

Fig. 13.2 (**a**) Patient with L maxillary sinus recirculation undergoing in-office removal of bony/mucosal strut separating the surgical antrostomy from a posterior fontanelle using a straight through-cutting instrument. (**b**) Large contiguous maxillary antrostomy encompassing both ostia after removal of the strut

endoscope is used to confirm completion of the antrostomy and may be particularly useful to verify that the natural ostium is included in the antrostomy to avoid future issues with maxillary recirculation. When addressing a mucocele, it is important to marsupialize the entire structure after draining the contents to prevent recurrence.

Balloon dilation can alternatively be used to enlarge the natural ostium in order to facilitate drainage. Purulence or debris within the sinus can be cleared using high pressure large volume irrigation by connecting a luer-lock syringe to a curved maxillary sinus suction. This technique is especially useful to clear fungal balls or allergic fungal mucin. Culture and pathology can be sent when indicated.

Ethmoid Sinus Disease

The role of office-based procedures to address the ethmoid sinuses is limited. For patients who have had prior ethmoidectomies, a microdebrider can be used to remove recurrent polypoid disease. When removing polypoid disease within the ethmoids, great care must be taken not to injure the orbit or anterior and posterior ethmoid arteries. If residual ethmoid partitions are noted, the microdebrider, through-cutting instruments, or rongeurs can be used to cut the bone, taking care to minimize removal of surrounding mucosa. The performance of a total ethmoidectomy with removal of all bony partitions can occasionally be performed in the office if needed. This will require sequential repeat administration of topical and local anesthetic as the procedure progresses posteriorly. Patients who have significant residual ethmoid partitions may be better served by having surgery in the operating room.

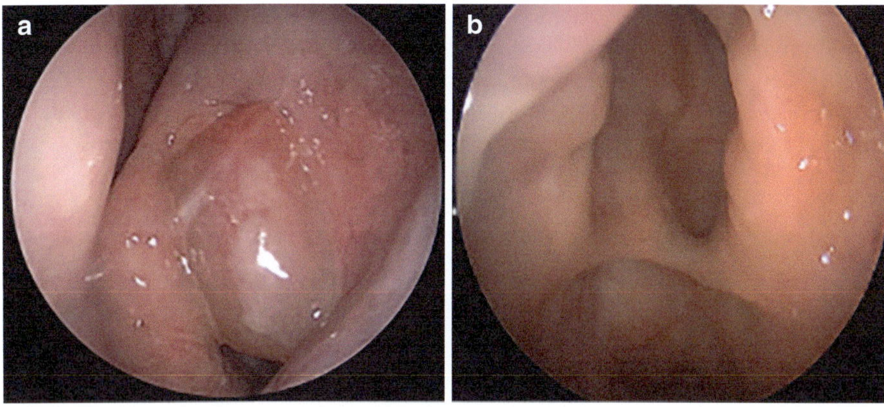

Fig. 13.3 (**a**) Preoperative endoscopy of polyps obstructing L frontal sinus outflow tract. (**b**) Postoperative endoscopy of patent L frontal sinus outflow tract one year after in-office surgery

Frontal Sinus Disease

Despite its challenging and narrow drainage pathway, certain frontal sinus issues can be addressed in the office. The most common indication is to address postoperative scarring and stenosis of the frontal sinus outflow tract, which is the cause of surgical failure in 25% of cases [6]. Alternative indications include recurrent frontal sinus disease or mucocele formation. Angled telescopes, 30°, 45°, or 70°, depending on the patient's anatomy, are essential for frontal sinus work and the use of image navigation can be a helpful adjunct. Any mucosal disease or residual ethmoid partitions narrowing the drainage pathway can be removed with through-cutting instruments or microdebrider (Fig. 13.3). Care must be taken to avoid injury to the posterior table of the frontal sinus and the anterior ethmoid artery. Patients who require additional drilling or extended Lothrop procedures should be taken to the operating room. In the immediate postoperative period, frontal sinus instruments may be used to gently debride material from the outflow tract to restore patency and prevent further scarring. Frontal sinus balloon dilation is a useful adjunct that can also be used with or without surgical navigation, or with transillumination.

After enlarging the frontal sinus outflow tract, high pressure irrigation delivered via a curved frontal sinus suction can be used to clear any residual debris. Once the outflow tract is sufficiently enlarged, a steroid eluting stent may be placed to prevent recurrent stenosis [11].

Sphenoid Sinus Disease

Because of its posterior location and proximity to critical neurovascular structures, the sphenoid sinus is more challenging under local anesthesia, but the straight access from the nasal cavity makes it accessible. Certain sphenoid sinus lesions can be addressed with an office-based procedure, especially in patients who have undergone prior ESS. Indications include recurrent polyposis, isolated sphenoid sinus opacification, mucocele, and fungus ball. Lesions with bony dehiscence of the lateral or posterior sphenoid walls can still be safely performed in the office, but if the surgeon is uncomfortable due to the potential involvement of critical neurovascular structures, they should be performed in the operating room.

The sphenoid sinus may be accessed via two routes: trans-nasally (medial to the middle and superior turbinates) or trans-ethmoidally (lateral to the middle turbinate through the posterior ethmoids). In patients who have not previously undergone ESS with total ethmoidectomy, the trans-ethmoid approach would require a total or posterior ethmoidectomy first, which is more difficult to perform in-office. The trans-nasal approach can be utilized by lateralizing the middle and superior turbinates to find the sphenoid ostium 1.5 cm superior to the choana. Placing additional pledgets to decongest this area significantly improves exposure and visualization. The inferior 1/third of the superior turbinate can be trimmed with straight through-cut forceps to improve visualization of the ostium, although the senior author prefers to preserve the entire superior turbinate. A Freer or Cottle elevator is used to gently palpate and enlarge the sphenoid ostium, followed by a sphenoid punch to remove the anterior face of the sphenoid. The sphenoidotomy can be extended through the posterior ethmoid sinuses to the lateral face of the sphenoid while preserving the superior turbinate, termed the Superior Turbinate Straddling Sphenoidotomy [12].

In the office setting, one should avoid the posterior septal branch of the sphenopalatine artery running inferiorly along the anterior face of the sphenoid in order to prevent bleeding. If performing an in-office sphenoidotomy, it is important to have the means to perform cauterization of this vessel readily available. Debris or polyps within the sinus can be removed by suction, forceps, or irrigation, taking care to avoid contact or injury to the lateral sphenoid walls and surrounding structures. A microdebrider is not used beyond the face of the sphenoid sinus itself to avoid damage to critical neurovascular structures.

Mucocele Drainage

Mucoceles are obstructed sinus cells or cavities that expand over time, frequently causing bony erosion and exerting pressure on adjacent structures. Risk factors for development include chronic rhinosinusitis, prior surgery, facial trauma, and allergy, and idiopathic mucocele development is also common [8]. The frontal and ethmoid sinuses are the most likely to develop mucoceles, but they can occur throughout the sinonasal cavities. When accessible, the vast majority of mucoceles can successfully be drained in the office [13]. Obtaining cross-sectional imaging preoperatively is important for diagnosis and to identify any bony dehiscences of surrounding neurovascular structures. Surgically, the goal is to create as large of a drainage pathway as safely possible and to marsupialize the entire lesion to minimize the risk of recurrence.

The frontal sinus is most frequently affected by mucocele formation and may be the most challenging to address. When there is anterior and inferior extension into the ethmoid cavity, these lesions are more easily accessed in the office under local anesthesia. The presence of posterior table or orbital roof erosion must be noted, although they are not necessarily contraindications to an office-based procedure.

Although less common, maxillary sinus mucoceles are easily drained in the office setting, even in patients who have not had prior sinus surgery. It is important to differentiate maxillary sinus mucoceles from mucus retention cysts, which are incidentally found and rarely expand or cause symptoms. Medial expansion of mucoceles into the nasal cavity often thins the medial wall of the maxillary sinus, making entry into the sinus easier than usual via the inferior meatus. If this modality is employed, it is important to connect the antrostomy with the natural ostium or keep it sufficiently far away to decrease the risk of mucus recirculation. If significant medial expansion has not occurred, a traditional maxillary antrostomy via the middle meatus may be performed.

Ethmoid mucoceles can be addressed in the office setting when they are sufficiently anterior or if the patient has undergone prior surgery, allowing access to the posterior ethmoid cavity. Ethmoid mucoceles frequently thin the bone of the adjacent orbit or skull base, thus careful review of preoperative imaging is essential.

Sphenoid sinus mucoceles are the least common, but may be addressed with an office-based procedure, especially if the patient has undergone prior surgery. The trans-nasal or trans-ethmoid approaches to the sphenoid sinus can be employed, as discussed above.

Balloon Sinus Dilation

Balloon sinus dilation is a useful tool when performing office-based procedures for the treatment of chronic rhinosinusitis. We will cover some aspects of balloon dilation in this section, but more details regarding balloon sinuplasty are available in Chap. 12 of this text. The minimally invasive nature of balloon dilation as compared with traditional ESS makes it well tolerated under local anesthesia. Balloon dilation systems can be used to enlarge the ostia of the maxillary, sphenoid, and frontal sinuses, but cannot directly address the ethmoid sinus.

Data regarding the use of balloon dilation demonstrates significant quality of life improvements in patients with CRS, although the majority of patients studied had relatively mild disease with a mean preoperative Lund-Mackay score of 7.7, compared with an average of 13 for all-comers undergoing treatment for CRS [14]. The Clinical Consensus Statement on sinus balloon dilation released by the American Academy of Otolaryngology—Head and Neck Surgery Foundation states that balloon dilation can improve quality of life in patients with limited CRS without nasal polyps. However, there was consensus that it should not be used in the absence of a preoperative CT scan demonstrating findings consistent with sinusitis [15]. There is no role for balloon dilation in patients who do not meet the formal diagnostic criteria for *CRS or recurrent acute sinusitis.*

Understanding the appropriate indications for balloon sinus dilation makes it a valuable tool for office-based surgery. Patients with nasal polyps or extensive disease, especially involving the ethmoid sinuses, are more likely to benefit from traditional ESS. Patients with relatively mild CRS without nasal polyps who have symptoms refractory to medical therapy may benefit from in-office balloon dilation of the affected sinuses. In the senior author's experience, balloon dilation serves a more valuable role in addressing postoperative stenosis of sinus ostia. The frontal sinus outflow tract is narrow and has a propensity to stenose. In patients who develop recurrent symptoms secondary to frontal sinus stenosis, balloon dilation can be used to reestablish the drainage pathway while minimizing trauma to the surrounding mucosa. The same technique can be applied to the maxillary or sphenoid sinuses.

Under direct visualization using a rigid endoscope, the ostium is cannulated with the guidewire in an atraumatic fashion. When addressing the frontal sinus, transillumination or image navigation can be used to verify appropriate placement. The balloon is then advanced over the guidewire until it is located at the level of the ostium, in its most narrow location (Fig. 13.4; see video, Video 13.1). Once

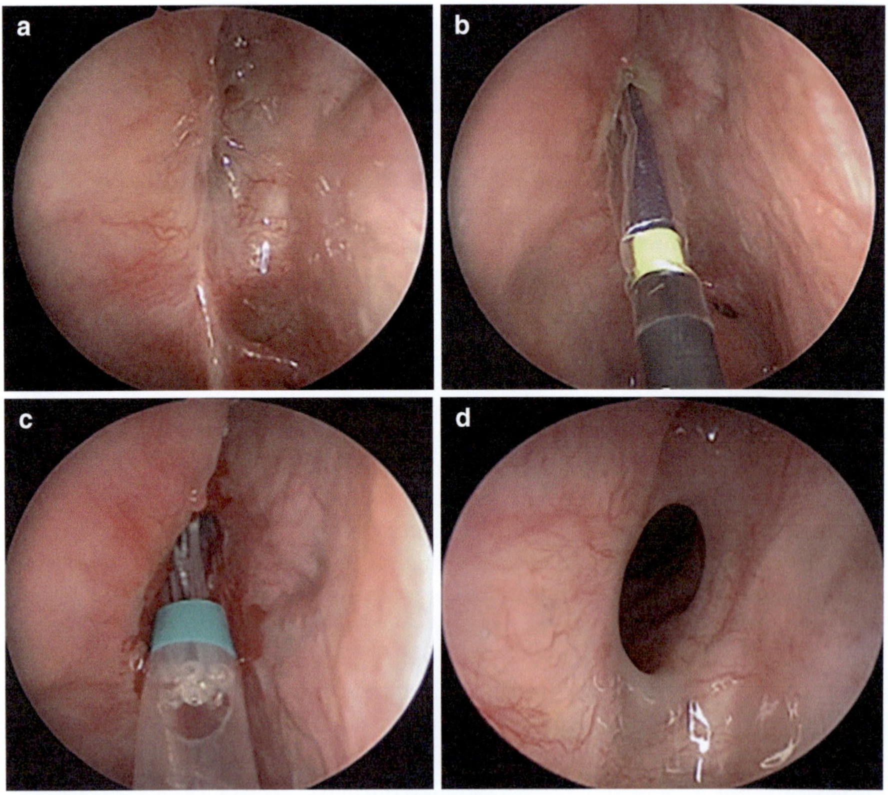

Fig. 13.4 (**a**) Stenotic R frontal sinus outflow tract after prior ESS (**b**) In-office balloon dilation (**c**) Steroid eluting stent placement (**d**) Patent frontal sinus outflow tract 6 months postoperatively

appropriate placement is confirmed, the balloon is inflated for several seconds according to manufacturer instructions. If the outflow tract remains stenotic, the balloon can be advanced and a second dilation can be performed. Providers who utilize sinonasal balloons must understand the manufacturer and FDA regulations regarding reuse of the devices.

Outcomes

While there is extensive evidence to support the benefits of ESS for patients with CRS refractory to medical therapy, there is a paucity of data isolated to office-based surgical procedures. Goyal and Hwang report the outcomes of 52 office-based procedures performed by a single surgeon under local anesthesia, which were well tolerated without complication [16]. The majority of these procedures were performed for recurrent disease following traditional ESS for CRS.

Office-based revision ESS has been demonstrated to have encouraging outcomes in a pilot study of five CF patients who previously underwent full-house ESS. All were noted to have significant improvements in quality of life and Lund-Mackay scores [7]. Drainage of mucoceles in-office is well tolerated with excellent outcomes. Barrow and DelGaudio reported on the office-based drainage of 36 mucoceles. All were successfully accessed under local anesthesia except for one. Five patients (14%) required additional future surgery to address septated mucoceles or recurrence [13]. These results are similar to those reported for operating room drainage of mucoceles.

Office-based balloon dilation has been demonstrated to improve sinonasal quality of life in patients with CRS refractory to medical therapy after one-year follow-up [17–19]. While balloon sinus dilation has been associated with clinically significant improvements in quality of life metrics, these studies lack a wide distribution of CRS patients or those with more severe forms of disease [14]. Proper patient selection for appropriate use of the balloon sinuplasty technique is essential, as patients with significant sinonasal disease are likely to benefit more from traditional ESS. In the authors' experience, balloon sinus dilation is most useful as an adjunct for patients with CRS who have mucosal scarring and a narrowed ostium following traditional ESS. In two pilot studies, this has been demonstrated to be a safe and effective technique following frontal sinusotomy in the operating room [20, 21].

Increasing competition to secure time in the operating room and the increased cost of operating room services makes the performance of in-office procedures highly palatable for both patients and physicians. Members of the rhinology community have already demonstrated that they regularly perform office-based procedures. The prevalence of office-based endoscopic sinus surgery is likely to increase with time because it is cost effective and improves the patient experience. An emphasis should be placed on proper patient selection and safe technique.

Tips and Pearls

- Patient selection and realistic expectations are essential.
- Anxious patients with a low pain tolerance or those who require significant bone removal are better suited for procedures in the operating room.
- Decongestion of the nasal mucosa and delivery of both topical and injected local anesthetic must be used.
- Ideal candidates for office-based procedures are those with symptomatic inflammatory disease, but minimal residual bony septations, often after primary ESS.
- The most common indications for office-based surgery include recurrent nasal polyposis, maxillary/frontal sinus ostium stenosis, mucocele, and maxillary sinus recirculation syndrome.
- Pediatric endoscopes and instruments may allow for improved access with less patient discomfort.
- Balloon sinus dilation and steroid eluting stents are valuable tools that can easily be used in the office for patients with ostial stenosis and residual symptoms after initial surgery.

References

1. Smith KA, Orlandi RR, Oakley G, Meeks H, Curtin K, Alt JA. Long-term revision rates for endoscopic sinus surgery. Int Forum Allergy Rhinol. 2019;9(4):402–8. 1 [cited 2022 Jun 21] [Internet] https://onlinelibrary.wiley.com/doi/full/10.1002/alr.22264
2. Wynn R, Har-El G. Recurrence rates after endoscopic sinus surgery for massive sinus polyposis. Laryngoscope [Internet]. 2004;114(5):811–3. [cited 2022 Jun 21]. https://doi.org/10.1097/00005537-200405000-00004.
3. Rickert S, Banuchi VE, Germana JD, Stewart MG, April MM. Cystic fibrosis and endoscopic sinus surgery relationship between nasal polyposis and likelihood of revision endoscopic sinus surgery in patients with cystic fibrosis [Internet]. www.jamaarchivescme.com
4. Lee JT, DelGaudio J, Orlandi RR. Practice patterns in office-based rhinology: survey of the American Rhinologic Society. Am J Rhinol Allergy [Internet]. 2019;33(1):26–35. [cited 2022 Jun 21]. https://doi.org/10.1177/1945892418804904.
5. Prickett KK, Wise SK, DelGaudio JM. Cost analysis of office-based and operating room procedures in rhinology. Int Forum Allergy Rhinol. 2012;2(3):207–11.
6. Ramadan HH. Surgical causes of failure in endoscopic sinus surgery. Laryngoscope [Internet]. 1999;109(1):27–9. [cited 2022 Jun 21]. https://doi.org/10.1097/00005537-199901000-00006.
7. Spielman DB, Gudis DA. Office-based sinus surgery for cystic fibrosis chronic rhinosinusitis. ORL. 2021;83(2):93–6. [Internet] [cited 2021 May 21] https://pubmed.ncbi.nlm.nih.gov/33333509/
8. Patel ZM, Wise SK, DelGaudio JM, Adelson RT. Office-based rhinology: principles and techniques. In Office-Based Rhinology. Patel ZM, Wise SK, DelGaudio JM (eds). Plural Publishing. San Diego, CA. 2013;1–168.
9. Kane KJ. Recirculation of mucus as a cause of persistent sinusitis. Am J Rhinol. 1997;11(5):361–9.
10. DelGaudio JM, Ochsner MC. Office surgery for paranasal sinus recirculation. Int Forum Allergy Rhinol. 2015;5(4):326–8. [cited 2022 Jun 24] [Internet] https://pubmed.ncbi.nlm.nih.gov/25611335/

11. Goshtasbi K, Abouzari M, Abiri A, Yasaka T, Sahyouni R, Bitner B, et al. Efficacy of steroid-eluting stents in management of chronic rhinosinusitis after endoscopic sinus surgery: updated meta-analysis. Int Forum Allergy Rhinol. 2019;9(12):1443–50.
12. DelGaudio JM. The superior turbinate straddling sphenoidotomy. Int Forum Allergy Rhinol. 2015;5(5):445–7. [Internet] [cited 2022 Jun 29]. https://doi.org/10.1002/alr.21477.
13. Barrow EM, DelGaudio JM. In-office drainage of sinus Mucoceles: an alternative to operating-room drainage. Laryngoscope. 2015;125(5):1043–7. [Internet]. [cited 2022 Jun 29]. https://doi.org/10.1002/lary.25042.
14. Levy JM, Marino MJ, Mccoul ED. Paranasal sinus balloon catheter dilation for treatment of chronic rhinosinusitis: a systematic review and meta-analysis. Otolaryngol Neck Surg. 2016;154(1):33–40. [cited 2022 Jun 28] [Internet] http://otojournal.org
15. Piccirillo JF, Payne SC, Rosenfeld RM, Baroody FM, Batra PS, DelGaudio JM, et al. Clinical consensus statement: balloon dilation of the sinuses. Otolaryngol Neck Surg. 2018;158(2):203–14.
16. Goyal P, Hwang PH. In-office surgical treatment of sinus disease: office-based surgical procedures in rhinology. Oper Tech Otolaryngol Neck Surg. 2006;17(1):58–65.
17. Karanfilov B, Silvers S, Pasha R, Sikand A, Shikani A, Sillers M. Office-based balloon sinus dilation: a prospective, multicenter study of 203 patients. Int Forum Allergy Rhinol [Internet]. 2013;3(5):404–11. [cited 2022 Jun 28] https://pubmed.ncbi.nlm.nih.gov/23136057/
18. Sikand A, Silvers SL, Pasha R, Shikani A, Karanfilov BI, Harfe DT, et al. Office-based balloon sinus dilation: 1-year follow-up of a prospective, multicenter study. Ann Otol Rhinol Laryngol. 2015;124(8):630–7.
19. Stolovitzky JP, Mehendale N, Matheny KE, Brown WJ, Rieder AA, Liepert DR, et al. Medical therapy versus balloon sinus dilation in adults with chronic rhinosinusitis (MERLOT): 12-month follow-up. Am J Rhinol Allergy [Internet]. 2018;32(4):294–302. [cited 2022 Jun 28] https://pubmed.ncbi.nlm.nih.gov/29781286/
20. Eloy JA, Friedel ME, Eloy JD, Govindaraj S, Folbe AJ. In-office balloon dilation of the failed frontal sinusotomy. Otolaryngol Head Neck Surg. 2012;146(2):320–2. [cited 2022 Jun 26] [Internet] https://journals.sagepub.com/doi/full/10.1177/0194599811425885?casa_token=5Rsl5J-y83cAAAAA%3AbfiA594JnkQ7f3MuKo-YtRDAQaXVV6kAzWL6-EJ4lN1PirvMKeTDdqfx6G0k7M8PFkpx3RGht8o
21. Luong A, Batra PS, Fakhri S, Citardi MJ. Balloon catheter dilatation for frontal sinus ostium stenosis in the office setting. Am J Rhinol. 2008;22(6):621–4. [cited 2022 Jun 26] [Internet] https://pubmed.ncbi.nlm.nih.gov/19178802/

In-Office Navigation for Recalcitrant Chronic Rhinosinusitis

14

Nora W. Perkins

Key Points
- Advances in endoscopic sinus surgery have allowed surgeons to apply rhinologic procedures to the office setting.
- Image guidance is a useful adjunct that can be applied to patients in-office to allow more thorough in-office dissection.

Background

The advances in endoscopic sinus technologies in the twentieth and twenty-first centuries have allowed sinus surgeons to skillfully visualize and access all of the paranasal sinuses and generally avoid the need for open surgical sinus procedures [1]. Angled endoscopes of various sizes with large monitor video systems, a plethora of instrumentation choices, powered shavers, and navigation systems that allow those instruments and shavers to be tracked throughout the surgical procedure have become customary in the operating suite [1–3]. As these endoscopic sinus surgery technologies advanced, several factors directed surgeons to bring sinus procedures from the operating room into the office, including economic drivers like lower overall healthcare cost and direct to patient cost, ease and timeliness of procedure scheduling, access to operating room block time, patient preference to avoid general anesthesia and recover/return to work more quickly, surgeon preference, and improved surgical efficiency during and between procedures [2, 4–7].

N. W. Perkins (✉)
Albany ENT & Allergy Services, Albany, NY, USA
e-mail: nperkins@albanyent.com

J. T. Lee et al. (eds.), *Advances in Surgical and Medical Interventions for Recalcitrant Chronic Rhinosinusitis*,
https://doi.org/10.1007/978-3-031-89191-5_14

These technological advancements have also allowed surgeons to expand the breadth of their office-based surgical repertoire. There are numerous studies and reports of safety and feasibility for a diverse scope of sinus procedures in the office, including balloon sinus dilation, turbinate reduction, mucocele drainage and marsupialization, polypectomy, septoplasty, and traditional endoscopic sinus procedures (maxillary antrostomy, ethmoidectomy, etc.) [4, 5, 7–13].

As access to these technological advancements has expanded beyond the operating room, surgeons are able to perform office-based primary sinus procedures in patients with medically recalcitrant chronic rhinosinusitis, with or without nasal polyps, about 30–55% of who require some type of surgical treatment, and office-based revision surgical procedures in those patients with surgically recalcitrant chronic rhinosinusitis, who constitute about 4–20% of those patients who previously underwent primary surgery for CRS [2, 6]. With these tools at their disposal, surgeons may now reframe their surgical discussions with patients to include the office as a potential site of service and further challenge their own historical bias to ask themselves, "is there a reason this case cannot be done in the office setting?"

History of Sinus Navigation

Since its inception, developments in CT imaging, including patient access, speed of the study and higher resolution images, have allowed surgeons the ability to easily and effectively evaluate patient sinus anatomy and disease [1]. CT scanners are readily available in the community and often offered in the surgeon's own office, allowing for immediate imaging and interpretation in appropriately selected patients. These high-resolution images can easily be transferred into the navigation systems for all scheduled surgical patients and used if needed at the surgeon's choice.

Improvements in image-guidance systems, such as improvements in accuracy, ease of registration and setup, have contributed to the transition of navigation systems into the office-setting [1, 2, 7, 10]. Navigation systems can now be housed on the same tower as the video system, monitor and powered shaver, eliminating spatial barriers in the office setting. Although use of navigation in sinus procedures is not necessarily the industry standard, the American Academy of Otolaryngology—Head and Neck Surgery offered a position statement supporting the use of navigation in appropriate cases, which are determined at the discretion of the surgeon [14].

A 2016 survey of the American Rhinologic Society members shows that 10% of respondents were using office-based navigation systems at that time, with 63% noting that they were performing more office-based procedures over the prior 5-year period [9]. Extrapolating from that trend, it is likely that the number of surgeons using office-based navigation systems is higher now, nine years after that survey, and will continue to rise. While there has not been conclusive data that supports the use of navigation in reducing complications, some propose that it may assist in reducing the surgeons perceived surgical workload, improve speed and efficiency of cases, and provide surgeons the tools to complete a more thorough surgical dissection [1].

Techniques and Considerations

Patient Selection

Patient selection and in-office techniques are thoroughly described in Chap. 13 of this text. In brief, when selecting patients for in-office sinus procedures, there are many factors which should be considered. Firstly, surgeons should recognize that they themselves may have a bias toward choosing the operating room as the site of service. Most surgeons are most familiar and comfortable with the operating room and patients being under general anesthesia. That bias will impact the surgeon's recommendation to patients when considering the office as a potential site of service.

Patients themselves may have strong preferences about avoiding general anesthesia and prefer to have their sinus procedure performed in the office setting. Conversely, others may express significant anxiety about pain or awareness during an office-based procedure and request "to be knocked out." Those who self-report difficulty tolerating dental procedures or who have not had success with local anesthetic in the past may be poor candidates for in-office procedures. However, patients who express concern about anxiety or pain during the procedure can be reassured that the procedural pre-medication regimen adequately addresses anxiety concerns and the local anesthetic protocol will assure that they will have minimal pain or discomfort during the procedure. Some patients may express that they "want to be knocked out" for their procedure. It is reasonable to clarify that desire with the patient, as they typically are not requesting general anesthesia, but instead are expressing their wish to manage pain and anxiety during their procedure. Setting appropriate and realistic expectations with patients prior to the procedure is critical. Patients should be counseled that they will feel pressure, even when local anesthesia is working well to eliminate pain, and they will also hear portions of the procedure, like lateral out-fracturing of the inferior turbinate or medialization of the middle turbinate. In order to assure a predictable patient experience, surgeons should follow a standard anesthetic protocol, both with regard to anxiolytic and analgesic pre-procedure medication regimen and local anesthesia protocol. This is particularly important as a surgeon is beginning to transition procedures from the operating room to the office. Following a standard protocol will increase the likelihood of success, as the variables related to patient anxiety and comfort will be better managed, allowing the surgeon to focus on the procedure itself. Tables 14.1 and 14.2 detail the author's preferred anesthesia protocol and local anesthetic administration protocol, respectively.

Lastly, patients with medical comorbidities that increase risks related to general anesthesia, or those who are unable to stop anticoagulation medications, may be better candidates for local anesthesia with or without minimal anxiolysis in the office-setting [15–17].

Table 14.1 Anesthesia protocol for preceding and during in-office procedure

Anesthesia Protocol
Pre-medications—although these are optional, particularly for very minor, brief procedures where the surgeon can expect local anesthesia to be very effective (cryoablation, nasal airway obstruction procedures, placement of drug-eluding stents), I find this regimen to be very effective for the majority of my patients. This regimen helps assure that you will have a predictable patient, which allows the surgeon to perform the procedure in their customary fashion, with fewer unpredictable patient factors. This regimen also helps address patient concerns regarding anxiety during the procedure, which can impact their surgical site choice (OR vs. office). Assuring them that they will have a medication regimen to address anxiety and pain, and a local anesthesia protocol that will limit pain or discomfort can help appropriate patients feel more comfortable in choosing an office procedure and avoiding general anesthesia
Pre-Procedure Day 1—start Medrol Dose pack (only if inflammatory/polyp disease present)
If significant inflammation, polyp disease is present, earlier pre-treatment with oral steroid may be beneficial
Procedure Day (*consents signed prior to procedure day*)
Eat light breakfast or lunch (do not need to be NPO)
2 Hours prior to procedure
Oxymetazoline 2 sprays each side of nose every 30 min (2–3 doses)
60 minutes prior to procedure
Promethazine 25 mg
Triazolam 0.125 mg
Tramadol 50 mg (optional, may not be necessary for minor procedures)
MD Evaluation
If patient remains anxious, can take additional 1–2 Triazolam 0.125 mg
Post-Procedure Day 1
Start saline irrigations (+/– topical steroid)
Antibiotic if indicated
Oral steroid if indicated

Room Setup/Equipment

In-office sinus procedures can be performed in any ENT office exam room. The most basic room requirements include an ENT chair that will convert into the supine position, a video system and monitor to attach to sinus endoscopes, suction and the necessary equipment for the particular procedure. As the surgeon is expanding their breadth of in-office sinus procedures, a more extensive room setup may develop (Fig. 14.1). An advanced office-based procedure room will include a comfortable ENT chair that will go into the supine position and raise/lower for surgeon comfort, a video/monitor system to allow for endoscopic visualization, various 3 or 4 mm endoscopes (0, 30, 45, 70 degrees), a microdebrider or shaver system, an image-guidance navigation system, secondary suction, traditional FESS instruments (through cutting forceps, back biting forceps, mushroom punch, Kerrison forceps), balloon sinus dilation devices, irrigation devices, drug-eluting sinus implants, hemostatic agents, and cautery [10]. Staff may find benefit from having an additional instrument cart that is easily accessible during procedures (Fig. 14.2). This

Table 14.2 Local anesthesia protocol for in-office procedures

Local Anesthesia
2 Hours prior to procedure
Oxymetazoline 2 sprays each side of nose every 30 min (2–3 doses)
In office
Topical 4% lidocaine and Afrin (1:1) cotton pledgets—squeezed out to avoid dripping down the pharynx—placed along the floor of the nose between the septum and inferior turbinate
Leave in place for 7–10 minutes
Topical 4% Lidocaine and 1:1000 Adrenaline (1:1)
Small pledgets placed along middle turbinate root, anterior face of the middle turbinate, in middle meatus (if adequate spacing), medial to middle turbinate against septum
Long cotton pledgets along floor of the nose between inferior turbinate and septum
Squeeze out excess liquid to avoid dripping anesthetic into pharynx
Leave in placed for 7–10 min
1% or 2% Lidocaine with 1:200,000 epinephrine
Injection sites (27 g needle)
Inferior turbinate
Septum (particularly if spur or deviation present or anteriorly if instruments will be abutting septum)
Root of the middle turbinate, anterior face of the middle turbinate
Septum medial to middle turbinate (optional)
Injection sites (Spinal Needle or Reinforced Anesthesia Needle (Stryker ENT, Plymouth, MN)
Sphenoid rostrum (if surgical plan includes sphenoid)
Sphenopalatine (infero/lateral attachment of middle turbinate)
Polyp tissue

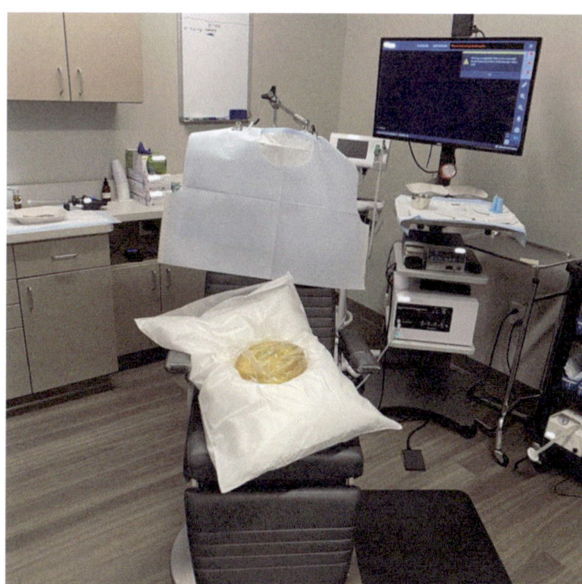

Fig. 14.1 Office-based procedure room setup—tower holds navigation system, microdebrider, and video monitor. The surgeon can stand or sit to the patient's right, with a chair in their preferred position. Staff can stand to the patient's left and assist in typical surgical fashion

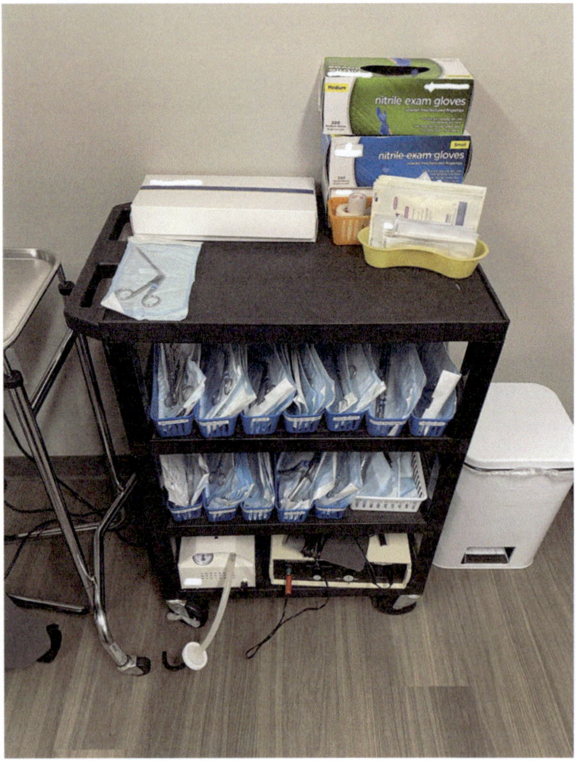

Fig. 14.2 Instrument cart—procedure pack and individually wrapped instruments, easily accessible to staff throughout the procedure

can reduce confusion during a procedure when an unanticipated instrument is needed and allows the surgeon to feel confident that all instruments are available if intra-operative treatment changes.

Navigation Systems

The utilization of navigation during sinus procedures in the office is increasing and will likely continue to rise as residents are increasingly trained with navigation systems in the OR for a variety of reasons; such as to facilitate teaching, improve supervising surgeon comfort/guidance and the perception of improved safety and completeness of surgery [2, 9]. Historically, navigation may have only been used in rare cases, like skull base or neoplastic surgeries, but as the devices became less cumbersome, easier for staff to set up and surgeons to use, and accuracy improved, navigation may now be used even for routine cases [1, 2]. Additionally, the smaller footprint of the navigation systems allowed for a natural transition of the technology into the office setting. These advances, coupled with surgeon, patient, and overall healthcare system preferences for in-office procedures, have complemented one another and allowed for an increasing number and complexity of cases to be performed in the office setting.

The current office-based sinus navigation system market includes the Acclarent TruDi Navigation System (Acclarent, Irvine, CA), the Karl Storz NAV1 Navigation System (Karl Storz, El Segundo, CA), the Medtronic StealthStation FlexENT Navigation System (Medtronic, Minneapolis, MN), and the Stryker Scopis ENT Navigation System (Stryker ENT, Plymouth, MN). Surgeon preference may dictate the system used; however, economic factors, trackable device options, and availability (what the surgeon has access to in their facility) may also be considered when choosing an in-office navigation system. These systems utilize either electromagnetic or hybrid, electromagnetic and optical, tracking technologies. They can be housed in a single unit with the monitor, video system, and other devices, like a powered shaver/microdebrider, and secondary suction.

Depending on the navigation system, there may be no cost associated with registering patients, so staff can be trained to upload CT images and register all scheduled patients, with cost only being incurred if the surgeon chooses to use navigation during the procedure. The navigation systems have various capabilities that allow the surgeon to pre-mark surgical targets, critical structures to be avoided and plan pathways into the targeted sinuses. These pre-planning software features allow the surgeon to map their surgical plan and can be particularly useful in the teaching setting. The Stryker Scopis system (Stryker, Plymouth, MN) features an augmented reality option, where the surgeon can pre-plan the surgical pathway and then utilize the hybrid optical and electromagnetic properties to follow the pre-planned surgical pathway to the targeted sinus. Other systems, like the Acclarent TruDi (Acclarent, Irvine, CA), have software that uses artificial intelligence to identify known structures and calculate likely surgical pathways.

Although specific trackable devices vary by manufacturer, devices such as suction, pointers, powered shavers/microdebriders, sinus balloons, and traditional sinus instruments can all be tracked. These capabilities have allowed surgeons to treat cases that may not have historically been considered for office-based surgery, such as revision sinus cases, synechiae and stenosis, drainage and marsupialization of mucoceles, polypectomy, and ethmoidectomy. Excision of limited neoplasms, like inverting papilloma, can also be considered with the assistance of navigation in the office setting. Video 14.1 shows a revision frontal sinus polypectomy using in-office navigation. A navigatable frontal sinus seeker is used to confirm the location of the frontal sinus ostium. A curved microdebrider is used to remove polyps within the frontal sinus. A steroid-eluting implant is then placed into the frontal sinus at the end of the procedure.

Monitoring

Patient monitoring is dependent on type of anesthesia (local, oral sedation, IV sedation) and varies by state. Surgeons should confirm their state monitoring requirements, as well as any state specific accreditation requirements. In our practice, we do not utilize IV sedation, and our sedation goal, according to the American Society of Anesthesiologists Continuum of Depth of Sedation, is Minimal Sedation

Anxiolysis, defined as “a drug-induced state during which patients respond normally to verbal commands. Although cognitive function and physical coordination may be impaired, airway reflexes, and ventilatory and cardiovascular functions are unaffected [18].” We routinely record pre and post procedure vital signs and monitor pulse oximetry throughout the procedures. Depending on patient comorbidities, state requirements, type of anesthesia, and surgeon preference, some surgeons may choose or be required to monitor blood pressure and EKG throughout their procedures [15, 17]. Surgeons should be prepared for potential complications related to anesthesia, including allergic reaction and medication toxicity, and be prepared to manage immediate complications.

Patient Comfort

To create a comfortable experience for patients, the surgeon and staff should consider playing relaxing music, or music of the patients choosing, and covering the eyes to limit irritation from bright endoscopic lights and anxiety caused by seeing surgical instruments. Instruct patients to wear comfortable clothing, and place them in a comfortable position, with a pillow or other support under the lower legs and a gel pillow under their head. If the room is small, and becomes warm due to equipment and staff, having a fan to keep the patient comfortable can also be helpful. Although ultimately patient position is the surgeon’s preference, placing patients in a supine position may limit drainage into the oropharynx, as secretions will pool in the nasopharynx and can be easily suctioned.

Staff Training

In order to successfully perform office-based rhinology procedures and particularly office-based image guidance, it is imperative to train nursing and medical staff on the surgical equipment, navigation systems, typical order of surgical procedures and surgeon preferences. It is also important to remind staff that the patients are awake throughout the procedure, so using gentle terms to describe surgical instruments (asking for the local anesthetic, not the needle or injection) can alleviate patient anxiety. Also, if a complication or unforeseen event occurs, it is critical for staff to avoid comments that may increase patient anxiety. Although many surgeons may prefer a dedicated staff member, or champion, to assist in their cases, cross-training throughout many staff can help reduce challenges related to illness, vacation or staff changes. Regular staff training and retraining, as well as “mock” cases and navigation system troubleshooting guides can improve staff confidence and comfort during procedures. The author’s preferred procedure protocol is detailed in Table 14.3.

Table 14.3 Surgical technique, room set-up, and required prerequisite skills to perform in-office procedures

Surgical Technique/How I Do It:

- Room setup/Equipment
  - Dark room, Relaxing music, eye covering, comfortable clothing, supine position with gel donut under head and pillow under knees, fan, blankets
- Patient positioning
  - Surgeon preference
    - Supine
      - Traditional operating position for Surgeon
      - Potentially less drainage into nasopharynx/oropharynx (secretions pool in nasopharynx—can be suctioned)
      - May need to add leg/knee support/pillow for low back comfort
    - Semi-recumbant
      - Non-standard operating position for Surgeon
      - Potentially more drainage into nasopharynx/oropharynx
    - Seated
      - Potentially less drainage into nasopharynx/oropharynx
      - Non-standard operating position for Surgeon
  - Surgeon position—standing or sitting
- Staff training
  - Staff should become "super-users" with navigation systems—able to troubleshoot problems, upload images, set up for surgeon preferences
  - Perform mock cases with all staff—familiarity with instruments, familiarity with progression/flow of common procedures, ability to setup/access instrumentation during procedure
  - Staff champion—able to lead new trainees/staff in cross-training, the "go-to" person for questions
  - Nursing –
    - Call patient about 7–14 days prior to procedure. Review their medications (current), as well as prescriptions for pre-medications that will be sent to pharmacy (triazolam, promethazine, +/− tramadol, methylprednisolone).—procedure protocols—similar to OR (stopping NSAIDs, ASA), review timing of pre-medication regimen, expected length of procedure/visit, confirm transportation/responsible person (mandatory if taking pre-medication, option if local anesthetic only)
- Post-procedure protocols—POD #1 telephone call

Reported Outcomes/Evolving Practice Patterns

Lee et al. reported 2016 survey results from the American Rhinological Society in 2019 and found an increasing trend toward in-office rhinologic procedures, both for academic and private practice physicians [5]. At that time, about 10% of surveyed physicians were using navigation in the office setting, but 77% were performing polypectomy in the office, 56% were performing balloon ostial dilations in the office, and about 1/3 of respondents performed more traditional FESS procedures (maxillary antrostomy, ethmoidectomy. Sphenoidotomy, frontal sinusotomy) in the office setting [5]. There are numerous feasibility, safety, and outcome durability studies supporting the success of balloon ostial dilation, steroid eluting implant placement, management of mucoceles, correction of recirculation, and recalcitrant frontal sinus disease in the office setting [8, 9, 11–13, 19–21].

With the vast technological advances available to surgeons in the office setting, the reduced healthcare costs, and the encouraging safety and feasibility reports, there is likely to be a continued shift away from the operating room and toward the office as the primary choice for site of service.

Tips and Pearls

- Set realistic patient expectations regarding anxiety, pain/discomfort.
- Set up the room optimally for your procedure prior to patient arrival.
- Modern navigation systems have a small footprint, but ensure that you have adequate space for monitors and navigation systems and that they are set up appropriately for visualization during the entirety of the procedure.
- Try to limit case times to less than 1 h from start to finish, longer cases can lead to increased discomfort with prolonged patient immobility. This should, when able, include set-up time.

References

1. Tajudeen B, Kennedy D. Thirty years of endoscopic sinus surgery: what have we learned? World J Otorhinolaryngol Head Neck Surg. 2017;3(2):115–21.
2. Marino M, Citardi M, Yao W, Luong A. Image guidance in endoscopic sinus surgery: where are we heading? Curr Otolaryngol Rep. 2017;5:8–15.
3. Tang D, Lobo B, D'Anza, et al. Advances in microdebrider technology: improving functionality and expanding utility. Otolaryngol Clin N Am. 2017;50:589–98.
4. Albritton F, Casiano R, Sillers M. Feasibility of in-office endoscopic sinus surgery with balloon sinus dilation. Am J Rhinol Allergy. 2012;26(3):243–8.
5. Lee J, DelGaudio J, Orlandi R. Practice patterns in office-based rhinology: survey of the American Rhinologic Society. Am J Rhinol Allergy. 2019;33(1):26–35.
6. Unsal A, Gregory N, Rosenstein K. Current opinions in office-based rhinology. Curr Opin Otolaryngol Head Neck Surg. 2018;26:8–12.
7. Varshney R, Lee J. New innovations in office-based rhinology. Curr Opin Otolaryngol Head Neck Surg. 2016;24:3–9.
8. Anderson Eloy J, Shukla P, Choudhry O, et al. In-office balloon dilation and drainage of frontal sinus mucocele. Allergy Rhinol. 2013;4:36–40.
9. Barrow E, DelGaudio J. In-office drainage of sinus Mucoceles: an alternative to operating-room drainage. Laryngoscope. 2015;125:1043–7.
10. Saini A, Citardi M, Yao W, Luong A. Office-based sinus surgery. Otolaryngol Clin N Am. 2019;52:473–83.
11. Scott J, Sowerby L, Rotenberg B. Office0based rhinologic surgery: a modern experience with operative techniques under local anesthetic. Am J Rhinol Allergy. 2017;31(2):135–8.
12. Sikand A, Silvers S, Pasha R, et al. Office-based balloon sinus dilation: 1-year follow-up of a prospective, multicenter study. Ann Otol Rhinol Laryngol. 2015;124(8):630–7.
13. Thamboo A, Patel Z. Office procedures in refractory chronic rhinosinusitis. Otolaryngol Clin N Am. 2017;50:113–28.
14. AAO-HNS. Position statement: intra-operative use of computer aided surgery; 2014. https://www.entnet.org/resource/position-statement-intra-operative-use-of-computer-aided-surgery/. Accessed 2 Jul 2022.
15. Chang M, Jitaroon K, Nguyen T, et al. Hemodynamic changes in patients undergoing office-based patients undergoing office-based sinus procedures under local anesthesia. Int Forum Allergy Rhinol. 2020;10:114–20.

16. Higgins T, Ocal B, Adams R, Wu A. In-office balloon sinus ostial dilation with concurrent antiplatelet and anticoagulant therapy for chronic rhinosinusitis without nasal polyps. Ann Otol Rhinol Laryngol. 2020;129(3):280–6.
17. Schmalbach C. Patient safety and anesthesia considerations for office-based otolaryngology procedures. Otolaryngol Clin N Am. 2019;52:379–90.
18. American Society of Anesthesiologists. Continuum of depth of sedation: definition of general anesthesia and levels of sedation/analgesia; 2019. https://www.asahq.org/standards-and-guidelines/continuum-of-depth-of-sedation-definition-of-general-anesthesia-and-levels-of-sedationanalgesia/. Accessed on 5 Jul 2022.
19. Castro A, Furtado M, Rego A, et al. Long term outcomes of balloon sinuplasty for the treatment of chronic rhinosinusitis with and without nasal polyps. Am. J Otolaryngol. 2021;42:1.
20. DelGaudio J, Ochsner M. Office surgery for paranasal sinus recirculation. Int Forum Allergy Rhinol. 2015;5:326–8.
21. Sikand A. Introduction to an office-based sinus surgery technique. Op Tech Otolaryngol Head Neck Surg. 2011;22(3):246–52.

In Office Polypectomy for Recalcitrant Chronic Sinusitis with Polyposis (CRSwNP) Patients

15

Bader M. Alim, Juan Carlos Hernaiz-Leonardo, and Amin R. Javer

Key Points

- Disease recurrence in patients with chronic rhinosinusitis with nasal polyposis (CRSwNP) is common.
- Surgical revision under general anesthesia is not always feasible due to high anesthetic risk, long wait times, or other factors.
- In-office procedures using powered instrumentation can significantly improve symptoms and reduce the need for oral steroids or other medications in refractory cases.
- Adequate patient selection is key for a successful outcome and thorough communication before, during and after the procedure will aid in patient comfort.
- In-office polypectomies are effective in the short and medium term, but they are not definitive treatments for recalcitrant CRSwNP.
- Adequate medical management and close follow-up will help maintain good symptomatic control in this challenging-to-treat subpopulation.

Supplementary Information The online version contains supplementary material available at https://doi.org/10.1007/978-3-031-89191-5_15.

B. M. Alim
Department of Otolaryngology—Head and Neck Surgery, Prince Mohammed Bin Abdul-Aziz Hospital, National Guard Health Affairs, Madina, Saudi Arabia

J. C. Hernaiz-Leonardo · A. R. Javer (✉)
Department of Otolaryngology—Head and Neck Surgery, University of British Columbia, Vancouver, BC, Canada
e-mail: hernaiz@student.ubc.ca

J. T. Lee et al. (eds.), *Advances in Surgical and Medical Interventions for Recalcitrant Chronic Rhinosinusitis*,
https://doi.org/10.1007/978-3-031-89191-5_15

Background

Chronic rhinosinusitis (CRS) refers to inflammation of the nasal cavity and paranasal sinuses with symptoms lasting more than 12 weeks [1]. The incidence of chronic rhinosinusitis with nasal polyposis (CRSwNP) varies according to the geographical location where studies are done and ranges from 2.7% to 33%. It has a high association with bronchial asthma (BA), aspirin exacerbated respiratory diseases (AERD) and allergic fungal rhinosinusitis (AFRS) [2, 3]. CRSwNP patients whose disease is poorly responsive to medical therapies and have persistent signs and symptoms of nasal blockage and disturbed sense of smell may need to undergo endoscopic sinus surgery in order to decrease the inflammatory burden of the disease, alleviate obstructive nasal symptoms, and facilitate medication delivery to the sinonasal cavity. CRSwNP patients with recalcitrant symptoms despite appropriate medical and surgical therapy have an essential need for close monitoring and rapid interventions to optimize symptom control.

As the waiting time for full-house functional endoscopic sinus surgery (FESS) can be lengthy in the public health care systems in many parts of the world, there is a need for solutions that can provide relief for CRSwNP patients with nasal obstruction as their main symptom. Prior to current advancements in endoscopic techniques, office-based procedures were carried out using headlight illumination and cold steel instruments, such as snares and blakesley forceps, often leading to unacceptable bleeding, mucosal stripping and most importantly poor outcomes [4]. With the advent of advanced endoscopic surgical technologies and powered instrumentation carefully designed for use in the clinical setting, together with a heightened awareness toward delivering cost-effective healthcare, office-based procedures have become an integral part of tertiary rhinology practices [5]. In-office microdebrider assisted polypectomy is one of those technologies that provides a viable option for keeping the recalcitrant CRSwNP patient under adequate control.

In this chapter we describe and share our experience with microdebrider assisted in-office polypectomy for patients with recalcitrant CRSwNP.

Indications for in-Office Polypectomy

1- Patients with grade 2–4 nasal polyp score (polyps extending beyond the middle meatus) who have failed previous medical (topical and short- and long-term courses of oral antibiotic and steroids) and surgical (in-office polypectomy or FESS) management.
2- Recalcitrant CRSwNP patients unable to undergo general anesthesia secondary to high-risk medical comorbidities and/or pregnancy.
3- Recalcitrant CRSwNP patients awaiting elective FESS on long wait lists in the public health care system.

The main goal of in-office polypectomy in the aforementioned group is to decrease the inflammatory burden of their disease, improve nasal airflow, and create a wider passageway for improved access and distribution of topical medications.

Surgical Technique (Video 15.1)

Room Setup, Patient Positioning, and Local Anesthesia Protocol

All patients are formally consented for the procedure, during which time all potential risks and complications, including intra- and post-procedure epistaxis, syncope, risk of infection, possibility of recurrence, possibility of cardiac events, etc., are explained.

Patients are positioned on an operating room bed in a sitting position at approximately 60–70 degrees of head elevation. Patients are advised to wear light clothing and all heavy jackets and sweaters are removed. The front of the patient is covered with a towel around the neck and a blue pad so as not to soil their clothes. Pulse oximetry is continually monitored prior to, during and after the procedure. The setup is similar to the operating room, in that the surgeon stands on the right side of the patient while the endoscopic tower is positioned on the left side of the patient and directly facing the operating surgeon in an ergonomically favorable position. Two suctions are available where one is connected to the microdebrider and the second one is connected to a yankauer tip which is given to the patient so that all blood, saline, and debris can be easily expectorated per orally by the patient throughout the procedure. A second monitor is positioned across from the patient so that patients who want to watch the procedure can do so. We have noticed that patients who view their procedure often get distracted and handle the procedure much better than those who don't.

The microdebrider is ideally set at 3000 rotations per minute (RPM) and in the XPS mode. We find that the XPS mode allows better control of the debrider blade for the surgeon. Ten minutes prior to the beginning of the procedure, 5 ml of a mixture of 4% topical lidocaine and 0.05% of oxymetazoline is sprayed into both nostrils using a mucosal atomization device (MAD). This allows for topical decongestion and anesthesia for the sinonasal mucosa. Subsequently, one to two 0.05% oxymetazoline/4% lidocaine soaked neuropatties are gently placed into each nostril. The authors avoid the use of injections containing epinephrine as they can lead to reflex tachycardia and increases in blood pressure, which can further lead to increased bleeding and anxiety [6]. At this point, the patient is considered ready to undergo an in-office polypectomy.

In-Office Polypectomy

Under endoscopic guidance using straight and angled endoscopes and powered microdebrider. The authors prefer the HOPKINS® 3.0 mm, 0-degree and 30-degree rigid endoscope (KARL STORZ, Tuttlingen, Germany), and the Straightshot™ M5 microdebrider (Medtronic. Minnesota, USA) with a suction irrigation system.

The polypectomy procedure begins with removal of all polyps along the nasal floor until the choanae can be fully visualized. If possible, starting posteriorly may be beneficial to minimize blood soiling at the tip of the instrument. Progress by removing all polyps surpassing and covering the head of the middle turbinate until the axilla can be clearly visualized. We again recommend working from posteriorly to anteriorly as much as is feasible and working from inferiorly to superiorly. Once this is accomplished, continue to gently remove middle meatal polyps, and if possible, remove any polyps extending out of the maxillary sinus ostium until the sphenoid and maxillary ostia can be visualized. Debulking of polyps can continue superiorly at this point within the ethmoid cavity, taking care to avoid the skull base. This can be done with direct visualization of landmarks or with the use of navigation systems. Debride all polyps medial to the middle turbinate to clear the olfactory cleft as well as remove polyps hanging from the sphenoethmoidal recess.

Once the procedure is completed, patients are cleansed of all blood around their nares, a moustache dressing is placed under the nose to avoid the patient from having to wipe their nose continually while going home. Patients are asked to start lavaging their nose and sinuses with corticosteroid impregnated nasal rinses (2 mL of 0.5 mg/mL budesonide ampoules in 240 mL of saline, 120 ml in each side) twice a day until their first post-procedure follow-up visit at 6 weeks.

Reported Outcomes

There have been multiple publications examining outpatient polypectomy outcomes. A recent publication by Viera-Artiles et al. on 44 patients showed a 64% reduction in SNOT-22 scores with one patient experiencing severe bradycardia and bradypnea [7]. We have reported our published results [8] on a total of 68 patients who received office-based polypectomy, with a mean age of 49 years. There was an equal distribution of males and females (Table 15.1). Fifty-three patients (78%) had previously received FESS. Twenty-one patients (31%) had previously received both FESS and an office-based polypectomy. Office polypectomies were selected for

Table 15.1 Subject characteristics

Subject variables ($n = 68$)	
Age (years)	49 ± 13
Males	34 (50)
CRSwNP	37 (54)
AFRS	31 (46)
Samter's triad	2 (3)
Previous FESS	50 (74)
Previous polypectomy	22 (32)

AFRS allergic fungal rhinosinusitis, *CRSwNP* chronic rhinosinusitis with polyposis, *FESS* functional endoscopic sinus surgery these patients because 53 (78%) had recurrent polyps refractory to medical and/or surgical treatment.

A total of 54 (79%) patients reported prior use of nasal steroid sprays and 25 (37%) reported use of oral steroids. Patients who had not used nasal steroid sprays previously were started on topical budesonide (Pulmicort ampoules; 2 mL of 0.5 mg/mL) administered in the Mygind's position using a Mucosal Atomization Device (MAD; Wolfe Tory Medical, Inc., Salt Lake City, UT) immediately after office polypectomy. These patients had their polypectomies performed during their first clinic consultation to provide immediate relief of nasal obstruction and to allow access of topical nasal steroid into the sinus cavities.

Patients presented with a mean pre-polypectomy grade of 2.2 ± 0.8 on the left and 2.4 ± 0.7 on the right. The resected polyps were non-fibrous in 56 patients (82%) and fibrous in 12 patients (18%). The consistency of the polyps was evaluated by the senior author (ARJ). Resections were completed in a mean of 3 min per side. Resection primarily occurred within the ethmoid sinus (45%) and nasal cavities (36%). There were 6 (9%) polyps resected within the spheno-ethmoid recess and 3 (4%) antrochoanal polyps originating from the maxillary sinus.

Post-procedure, polyps were reduced to a mean grade of 0.7 ± 0.5 on the left nasal cavity and 0.7 ± 0.5 on the right nasal cavity (Fig. 15.1). Paired Student t test

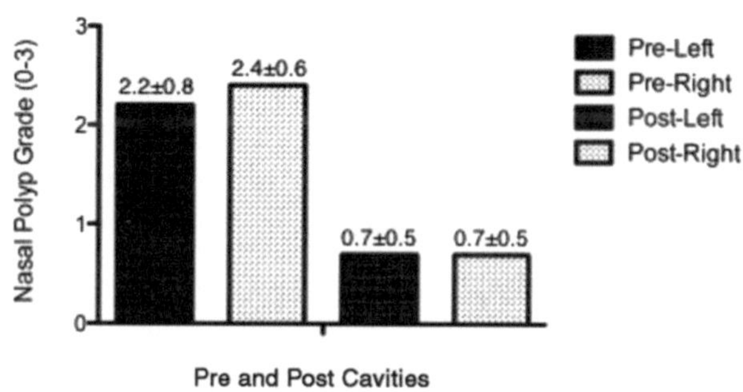

Fig. 15.1 Pre vs. post polypectomy grade of nasal polyps [8]

Table 15.2 Procedural details

Areas performed	Frequency (%)
Nasal	43 (36%)
Ethmoid	53 (45%)
Sphenoid	8 (7%)
Maxillary	9 (8%)
Frontal	6 (4%)
Consistency ($n = 68$)	Frequency (%)
Fibrous	12 (18%)
Non-fibrous	56 (82%)
Time (minutes)	Mean (range)
Left	3.0 (1.6–10.0)
Right	3.0 (2.0–10.0)

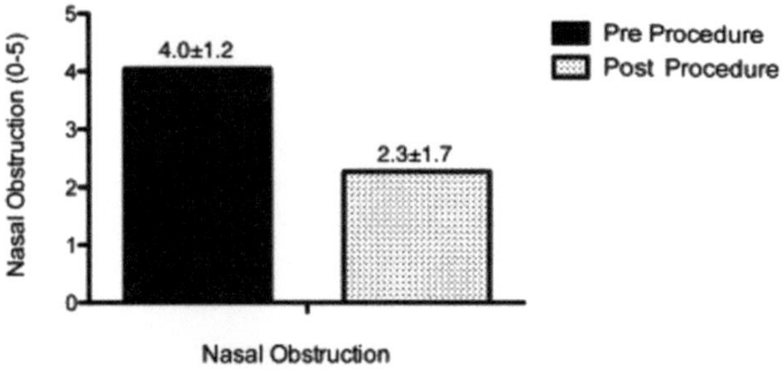

Fig. 15.2 Pre vs. post polypectomy nasal obstruction [8]

comparing nasal polyp score indicated a significant difference between pre-procedure and post-procedure grade for left and right sides, respectively ($p < 0.001$; 95% confidence interval [CI], 1.3–1.6; $p < 0.001$; 95% CI, 1.4–1.8) (Table 15.2, Fig. 15.1). Patients reported reduced nasal obstruction (4.0 ± 1.2 vs 2.3 ± 1.7) when comparing pre-procedure and post-procedure responses (Fig. 15.2).

Tips and Pearls

- It is critical to choose the appropriate patient for an awake procedure. A patient who is extremely anxious may not be a good candidate for an awake procedure.
- Build a strong positive relationship with the patient. Gaining the patients' trust will help immensely in minimizing the anxiety that is sometimes inevitable in such situations.
- Explain each and every step before starting the procedure so that the patient is not surprised by what happens during the procedure. For example, explaining that there may be some amount of blood mixed with saline that might go posteriorly down the throat for which the yankauer suction may be used to suction these contents.
- It is important to inform the patient that topical anesthesia may also numb their throat and give them a sensation of difficulty breathing, but reassurance that that is a normal sensation and that they will be able to breath without difficulty is very important.
- During the polypectomy, it is vital that the surgeon avoid touching normal tissue with the tip of the debrider blade. The septum, inferior and middle turbinate can be exquisitely sensitive and can bleed profusely if mistakenly injured by a functioning debrider blade. It is important to advance the operating tip of the debrider directly toward the polyps while at the same time keeping the blunt, non-window end of the debrider toward normal mucosa.
- Hold your scope as close to the tip of the debrider blade without soiling the tip of the scope to allow accurate localization of where the functional tip is facing. As much as possible avoid holding the scope too far back and showing the long shaft of the blade.
- During, and at the end of the procedure, suction the nasal cavity all the way down to the choana, suction the middle meatus to remove all clots from the maxillary and sphenoid sinuses, and avoid any type of nasal packing.

- At the end of the procedure, it is wise to place an oxymetazoline/lidocaine soaked neuropattie into the middle meatus and in areas where debridement was carried out to control any oozing.

References

1. Desrosiers M, Evans GA, Keith PK, et al. Canadian clinical practice guidelines for acute and chronic rhinosinusitis. J Otolaryngol Head Neck Surg. 2011;40:S99–S193.
2. Chen Y, Dales R, Lin M. The epidemiology of chronic rhinosinusitis in Canadians. Laryngoscope. 2003;113:1199–205.
3. Orlandi RR, Kingdom TT, Smith TL, Bleier B, et al. International consensus statement on allergy and rhinology: rhinosinusitis 2021. Int Forum Allergy Rhinol. 2021;11(3):213–739.
4. Hackman TG, Ferguson BJ. Powered instrumentation and tissue effects in the nose and paranasal sinuses. Curr Opin Otolaryngol Head Neck Surg. 2005;13:22–6.
5. Lee JT, DelGaudio J, Orlandi RR. Practice patterns in office-based rhinology: survey of the American rhinologic society. Am J Rhinol Allergy. 2019;33(1):26–35.
6. Alsaleh S, Manji J, Javer A. Optimization of the surgical field in endoscopic sinus surgery: an evidence-based approach. Curr Allergy Asthma Rep. 2019;19(1):8.
7. Viera-Artiles J, Corriols-Noval P, López-Simón E, González-Aguado R, Lobo D, Megía R. In-office endoscopic nasal polypectomy: prospective analysis of patient tolerability and efficacy. Eur Arch Otorrinolaringol. 2020;277(12):3341–8.
8. Gan EC, Habib A-RR, Hathorn I, Javer AR. The efficacy and safety of an office-based polypectomy with a vacuum-powered microdebrider. Int Forum Allergy Rhinol. 2013;3:890–5.

16 Steroid Eluting-Implants

Firas Sbeih, Jonathan Tyes, and Troy Woodard

Key Points

- The delivery of corticosteroids to the paranasal sinuses is crucial in the management of chronic rhinosinusitis.
- Various implants are available to sinus surgeons both in the operating room and in the clinic.
- The type and location of the implant should be tailored to each individual patient.
- Patient selection is crucial for successful placement and positive outcomes.
- More randomized controlled trials are needed to further define the role of steroid eluting stents in the treatment paradigm of chronic rhinosinusitis.

Background

Chronic rhinosinusitis (CRS) is an inflammatory disease of the paranasal sinus mucosa [1]. CRS can be challenging to manage, especially because endoscopic sinus surgery does not address the underlying pathophysiology [2]. Corticosteroids play a key role in the treatment paradigm and are crucial to successful postoperative

Supplementary Information The online version contains supplementary material available at https://doi.org/10.1007/978-3-031-89191-5_16.

F. Sbeih
Department of Otolaryngology, University of Florida, Jacksonville, FL, USA
e-mail: Firas.Sbeih@jax.ufl.edu

J. Tyes
School of Medicine, University of Louisville, Louisville, KY, USA

T. Woodard (✉)
Head and Neck Institute, Cleveland Clinic Foundation, Cleveland, OH, USA

J. T. Lee et al. (eds.), *Advances in Surgical and Medical Interventions for Recalcitrant Chronic Rhinosinusitis*,
https://doi.org/10.1007/978-3-031-89191-5_16

outcomes. Oral corticosteroids, while beneficial, have undesirable systemic risks and side effects such as weight gain, hyperglycemia, osteoporosis, cataracts, mood changes, suppression of the hypothalamic-pituitary-adrenal axis, and even aseptic necrosis of the joint [3]. Therefore, topical corticosteroid administration to the paranasal sinuses is integral to long-term disease management and successful outcomes. Multiple methods exist for topical corticosteroid administration which vary from corticosteroid nasal drops, corticosteroid nasal sprays, corticosteroid nasal irrigations, nebulization, and steroid eluting stents [4]. Some of these methods can have limitations due to dependence on technique of administration, compliance, and access to therapy [5, 6].

Steroid eluting stents have emerged as an exciting option for patients as they provide controlled local corticosteroid delivery without the need for daily administration of a nasal spray or irrigation. After the safety and efficacy of the PROPEL implant was studied in three clinical trials, it became the first steroid eluting stent to gain FDA approval in 2011 [7–9]. The PROPEL stent has a spring-like shape with a self-expanding design that allows it to sit in the ethmoid cavity after deployment. This bio-absorbable implant releases 370 μg of Mometasone Furoate in a controlled manner over the 30 days during which the implant dissolves [10]. Since 2011, several other steroid eluting implants have gained FDA approval such as the PROPEL family products (Propel mini, Propel contour) as well as SINUVA [11]. Each of these implants has different preferred locations and potential indications that surgeons must be intimately be familiar with prior to use.

Given the various treatment options available to sinus surgeons, an in-depth understanding of steroid eluting stents is necessary to provide adequate counseling and evidence-based recommendations to patients. This chapter will provide a comprehensive review of steroid eluting stents with a focus on indications, outcomes, and safety results. Additionally, surgical techniques will be discussed in various clinical settings to allow the surgeon to be equipped for placement in the operating room and in the clinic.

Indications

The use of steroid eluting stents has been described in multiple clinical scenarios. One common scenario is stent placement intraoperatively or within a few days after surgery to administer steroids in the immediate postoperative period. In the immediate postoperative setting, steroid eluting stents also function as a stent to separate the healing tissue and prevent the formation of scarring/synechiae. The implant also helps ensure that the middle turbinate stays medialized. Finally, the sustained local delivery of steroids to the paranasal sinuses allows for better control of the mucosal inflammatory response leading to improved healing results [12]. The PROPEL (ethmoid), PROPEL mini (frontal sinus), and PROPEL contour (frontal sinus) are typically used in this context (Fig. 16.1] Videos 16.1 and 16.2 illustrate placement of the steroid-eluting implants in the ethmoid and frontal sinuses, respectively, immediatley after endoscopic sinus surgery.

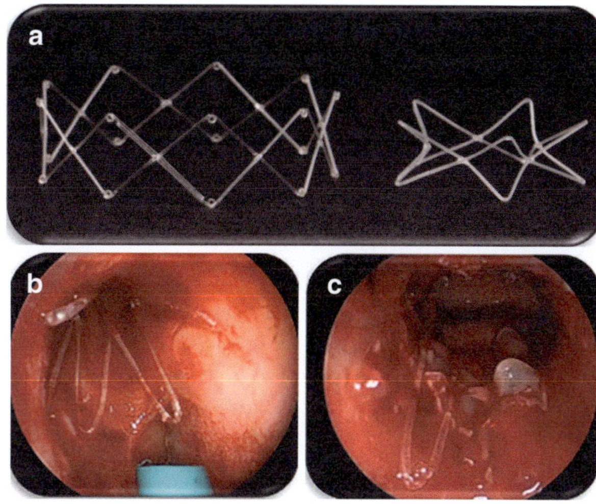

Fig. 16.1 (**a**) Photo of steroid-eluting implants: PROPEL and CONTOUR. (**b**) Endoscopic image of the hourglass shaped steroid-eluting implant (CONTOUR) placed in the frontal sinus. (**c**) Endoscopic inage of the cylindrical shaped steroid-eluting implant (PROPEL MINI) placed in the frontal sinus. Images reprinted with permission from Medtronic ENT

Another common clinical scenario relates to patients with chronic rhinosinusitis with nasal polyposis who have undergone prior surgery. The SINUVA implant, which releases 1350 μg of mometasone over the course of 90 days, is used for patients with a history of previous endoscopic sinus surgery who develop recurrent ethmoid polyps. The recurrence of polyps after endoscopic sinus surgery can be frustrating to the patient and the surgeon. The return of nasal polyposis could be related to a myriad of reasons including sub-optimal delivery of corticosteroids to the diseased mucosa, anatomic reasons such as middle turbinate lateralization, sinus ostium narrowing, crusting, or synechiae [13]. Other reasons for treatment failure could be related to the technique of topical therapy administration, and in some cases patient's compliance with the treatment regimen [5]. For this patient population, a steroid eluting implant could be a great option especially since it can be placed in clinic bypassing the need for general anesthesia [14].

In Video 16.3, the patient presented to the senior author with a history of asthma-exacerbated respiratory disease with two prior functional endoscopic sinus surgeries and was non-compliant with corticosteroid rinses. The patient had significant nasal congestion, discolored drainage, and hyposmia. A SINUVA implant was placed into the ethmoid sinus cavities bilaterally aiming to place it posteriorly and superiorly. At the 3 month endoscopy, there was a significant reduction in the polyps in both ethmoid cavities and the ostiomeatal complex appears open bilaterally. Lavigne et al. demonstrated the safety and efficacy of the SINUVA implant in a prospective multicenter study of 12 patients. At the 6 month evaluation, 64% of the patients in the study were no longer candidates for revision surgery [14].

For patients who have never undergone endoscopic sinus surgery, there is a steroid eluting implant option that could be placed in the middle meatus known as the LYR-210. The LYR-210 implant remains an investigational product. At the time of the drafting of this chapter, this device has not yet been FDA approved but has undergone phase 1, phase 2, and phase 3 clinical trials [15, 16]. The LYR-210 implant is a biocompatible mesh that conforms and adapts to the shape of the middle meatus providing a steady daily dosing of Mometasone Furoate for up to 24 weeks (total of 7500 μg of mometasone) [17]. In Video 16.4, the senior author demonstrates in-office placement of the LYR-210 implant into the left middle meatus.

Surgical Technique

A prerequisite to successful placement of a steroid eluting stent is mastery of endoscopic sinonasal anatomy and surgical techniques. For stents that are placed intraoperatively, the key is to ensure completion of the ethmoidectomy and/or frontal sinusotomy. Placing the implant in the frontal recess is more technically challenging than the ethmoid cavity. An angled scope is needed to visualize the frontal cavity and place the stent. The senior author recommends that the guide catheter be aimed at the frontal sinus opening. The implant is then deployed slightly through the frontal os while the guide catheter is being withdrawn simultaneously. The final result is a spring-like implant stenting the frontal sinus opening with the outer limbs contacting the lamina and middle turbinate. Intraoperative placement into the ethmoid cavity is more straightforward. A zero degree endoscope can be used. The surgeon should aim to place the implant more posteriorly and superiorly into the ethmoid cavity so that when the implant is deployed, the implant sits in a position that stents the middle turbinate medially and does not impede the maxillary antrostomy opening.

In-office endoscopic nasal procedures can be more technically challenging which makes the preparation for the procedure crucial. Patient counseling on what to expect with a procedure is essential to help ease nerves and build expectations. Patient selection is important as not all patients would be tolerant of in-office procedures due to lower pain thresholds or anxiety. Patients who struggle with routine nasal endoscopy during office visits would not be good candidates. Additionally, some patients with certain anatomical variants might not be candidates for in-office procedures. Severe nasal polyps, a deviated nasal septum, or synechiae may make it very challenging to get the implant into the middle meatus.

Excellent topical anesthesia and decongestion are necessary for successful implant placement. To accomplish this, we recommend 0.05% Afrin mixed with 4% lidocaine pledgets that are placed along the nasal floor and into the middle meatus. These are left in place for at least 5 min and by that time the patient should start to report palatal numbness at which time the pledgets can be removed. Injection of an anesthetic is not necessary in our experience. After removal of the pledgets, the surgeon should perform a quick nasal endoscopy to assess if in-office placement is feasible and ensure adequacy of numbing. If there is good access to the middle meatus, then depending on the type of implant being placed, the surgeon should consider whether an angled scope is needed. In our experience, a 30 degree rigid endoscope is favored as it provides better visualization of the middle meatus and better understanding of the surrounding anatomy. In Video 16.3, the senior author demonstrates the positioning of the SINUVA implant into the middle meatus of a patient with recurrent nasal polyposis. Video 16.4 demonstrates the technique for placement of the LYR-210 implant into a patient who has never undergone prior endoscopic sinus surgery.

Reported Outcomes

As mentioned earlier in the chapter, the PROPEL implant was the first steroid eluting stent to gain FDA approval in 2011. The approval came after the device was studied in three clinical trials, two of which were randomized controlled double blinded studies [7–9]. In all three studies, patients were not permitted to have oral or topical corticosteroid therapy in the first 30 days. The two randomized controlled trials utilized intra-patient controls. In the pilot study which was carried out at 4 clinical sites, 38 patients who served as their own controls had the PROPEL implant or a non-drug-eluting implant placed into the ethmoid sinuses [7]. Five patients in the pilot study received the PROPEL implant bilaterally to evaluate for systemic steroid absorption. In those five patients, there was no suppression of the hypothalamic-pituitary-adrenal axis and the levels of Mometasone Furoate were undetectable in the bloodstream. The pilot study was then followed by two clinical trials, the ADVANCE trial and the ADVANCE II trial, both of which were multicenter clinical trials [8, 9].

The ADVANCE trial took place in 2009 with fifty patients enrolled at seven tertiary centers between the period of March 2009 and June 2009 [8]. Patients were all candidates for either primary FESS or a revision FESS and deemed candidates for the PROPEL implant in the ethmoid cavity at the conclusion of surgery. Of the 50 patients enrolled, 40 received the PROPEL stent bilaterally while 10 received it unilaterally. The trial had excellent follow-up rates with 100% follow-up rate at the 30 day mark, 98% follow-up at day 60, and 90% follow-up at the 6-month mark. At day 30, 85% of the placed stents were dissolved and at day 60 only 0.2% were remaining [8]. Additionally the study confirmed the safety of the implant with no ocular complications noted. Objective and subjective efficacy metrics were also employed in the study. At day 30, only one sinus had evidence of adhesions corresponding to 1.1% rate compared to 5.3% in the pilot study by Murr, et al. [7, 8]. In the ADVANCE trial, lateralization of the middle turbinate only occurred in 4.4% of patients (4 of 90 sinuses).

The ADVANCE II clinical trial was a prospective, randomized, double blinded, multi-center trial which included 105 patients enrolled between December 2009 and July 2010 [9]. Intra-patient controls were used in this study. Efficacy was assessed by having three blinded sinus surgeons review post-operative endoscopy videos. There was significant reduction in nasal polyposis in the treatment group compared to the control group (18.8% vs 34.1%, $P = 0.002$). The treatment group also had a relative reduction of 29% in the need for post-operative interventions at day 30. Safety assessments were also performed and there were no changes from baseline in intraocular pressure measurements or lens opacities consistent with the prior trials studying the PROPEL implant.

In 2012, Han et al. performed a meta-analysis of the two randomized controlled trials (Pilot study and ADVANCE II) producing level 1A evidence of the safety and efficacy of the PROPEL implant [18]. This pooled results from 143 patients that were enrolled who served as intra-patient controls. The results of the meta-analysis showed that the study group had a statistically significant relative reduction in postoperative interventions by 35% ($P = 0.0008$), nasal polyps by 46% ($P < 0.0001$), and need for oral steroids by 40% ($P = 0.0023$). Additionally, compared to the control group, the treatment group had a 75% relative reduction in middle turbinate lateralization ($P = 0.0225$) and 70% relative reduction in significant adhesions ($P = 0.0013$).

The SINUVA implant was first studied in a prospective, multicenter, nonrandomized clinical trial involving 12 enrolled patients who had the implant placed in a clinic setting [14]. All recruited patients had a history of chronic rhinosinusitis with prior FESS and were refractory to medical therapy. Of the 12 patients (24 sinuses), successful placement was completed in 21 of the 24 sinuses. One patient had improper positioning of the implant bilaterally and hence it was eventually removed. The other patient had severe septal deviation so only one side could be implanted. The mean SNOT-22 score was significantly improved after treatment from 2.19 at baseline to 0.90 at the 1 month follow-up ($P = 0.001$), and the improvement was sustained at the 6-month follow-up with the mean SNOT-22 score being 1.03 ($P = 0.0012$). At the 6-month follow-up, it was determined that 64% of the patients were no longer candidates for revision FESS [14].

In contrast, the LYR-210 implant is a potential treatment option for patients with chronic rhinosinusitis refractory to medical therapy with no history of prior sinus surgery. In a Phase I clinical trial, 20 patients were enrolled to primarily assess the safety of the implant [15]. There were 16 adverse events reported during the duration of the study, but only one adverse event was considered serious. The serious adverse event was related to a patient experiencing angina pectoris which was deemed an exacerbation of a pre-existing condition. The other 15 adverse events were all considered mild to moderate in nature and those included facial pain, sinusitis, procedural headache, nasal discomfort, and nasal odor. However, there were no local nasal adverse events such as ulceration, septal perforation, mucosal erosion, nasal dryness, nasal irritation, or epistaxis. Additionally, there was no effect on intraocular pressures or serum cortisol levels in any of the patients. The LYR-210 implant also demonstrated efficacy based on results of the SNOT-22 questionnaire at various intervals during the study. At the 24-week mark, and the 25-week mark (1 week post-removal of the implant), 70% of the patients had >8.9 points improvement in their SNOT-22 scores [15].

The LYR-210 implant was further evaluated in a multi-center, randomized, blinded, controlled phase 2 clinical trial involving 67 patients known as the LANTERN trial [16]. The study was intended to include more patients but recruitment was halted due to the COVID-19 pandemic. Patients were randomized into three treatment arms: (1) 2500 μg of Mometasone Furoate; (2) 7500 μg of

Mometasone Furoate; and (3) control arm. Similar to the phase 1 trial, there was only a single serious adverse event [15, 16]. This was related to a patient who experienced acarodermatitis which was determined to be unrelated to the LYR-210 implant. Other adverse reactions included headache, congestion, facial pain, rhinitis, rhinorrhea, epistaxis, and oropharyngeal pain. Intraocular pressures were also checked and none of the patients in the study developed increased intraocular pressures. Serum cortisol levels were checked and there were no significant changes at weeks 4, 12, or 24.

The LANTERN trial also demonstrated the efficacy of the LYR-210 implant, especially the 7500 μg of Mometasone Furoate (MF). Compared to the control arm, the LYR-2107500 μg MF cohort had statistically significant reductions in the cardinal symptoms of chronic rhinosinusitis as well as in SNOT-22 scores. This improvement persisted at the 24-week follow-up. All patients who received the LYR-2107500 μg MF implant reached the minimum clinically important difference (MCID) in improvement in their SNOT-22 scores at the 24-week follow-up. While the LYR-210 implant has had promising results, further studies are needed to validate its role in the chronic rhinosinusitis treatment paradigm. Phase III trials (ENLIGHTEN 1 and 2) are ongoing [19, 20].

Tips and Pearls

- Patient selection is a key factor in the success of in-office procedures. Patients who tolerate endoscopy and other in-office procedures are good candidates.
- Topical decongestant and anesthesia is fundamental to the success of implant placement.
- 0.05% Afrin mixed with 4% tetracaine pledgets are placed along the nasal floor and into the middle meatus. Injection is typically not necessary.
- A 30 degree rigid endoscope provides better visualization into the middle meatus.

References

1. Hulse KE, Stevens WW, Tan BK, Schleimer RP. Pathogenesis of nasal polyposis. Clin Exp Allergy. 2015;45(2):328–46.
2. Leung RM, Kern RC, Conley DB, Tan BK, Chandra RK. Osteomeatal complex obstruction is not associated with adjacent sinus disease in chronic rhinosinusitis with polyps. Am J Rhinol Allergy. 2011;25(6):401–3.
3. Strehl C, Buttgereit F. Langzeittherapie mit Glukokortikoiden: Gibt es eine sichere Dosierung? Internist. 2016;57(9):934–9.
4. Tai J, Lee K, Kim TH. Current perspective on nasal delivery systems for chronic rhinosinusitis. Pharmaceutics. MDPI AG. 2021;13:1–21.
5. Nabi S, Rotenberg BW, Vukin I, Payton K, Bureau Y. Nasal spray adherence after sinus surgery: problems and predictors. J Otolaryngol Head Neck Surg. 2012;41(SUPPL. 1)
6. Beule A, Athanasiadis T, Athanasiadis E, Field J, Wormald PJ. Efficacy of different techniques of sinonasal irrigation after modified Lothrop procedure. Am J Rhinol Allergy. 2009;23(1):85–90.

7. Murr AH, Smith TL, Hwang PH, Bhattacharyya N, Lanier BJ, Stambaugh JW, et al. Safety and efficacy of a novel bioabsorbable, steroid-eluting sinus stent. Int Forum Allergy Rhinol. 2011;1(1):23–32.
8. Forwith KD, Chandra RK, Yun PT, Miller SK, Jampel HD. ADVANCE: a multisite trial of bioabsorbable steroid-eluting sinus implants. Laryngoscope. 2011;121(11):2473–80.
9. Marple BF, Smith TL, Han JK, Gould AR, Jampel HD, Stambaugh JW, et al. Advance II: a prospective, randomized study assessing safety and efficacy of bioabsorbable steroid-releasing sinus implants. Otolaryngol Head Neck Surg (United States). 2012;146(6):1004–11.
10. Kennedy DW. The PROPEL™ steroid-releasing bioabsorbable implant to improve outcomes of sinus surgery. Expert Rev Respir Med. 2012;6:493–8.
11. Han JK, Kern RC. Topical therapies for management of chronic rhinosinusitis: steroid implants. Int Forum Allergy Rhinol. 2019;9:S22–S6. John Wiley and Sons Inc.
12. Campbell RG, Kennedy DW. What is new and promising with drug-eluting stents in sinus surgery. Curr Opin Otolaryngol Head Neck Surg. 2014;22:2–7.
13. Ramadan HH. Surgical causes of failure in endoscopic sinus surgery. Laryngoscope. 1999;109(1):27–9.
14. Lavigne F, Miller SK, Gould AR, Lanier BJ, Romett JL. Steroid-eluting sinus implant for in-office treatment of recurrent nasal polyposis: a prospective, multicenter study. Int Forum Allergy Rhinol. 2014;4(5):381–9.
15. Douglas RG, Psaltis AJ, Rimmer J, Kuruvilla T, Cervin A, Kuang Y. Phase 1 clinical study to assess the safety of a novel drug delivery system providing long-term topical steroid therapy for chronic rhinosinusitis. Int Forum Allergy Rhinol. 2019;9(4):378–87.
16. Cervin A, Rimmer J, Wrobel A, Abelak Y, Brayton L, Kuang Y. Long-acting implantable corticosteroid matrix for chronic rhinosinusitis: results of LANTERN phase 2 randomized controlled study. Int Forum Allergy Rhinol. 2022;12(2):147–59.
17. Sharma U, Concagh D, Core L, Kuang Y, You C, Pham Q, et al. The development of bioresorbable composite polymeric implants with high mechanical strength. Nat Mater. 2018;17(1):96–102.
18. Han JK, Marple BF, Smith TL, Murr AH, Lanier BJ, Stambaugh JW, et al. Effect of steroid-releasing sinus implants on postoperative medical and surgical interventions: an efficacy meta-analysis. Int Forum Allergy Rhinol. 2012;2(4):271–9.
19. Hopkins C, Browne JP, Slack R, Lund V, Brown P. The Lund-Mackay staging system for chronic rhinosinusitis: how is it used and what does it predict? Otolaryngol Head Neck Surg. 2007;137(4):555–61.
20. Kennedy JL, Hubbard MA, Huyett P, Patrie JT, Borish L, Payne SC. Sino-nasal outcome test (SNOT-22): a predictor of postsurgical improvement in patients with chronic sinusitis. Ann Allergy Asthma Immunol. 2013;111(4):246–51.e2

Cryoablation and Radiofrequency Ablation of Posterior Nasal Nerve

17

Neil N. Patel and Patricia A. Loftus

Key Points

- In patients with chronic rhinitis, cryoablation and radiofrequency ablation of the posterior nasal nerve (PNN) have been shown to be safe and effective in decreasing symptoms of rhinitis, particularly rhinorrhea.
- The PNN can be accessed by hand-held devices that use thermal energy to disrupt nerve fibers in the posterior aspect of the middle meatus.
- These new techniques have supplanted the need for more invasive procedures such as vidian neurectomy and can be performed in an office setting.
- Given the relative novelty of cryoablation and radiofrequency ablation of the PNN, long-term studies on the durability of these therapies on the order of years are lacking; however, symptom improvement has been measured to last 12–24 months.

Background

Chronic rhinitis is a common condition affecting roughly 60 million Americans [1, 2]. It can be classified as allergic or non-allergic based on IgE testing, yet both types present with four cardinal symptoms: nasal congestion, rhinorrhea/postnasal drip, nasal pruritus, and sneezing [1]. Chronic rhinitis has been shown to negatively impact job performance, quality of life, and overall psychosocial wellbeing [3].

Supplementary Information The online version contains supplementary material available at https://doi.org/10.1007/978-3-031-89191-5_17.

N. N. Patel · P. A. Loftus (✉)
Department of Otolaryngology—Head and Neck Surgery, University of California San Francisco, San Francisco, CA, USA
e-mail: Neil.Patel3@ucsf.edu; Patricia.Loftus@ucsf.edu

J. T. Lee et al. (eds.), *Advances in Surgical and Medical Interventions for Recalcitrant Chronic Rhinosinusitis*,
https://doi.org/10.1007/978-3-031-89191-5_17

While medical management in the form of intranasal saline, intranasal corticosteroids, oral/topical antihistamines, and/or oral/topical decongestant is the first-line therapy, not all patients respond well to medical therapy alone. In these recalcitrant cases or in cases where patients cannot comply with medical therapy, procedural interventions can be considered. For nasal congestion, inferior turbinate reduction is an option For patients mostly suffering from rhinorrhea or postnasal drainage, interventions targeting the parasympathetic system in the nasal cavity may be helpful.

Reducing parasympathetic innervation in the nasal cavity results in reduced blood flow to the submucosa, improved stromal edema, and decreased submucosal gland secretion [4, 5]. Historically, surgical neurolysis, namely vidian neurectomy, was the intervention of choice to decrease the parasympathetic tone of the nasal cavity. However, due to the high rate of dry eye [4], more recent approaches have focused on distal branches of the nasal parasympathetic system, called the posterior nasal nerves (PNN), which can be accessed and lysed through the middle meatus in a procedure called a posterior nasal neurectomy [6–8]. Although the risk of dry eye is removed, this procedure still requires general anesthesia.

Advances in cryoablation and radiofrequency ablation have led to new technologies that offer minimally invasive PNN-targeted intervention while awake under local anesthesia. Therefore, these methods have ushered in a new wave of office-based procedures for patients with recalcitrant chronic rhinitis.

Anatomy and Physiology

The value of targeting the PNN with minimally invasive techniques is best appreciated by reviewing the anatomy of the nasal autonomic system. The greater superficial petrosal nerve (GSPN), a branch of the facial nerve, carries preganglionic parasympathetic nerve fibers and the deep petrosal nerve carries sympathetic nerve fibers. The vidian nerve is formed by the joining of the GSPN and the deep petrosal nerve. The parasympathetic fibers contained within the vidian nerve synapse at the pterygopalatine ganglion (PPG) and then disperse throughout the nasal cavity, hard palate, and the lacrimal gland. The parasympathetic activation of these nerves is responsible for vasodilation and secretomotor release of mucus.

In effect, vidian neurectomy leads to secretomotor denervation of nasal submucosal glands; however, it also leads to denervation of the ipsilateral lacrimal glands. Therefore, vidian neurectomy is associated with significant morbidity, resulting in loss of lacrimation in 30% to 50% of patients [4, 9]. In some circumstances, decrease in tear production can be so severe that it can lead to permanent vision loss [9]. Vidian neurectomy also causes decrease in sympathetic function, which in some patients can cause counterproductive rhinorrhea [10]. Furthermore, it is an invasive procedure that requires general anesthesia. For these reasons, vidian neurectomy never gained wide acceptance and other options for treating chronic rhinorrhea were continuously sought out.

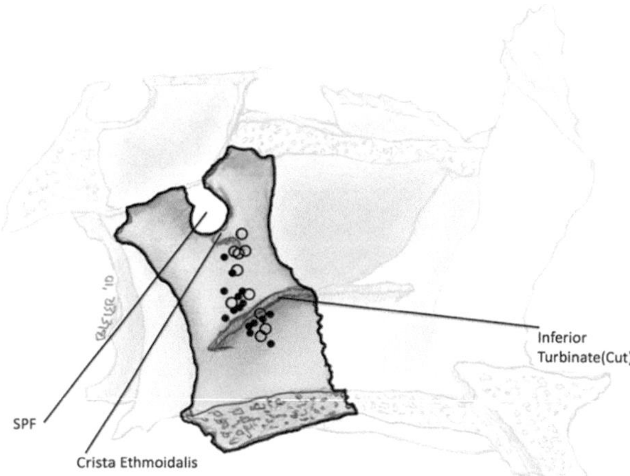

Fig. 17.1 Re-printed from Bleier et al. [11] The authors demonstrate an illustration of posterior nasal nerve fibers based on endoscopic dissection of cadaver heads. Shown are nerve fibers emanating from the palatine bone in the posterolateral region of the middle meatus. Closed dots demonstrate nerve fibers directly traversing the bone and open dots are distinct foramina in a representative patient observed by the study authors

Over the past decade, microanatomical and endoscopic assessments of the pterygopalatine fossa have elucidated the course of the postganglionic nerves. This allowed for targeted ablation of the postganglionic parasympathetic nerve fibers. After synapsing at the PPG, the parasympathetic branches take an anterior and posterior course to enter the nasal cavity. The posterior nerve fibers exit just inferior to the sphenopalatine foramen, in the posterior middle meatus (Fig. 17.1) [11]. This led to the idea of therapeutic surgical sectioning of these fibers, which were named the posterior nasal nerves (PNN) [6]. One option was direct identification and lysis of these nerves via an endoscopic posterior nasal neurectomy [6], but this is still a considerably invasive procedure that requires general anesthesia [7, 12]. Given the relative accessibility of the PNN in the middle meatus, devices capable of ablating the nerves in the office setting are now the most common procedural intervention to treat medically refractory rhinorrhea.

Principles of PNN Ablation

Cryotherapy and radiofrequency ablation devices use temperature changes, both cold and hot respectively, to disrupt the PNN. Selective reduction in the parasympathetic innervation reduces the secretory function of the end-organ submucosal glands and reduces vascular permeability in response to antigenic challenge. Various handheld devices are available on the market, and manufacturer instructions are provided by each supplier.

Cryotherapy

Cryoablation in the nose was first described in the 1970s [13, 14], but its applicability to chronic rhinitis was limited due to lack of endoscopic visualization and ergonomically infeasible delivery of cryogen [14]. Cryotherapy works by ablating soft tissue, including underlying nerves, with a predictable depth of penetration. Because the arterial blood supply is only minimally impacted, risk of tissue necrosis is reduced. Nitrous oxide serves as the most commonly used cryogen and is stored in a cartridge that loads into a disposable handheld device (Fig. 17.2). When triggered, the cryogen inflates a closed-end probe which is laid against the target mucosa. Heat from surrounding tissue is pulled into the probe causing transient tissue freezing. A variable temperature distribution exists in the frozen and unfrozen regions, with the lowest temperatures experienced at the cold application site. The probe's surface temperature reaches −80 to −60 °C. This affords a transient therapeutic temperature of −20 °C at a depth of 3 mm, which induces axonal damage while preserving the overlying mucosa viability. Freezing continues until heat provided by the body is in equilibrium to the heat extracted by the probe. The treatment is delivered at one or two non-overlapping positions in the PNN region.

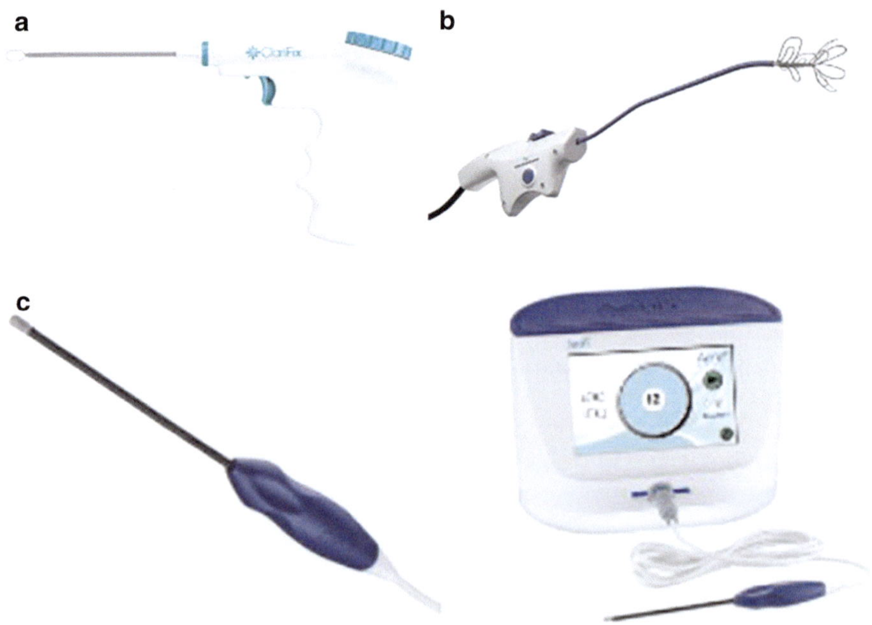

Fig. 17.2 Examples of hand-held devices currently available on the market. (**a**) ClariFix® (Stryker; ENT, Plymouth MN) which is a cryoablative technology. (**b**) NEUROMARK™ System (Neurent Medical; Oranmore, Galaway, Ireland), (**c**) RhinAer System® (Aerin Medical Inc.; Sunnyvale, CA) which are radiofrequency technologies

Radiofrequency Ablation

Radiofrequency energy-based devices are used in the nasal cavity as well as other regions of the head and neck, such as the palatine/lingual tonsils [15, 16]. Radiofrequency ablation technology targeting the PNN region has the differentiating feature of temperature modulation. A sensor at the tip of the instrument modulates the radiofrequency intensity to keep the therapeutic temperature generated at approximately 60 °C in order to minimize adjacent tissue damage, including the overlying mucosa. The energy for the device is generated by a console and is transmitted to a hand-held, disposable stylus (Fig. 17.2). The end of the stylus is placed against the target tissue at the PNN (Fig. 17.3), which then delivers temperature-controlled, bipolar, radiofrequency energy to the PNN region. The treatment is delivered at one to three non-overlapping positions in the PNN region.

In both ablative methods, the key treatment is second-degree nerve damage that results in loss of axon continuity, but preserves surrounding tissue. This means that the nearby sphenopalatine artery, connective tissue, and overlying mucosa are left intact. Despite this, procedure site disruption of mucociliary clearance leads to transient inflammation and, at times, symptoms of nasal obstruction and/or nasal dryness that clear 2–6 weeks after the procedure.

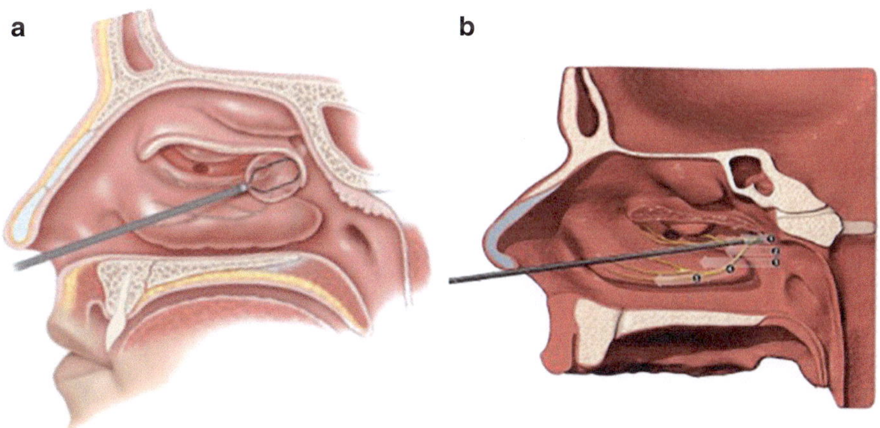

Fig. 17.3 Demonstration of (**a**) cryotherapy probe placement (ClariFix device) and (**b**) radiofrequency ablation stylus placement (RhinAer System)

Table 17.1 Indications and contraindications for posterior nasal nerve ablation

Indications	Contraindications
• Chronic rhinitis (allergic, non-allergic, or mixed) for >3 months • Dissatisfaction with medical management • Age > 18 years • Response to anti-cholinergic drugs	• Anatomical obstruction (septal deviation, polyps, tumor) • Severe epistaxis within the past 3 months • Rhinitis medicamentosa • Prior radiation that included the treatment area • Intolerance to anesthetic agents • Open intranasal wounds • Impaired mucosal wound healing (e.g., small vessel vasculitis)

Indications for PNN Ablation

Cryoablation and radiofrequency ablation are considered in patients with chronic rhinitis who have either failed medical management or are unable to comply with medical therapy. Because topical nasal regimens require long-term usage and often twice daily application, a significant cohort of patients fail medical therapy due to medication adherence alone. Indications for this intervention include adult patients who have medically refractory perennial rhinitis, moderate to severe chronic runny nose and/or nasal congestion, non-allergic chronic rhinitis, mixed allergic and non-allergic chronic rhinitis, and patients who demonstrate a response to anti-cholinergic drugs (Table 17.1).

Contraindications are primarily anatomical, as access to the sphenopalatine area is vital for correct treatment administration. Furthermore, given that the procedure is mostly performed in the office setting, tolerance of adequate topical analgesia and decongestion is necessary. Patients who are poor candidates for this intervention include those with anatomical obstruction (i.e., septal deviation), severe epistaxis, rhinitis medicamentosa, prior radiation, open nasal wounds, and intolerance to anesthetic/ decongesting agents (Table 17.1). In patients undergoing cryotherapy specifically, prior studies have excluded patients who have cold-temperature induced systemic disease, such as cryoglobulinemia, paroxysmal cold hemoglobinuria, cold urticaria, and Raynaud's disease [1].

Surgical Technique

This procedure is intended for clinic-based delivery with the use of local anesthesia, but can be performed under anesthesia as an adjunct procedure or sole procedure in select patient populations. Patients are seated in an upright position in a clinic chair with their head positioned on the headrest. The procedure is performed under endoscopic guidance using a 0-degree rigid scope, camera tower, and one of the devices available on the market which enable minimally invasive PNN ablation with cryotherapy or radiofrequency ablation (Fig. 17.2).

To begin, topical anesthesia, such as 4% lidocaine, and nasal decongestion, such as neo-synephrine or oxymetazoline, are applied topically to the middle meatus and anterior nasal cavity bilaterally with pledgets. Additional local anesthetic, such as 1% lidocaine with 1:100,000 epinephrine, is injected into the basal lamella, axilla of the middle turbinate, and/or the area of the sphenopalatine foramen. If cryotherapy is being used, pre-medication with gabapentin one hour prior to the start of the procedure has been shown to reduce acute headaches associated with this therapy [17].

The probe is introduced into the nasal cavity and guided to the target area (Fig. 17.3). The PNN is located in the posterior middle meatus, where the middle turbinate attaches to the lateral nasal wall. The treatment is delivered according to the device manufacturer protocol. With both types of ablation, multiple areas of the lateral nasal wall/sphenopalatine area may be targeted. An example video demonstrating in-office cryotherapy is included (Video 17.1) as well as a video depicting radiofrequency ablation of the PNN and posterior portion of the inferior turbinate (Video 17.2).

Reported Outcomes

Both cryotherapy [18] and radiofrequency ablation [19, 20] have been studied in patient-blinded, multicenter randomized controlled trials (RCTs) and have demonstrated clinical benefit. Due to minimal morbidity, a unique feature of cryoablation and radiofrequency ablative techniques is the ability to perform sham-controlled trials. In these patient-blinded, sham-controlled RCTs, both cryotherapy and radiofrequency ablation demonstrated improvement in chronic rhinitis symptoms as assessed by relative Total Nasal Symptom Score (rTNSS). In both RCTs, results were reported as percent of responders, defined as greater than or equal to 30% reduction of rTNSS from baseline at 3 months (Fig. 17.4). Using cryotherapy,

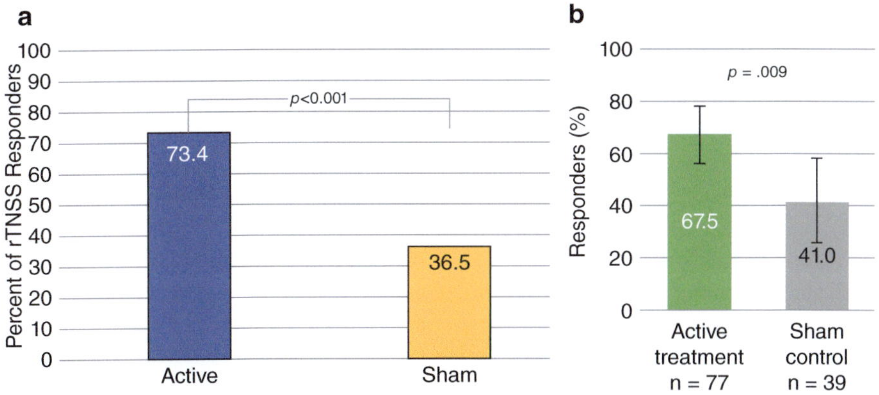

Fig. 17.4 Results of two sham-controlled, randomized controlled trials. Both trials defined greater than or equal to 30% reduction in rTNSS from baseline as the primary outcome measure, and both studies followed patients for 3 months. (**a**) Cryotherapy treatment (N = 64 treatment, N = 63 sham) [18] (**b**) Radiofrequency ablation (N = 77 treatment, N = 39 sham) [20]

73.4% versus 36.5% were identified as responders in the treatment versus sham groups, respectively ($p < 0.001$) [18]. Similarly, in a separate RCT, radiotherapy demonstrated 67.5% versus 41% responders in the treatment versus sham group, respectively ($p = 0.009$). For both technologies, other validated quality of life surveys have been reported as secondary outcomes and also demonstrated statistically significant improvement with treatment [21–23]. Of note, no study to date has performed a head-to-head comparison of these two technologies to determine superior therapeutic effect.

Both technologies enrolled similar patient populations in their studies, primarily utilizing rTNSS to identify those with long-standing rhinitis symptoms. Radiofrequency ablation trials additionally included patients with complaints of post-nasal drip and chronic cough, which are not included in the rTNSS. The RCTs of radiofrequency ablation determined that these two symptoms decreased after treatment [24]. Given that peripheral nerves have the ability to regrow, there is the concern that non-invasive PNN ablation may only provide transient relief. Thus far, studies in both cryoablation [25] and radiofrequency [24] PNN neurolysis have demonstrated a lasting response for up to 1–3 years [26].

In terms of adverse events, both technologies are well tolerated. The most commonly reported adverse events in a 2018 systematic review of PNN cryotherapy included epistaxis, nasal obstruction, nasal crusting, and ear blockage, none of which were reported as serious [27]. At the time of cryoablation, some patients complain of acute headache and/or tooth pain, akin to the colloquial "brain freeze" or "ice-cream headache," which can be alleviated with administration of gabapentin prior to cryotherapy [17]. In studies of radiofrequency ablation, adverse events were similarly mild, and include transient mild-to-moderate oropharyngeal pain, nasal soreness, epistaxis, and tooth pain [28]. Overall, there were no severe adverse events in the reported literature for either technology class.

Tips and Pearls

- For prevention of cryotherapy induced headache, premedicate with 600 mg of gabapentin at least 1 h in advance of the procedure and warn patients of possible transient "ice cream headache."
- Ensure complete release of cryotherapy from surrounding tissues prior to removal, and remove the probe slowly. Nasal breathing after administration may aid in release of the probe tip through warming.
- Avoid excess gel at the stylus tip for the radiofrequency ablation as this can impede visualization.
- Warn patients that radiofrequency ablation can result in transient burning smell during treatment.
- For both, ensure the nasal cavity is appropriately anesthetized prior to device introduction and insert the probe facing laterally so as to avoid trauma to nearby structures.
- Stop advancing the device when it reaches the basal lamella, an area which can provide immediate haptic feedback of target location.

- Warn patients that symptoms or rhinorrhea may worsen transiently during recovery prior to improvement.

References

1. Bernstein JA. Allergic and mixed rhinitis: epidemiology and natural history. Allergy Asthma Proc. 2010;31:365–9. https://doi.org/10.2500/aap.2010.31.3380.
2. Settipane RA, Charnock DR. Epidemiology of rhinitis: allergic and nonallergic. Clin Allergy Immunol. 2007;19:23–34.
3. Vandenplas O, et al. Impact of rhinitis on work productivity: a systematic review. J Allergy Clin Immunol Pract. 2018;6:1274–86. e1279. https://doi.org/10.1016/j.jaip.2017.09.002.
4. Robinson SR, Wormald PJ. Endoscopic vidian neurectomy. Am J Rhinol. 2006;20:197–202.
5. Konno A. Historical, pathophysiological, and therapeutic aspects of vidian neurectomy. Curr Allergy Asthma Rep. 2010;10:105–12. https://doi.org/10.1007/s11882-010-0093-3.
6. Ikeda K, et al. Effect of resection of the posterior nasal nerve on functional and morphological changes in the inferior turbinate mucosa. Acta Otolaryngol. 2008;128:1337–41. https://doi.org/10.1080/00016480801935525.
7. Ogawa T, Takeno S, Ishino T, Hirakawa K. Submucous turbinectomy combined with posterior nasal neurectomy in the management of severe allergic rhinitis: clinical outcomes and local cytokine changes. Auris Nasus Larynx. 2007;34:319–26. https://doi.org/10.1016/j.anl.2007.01.008.
8. Takahara D, Takeno S, Hamamoto T, Ishino T, Hirakawa K. Management of Intractable nasal hyperreactivity by selective resection of posterior nasal nerve branches. Int J Otolaryngol. 2017;2017:1907862. https://doi.org/10.1155/2017/1907862.
9. Lin PY, et al. Bilateral neurotrophic keratopathy complicating Vidian neurectomy. Am J Ophthalmol. 2001;132:106–8. https://doi.org/10.1016/s0002-9394(00)00958-2.
10. Golding-Wood PH. Observations on petrosal and vidian neurectomy in chronic vasomotor rhinitis. J Laryngol Otol. 1961;75:232–47. https://doi.org/10.1017/s0022215100057716.
11. Bleier BS, Schlosser RJ. Endoscopic anatomy of the postganglionic pterygopalatine innervation of the posterolateral nasal mucosa. Int Forum Allergy Rhinol. 2011;1:113–7. https://doi.org/10.1002/alr.20011.
12. Senanayake P, Wong E, McBride K, Singh N. Efficacy of Vidian neurectomy and posterior nasal neurectomy in the management of nonallergic rhinitis: a systematic review. Am J Rhinol Allergy. 2022;19458924221105933 https://doi.org/10.1177/19458924221105933.
13. Ozenberger JM. Cryosurgery for the treatment of chronic rhinitis. Laryngoscope. 1973;83:508–16. https://doi.org/10.1288/00005537-197304000-00007.
14. Terao A, Meshitsuka K, Suzaki H, Fukuda S. Cryosurgery on postganglionic fibers (posterior nasal branches) of the pterygopalatine ganglion for vasomotor rhinitis. Acta Otolaryngol. 1983;96:139–48. https://doi.org/10.3109/00016488309132884.
15. Friedman M, LoSavio P, Ibrahim H, Ramakrishnan V. Radiofrequency tonsil reduction: safety, morbidity, and efficacy. Laryngoscope. 2003;113:882–7. https://doi.org/10.1097/00005537-200305000-00020.
16. De Corso E, et al. Radiofrequency volumetric inferior turbinate reduction: long-term clinical results. Acta Otorhinolaryngol Ital. 2016;36:199–205. https://doi.org/10.14639/0392-100X-964.
17. Steele TO, et al. A preliminary report on the effect of gabapentin pretreatment on periprocedural pain during in-office posterior nasal nerve cryoablation. Int Forum Allergy Rhinol. 2020;10:159–64. https://doi.org/10.1002/alr.22456.
18. Del Signore AG, et al. Cryotherapy for treatment of chronic rhinitis: 3-month outcomes of a randomized, sham-controlled trial. Int Forum Allergy Rhinol. 2022;12:51–61. https://doi.org/10.1002/alr.22868.

19. Takashima M, et al. Temperature-controlled radiofrequency neurolysis for treatment of chronic rhinitis: 12-month outcomes after treatment in a randomized controlled trial. Int Forum Allergy Rhinol. 2022; https://doi.org/10.1002/alr.23047.
20. Stolovitzky JP, et al. Effect of radiofrequency neurolysis on the symptoms of chronic rhinitis: a randomized controlled trial. OTO Open. 2021;5:2473974X211041124. https://doi.org/10.1177/2473974X211041124.
21. Ow RA, O'Malley EM, Han JK, Lam KK, Yen DM. Cryosurgical ablation for treatment of rhinitis: two-year results of a prospective multicenter study. Laryngoscope. 2021;131:1952–7. https://doi.org/10.1002/lary.29453.
22. Chang MT, Song S, Hwang PH. Cryosurgical ablation for treatment of rhinitis: a prospective multicenter study. Laryngoscope. 2020;130:1877–84. https://doi.org/10.1002/lary.28301.
23. Lee JT, et al. Clinical and quality of life outcomes following temperature-controlled radiofrequency neurolysis of the posterior nasal nerve (RhinAer) for treatment of chronic rhinitis. Am J Rhinol Allergy. 2022;19458924221109987 https://doi.org/10.1177/19458924221109987.
24. Ehmer D, et al. Long-term outcomes following temperature-controlled radiofrequency neurolysis for the treatment of chronic rhinitis. Allergy Rhinol (Providence). 2022;13:21526575221096045. https://doi.org/10.1177/21526575221096045.
25. Gerka Stuyt JA, Luk L, Keschner D, Garg R. Evaluation of in-office cryoablation of posterior nasal nerves for the treatment of rhinitis. Allergy Rhinol (Providence). 2021;12:2152656720988565. https://doi.org/10.1177/2152656720988565.
26. Lee JT, Abbas GM, Charous DD, Cuevas M, Göktas Ö, Loftus PA, Nachlas NE, Toskala EM, Watkins JP, Brehmer D. Three-year outcomes after temperature-controlled radiofrequency ablation of the posterior nasal nerve for chronic rhinitis. Am J Rhinol Allergy. 2025;4:19458924251360889. https://doi.org/10.1177/19458924251360889. Epub ahead of print. PMID: 40760831.
27. Kompelli AR, Janz TA, Rowan NR, Nguyen SA, Soler ZM. Cryotherapy for the treatment of chronic rhinitis: a qualitative systematic review. Am J Rhinol Allergy. 2018;32:491–501. https://doi.org/10.1177/1945892418800879.
28. Ehmer D, et al. Temperature-controlled radiofrequency neurolysis for the treatment of rhinitis. Am J Rhinol Allergy. 2022;36:149–56. https://doi.org/10.1177/19458924211033400.

18 Inferior Turbinate Reduction

Stephen Leong, Michelle Yu, and Ashutosh Kacker

Key Points

- Nasal congestion is a common ailment that, while typically benign, can seriously detract from quality of life.
- The most common cause of chronic nasal congestion is enlargement of the erectile tissue of the inferior turbinates.
- Therapies such as topical or systemic corticosteroids, antihistamines, and decongestants can alleviate symptoms, but in cases of failure, surgical treatment of the inferior turbinate may be an option.
- Multiple techniques to reduce the turbinates have been developed, each with their own risks and benefits.

Supplementary Information The online version contains supplementary material available at https://doi.org/10.1007/978-3-031-89191-5_18.

S. Leong
Vagelos College of Physicians & Surgeons, Columbia University Irving Medical Center, New York, NY, USA
e-mail: sl3793@cumc.columbia.edu

M. Yu (✉)
Department of Otolaryngology—Head & Neck Surgery, NewYork-Presbyterian/Weill Cornell Medicine/Columbia University Irving Medical Center, New York, NY, USA
e-mail: miy7005@nyp.org

A. Kacker
Department of Otolaryngology – Head & Neck Surgery, New York-Presbyterian/Weill Cornell Medicine, New York, NY, USA
e-mail: ask9001@med.cornell.edu

J. T. Lee et al. (eds.), *Advances in Surgical and Medical Interventions for Recalcitrant Chronic Rhinosinusitis*,
https://doi.org/10.1007/978-3-031-89191-5_18

- Submucous resection generally has more lasting effects on nasal obstruction than extramucosal methods but preferred technique depends on surgeon preference, cost, resource availability, ease of use, and risk of postoperative complications.

Background

The inferior turbinates are scroll-like, mucosal structures attached to the lateral nasal wall that serve to filter, warm, and humidify air upon entry into the nasal cavity [1]. Inferior turbinate hypertrophy (ITH) is the most common cause of chronic nasal obstruction and has various etiologies including allergic rhinitis, vasomotor rhinitis, and rhinitis medicamentosa [1]. The first-line treatment for ITH is medical therapy with topical and/or oral antihistamines, corticosteroids, and/or decongestants; when these agents fail, surgical reduction is indicated [1].

The American Academy of Otolaryngology—Head and Neck Surgery recommends surgical inferior turbinate reduction (ITR) upon fulfillment of four criteria: (1) chronic nasal obstruction due to ITH, (2) failure of directed medical management with continued nasal symptoms, (3) failure of medical management of rhinitis medicamentosa, and (4) symptoms of obstructive sleep apnea [2]. In this chapter, we aim to review the different techniques for surgical ITR, and assess their relative pros, cons, and indications (Table 18.1).

Table 18.1 Pros and cons of listed techniques

Technique	Cost	Difficulty	Overall efficacy	Duration of effect
Complete turbinectomy	+	+	+++	+++
Laser cautery	+++	++	++	+
Electrocautery	+	+	+	+
Cryotherapy	++	+	+	+
Turbinate lateralization	+	+	+	+
Microdebrider turbinoplasty	+	++	+++	++
Coblation	++	++	+++	+++
Radiofrequency ablation	++	++	+++	++
Ultrasound turbinoplasty	++	++	+++	++

Extramucosal Surgical Techniques

The techniques described in this section achieve symptomatic control by either resecting inferior turbinate mucosa or reducing nasal obstruction without tunneling under the mucosa (i.e., turbinate lateralization). These techniques range from highly efficacious with high risk of complications (i.e., complete turbinectomy) to mostly ineffective with no significant complications (i.e., turbinate lateralization, cryotherapy). There is evidence to show that submucosal techniques have better long-term results than extramucosal techniques; overall many of the extramucosal techniques that will be discussed below have fallen out of favor and are no longer routinely used for ITR. However, some techniques, such as inferior turbinate lateralization, are used in conjunction with submucosal techniques for an additive effect on symptomatic control [3, 4].

Complete Turbinectomy

A complete turbinectomy may be performed using curved turbinate scissors and complete excision of all inferior turbinate tissue, leading to resolution of symptoms in the vast majority of cases [5]. However, complete turbinectomy is associated with unfavorable complications such as synechiae formation, significant postoperative pain, bleeding, and crusting [5]. Additionally, complete turbinectomy has been associated with empty nose syndrome (ENS), an iatrogenic condition where removal of turbinate tissue causes paradoxical nasal obstruction, impaired air sensation, and nasal dryness [6]. Because of the potentially significant functional burden of ENS, as well as the frequency of other complications following complete turbinectomy, this technique has largely fallen out of favor.

Laser Cautery

The most commonly used lasers for ITR are diode and CO_2 lasers; other lasers that may be used are argon, potassium-titanyl-phosphate (KTP), neodynium: YAG (Nd:YAG), and holmium: YAG (Ho:YAG) lasers [7]. Each laser type has specific pros and cons for ITR, which are beyond the scope of this chapter. Diode and CO_2 lasers are preferred for ITR because they accurately ablate tissue while producing hemostasis; these lasers are appropriate for use in endoscopic sinus surgery (ESS) as well [8]. Laser cautery of the inferior turbinates achieves symptomatic control through selective ablation of mucosa on the medial surface of the turbinate, thereby producing mucosal atrophy and turbinate reduction. The complications of laser cautery are relatively minimal due to its hemostatic, highly selective effect; bleeding and crusting have been observed in a small minority of patients [8]. Although symptom control may be achieved in the majority of patients, laser cautery does not appear to be as effective as other techniques, including submucosal techniques, because a relatively small amount of tissue is removed [7]. Laser cautery appears to be particularly ineffective for allergic rhinitis [7].

Electrocautery

Monopolar or bipolar cautery may be used to ablate turbinate tissue either on the mucosal surface or in a submucosal plane [5]. Typically, electrocautery is used on the mucosal surface because the amount of tissue damage is difficult to gauge when the electrode is inserted below the mucosa [8]. Both mucosal and submucosal cauterization are not highly effective in improving airflow, and both are associated with higher incidence of complications including crusting and synechiae formation [8]. Thus, inferior turbinate electrocautery is typically not performed as an isolated technique, but may be used in tandem with other submucosal techniques, and often with a more minimal, mucosal-sparing method.

Cryotherapy

Cryotherapy for inferior turbinate reduction utilizes nitrous oxide or liquid nitrogen to rapidly cool the turbinate, thus inducing necrosis and scarring in a minimally invasive fashion [8]. Though symptom control may be achieved in the short term, these effects do not persist; thus, this technique has largely been abandoned.

Turbinate Lateralization

Using a flat elevator or long nasal speculum, the turbinates may be fractured and pushed laterally to increase airflow within the nasal cavity [9]. Although the procedure is straightforward and associated with minimal morbidity, it has not been shown to reduce symptom burden when performed independently [9]. However, when performed in tandem with septoplasty or other methods of turbinate reduction, it may produce an added benefit in the relief of obstructive symptoms. Notably, turbinate lateralization is often performed in conjunction with submucosal resection; this technique will be discussed in following sections.

Submucosal Techniques

The goal of submucosal resection is removal of obstructive tissue while preserving the mucosal function of the inferior turbinate [8]. Thus, submucosal resection is typically not associated with nasal dryness or ENS. Two types of submucosal resection are used for ITR: intraturbinoplasty and extraturbinoplasty [8]. Both are performed under local anesthesia with lidocaine and epinephrine or neosynephrine.

Table 18.2 Complication risk of listed techniques

Technique	Minor bleeding	Major bleeding	Pain	Crusting	Necrosis	Nasal dryness	Synechiae
Complete turbinectomy	+++	++	+++	+++	+	+++	+++
Laser cautery	+	+	+	+	++	+	+
Electrocautery	+	+	++	++	++	++	++
Cryotherapy	+	+	+	+	++	+	+
Turbinate lateralization	+	+	+	+	+	+	+
Microdebrider turbinoplasty	++	+	+	+	+	+	+
Coblation	+	+	+	+	+	+	+
Radiofrequency ablation	+	+	+	+	+	+	+
Ultrasound turbinoplasty	+	+	+	+	+	+	+

Video 1 - ITR Microdebrider
Video 2 - ITR Coblation
Video 3 – ITR Radio Frequency

Intraturbinoplasty is achieved by tunneling devices into the inferior turbinate anteriorly and resecting erectile tissue along the length of the turbinate under endoscopic guidance [8]. Intraturbinoplasty is the most commonly used form of conventional turbinoplasty, and may be performed with a variety of tools including microdebrider, ultrasound, radiofrequency, and coblation. These specific techniques will be discussed in the following sections. Extraturbinoplasty is achieved by resecting the lateral erectile tissue and mucosa, elevating a medial mucosal flap, and rotation of the flap laterally to cover the exposed part of the inferior turbinate [8]. Both techniques achieve symptomatic control at high rates with relatively low complication rates; the most common side effects are bleeding and crusting (Table 18.2). Intraturbinoplasty is preferred over extraturbinoplasty because it is relatively easier to perform successfully. Additionally, turbinate lateralization may be performed in conjunction with intraturbinoplasty, and has an additive benefit in relief of nasal obstruction.

Microdebrider Turbinoplasty (Video 18.1)

The microdebrider is a critical tool in ESS, allowing for continuous suction with precise tissue removal [8]. Given its widespread use, the microdebrider is the most commonly employed tool for ITR following an ESS case. The microdebrider may be used for both intraturbinoplasty and extraturbinoplasty. For extraturbinoplasty, the microdebrider is used to resect the inferior and lateral aspects of the inferior turbinate; medialization of the turbinate may be required for appropriate access [10]. A Cottle elevator is then used to dissect the medial mucosa from underlying bone; the bone may be removed with a long Stevens tenotomy scissor. The medial mucosal flap is rotated laterally to cover the exposed part of the inferior turbinate. For intraturbinoplasty, a #15 blade is used to incise the anteromedial portion of the inferior turbinate; the microdebrider is then inserted into the submucosal pocket and used to debride soft tissue and turbinate bone [11]. Direct inspection with a 0 degree endoscopic is used to assess for bleeding; suction cautery may be used to achieve hemostasis. The incision into the inferior turbinate may be left open or closed with a simple interrupted suture. Complications of bleeding, crusting, and synechiae formation are minimal in both techniques, and symptomatic control is achieved in the vast majority of cases.

Coblation (Video 18.2)

Coblation is an ablative technique that uses bipolar radiofrequency in combination with saline irrigation to vaporize soft tissue [8]. Coblation can be used to perform intraturbinoplasty or extraturbinoplasty in a similar fashion to microdebrider resection. Coblation also produces postoperative fibrosis within the inferior turbinate, which prevents future hypertrophy by anchoring mucosa to the periosteum [8]. In multiple studies, coblation-mediated submucosal resection achieved symptomatic control in the vast majority of patients with minimal complications, and patients remained asymptomatic for durations of time exceeding 32 months [8]. Unlike microdebrider resection, traditional coblation cannot be used to resect turbinate bone; however, the Turbinator wand attachment was developed to add a cutting effect in addition to the thermal energy produced by traditional coblation [8]. Using the Turbinator wand, turbinate bone may be resected in addition to soft tissue, thereby allowing for significant reduction in turbinate size.

Radiofrequency Ablation (Video 18.3)

Radiofrequency energy is delivered submucosally to the inferior turbinate via a needle on a handheld device, ablating tissue with heat desiccation created by frictional energy. As the turbinate heals, the submucosal necrosis created by the ablation is replaced by fibroblasts and normal wound contraction leads to a reduction in turbinate volume. Temperatures range from 60° to 90 ° C in radiofrequency ablation as opposed to up to 800 °C with electrocautery or laser techniques [4]. A prospective, randomized, single-blinded, placebo-controlled trial in 32 patients conducted by Nease and Krempl showed that radiofrequency ablation is more effective in treating inferior turbinate hypertrophy than placebo [12]. Performance-wise, radiofrequency ablation is a comparable technique to coblation, but does not employ saline irrigation, and instead uses a radiofrequency electrode to directly heat soft tissue to 60–90° [13]. The efficacy of radiofrequency ablation is comparable to microdebrider resection, and the radiofrequency electrode produces a more targeted effect than coblation [8]. Like microdebrider resection, complications of bleeding, crusting, and synechiae are typically minimal.

Ultrasound Turbinoplasty

Ultrasound turbinoplasty is achieved with an ultrasonic nasal probe that is inserted submucosally. The low frequency ultrasound disrupts cavernous and connective tissue in the turbinate, thereby reducing the bulk of the soft tissue of the turbinate [14]. The technique can be performed under local anesthesia and is comparable in improving nasal obstruction to other techniques such as coblation, monopolar cautery, and radiofrequency turbinoplasty for at least 6 months from surgery [14]. This technique is well-tolerated under local anesthesia and has minimal complications, primarily consisting of pain and nasal discharge. Post-operative bleeding and synechiae are rare with this technique.

Tips and Pearls

- Surgical resection of the inferior turbinate may be performed for refractory inferior turbinate hypertrophy.
- A variety of techniques have been described, the most effective of which tend to be submucosal techniques given high efficacy with low complication rates.
- Submucosal techniques can be performed under local or general anesthesia as sole therapies or adjunctive procedures.
- Under local anesthesia, patient education and careful patient selection are necessary to set expectations and provide successful outcomes.

References

1. Berger G, Balum-Azim M, Ophir D. The normal inferior turbinate: histomorphometric analysis and clinical implications. Laryngoscope. 2003;113(7):1192–8. https://doi.org/10.1097/00005537-200307000-00015.
2. 125395. Clinical Indicators: Inferior Turbinate Surgery. American Academy of Otolaryngology-Head and Neck Surgery (AAO-HNS). Accessed June 25, 2022. https://www.entnet.org/resource/clinical-indicators-inferior-turbinate-surgery/
3. Passàli D, Passàli FM, Damiani V, Passàli GC, Bellussi L. Treatment of inferior turbinate hypertrophy: a randomized clinical trial. Ann Otol Rhinol Laryngol. 2003;112(8):683–8. https://doi.org/10.1177/000348940311200806.
4. Larrabee YC, Kacker A. Which inferior turbinate reduction technique best decreases nasal obstruction? Laryngoscope. 2014;124(4):814–5. https://doi.org/10.1002/lary.24182.
5. Rao SUP, Basavaraj P, Yempalle SB, Ramachandra AD. A prospective study of different methods of inferior turbinate reduction. J Clin Diagn Res JCDR. 2017;11(5):MC01–3. https://doi.org/10.7860/JCDR/2017/24861.9850.
6. Manji J, Nayak JV, Thamboo A. The functional and psychological burden of empty nose syndrome. Int Forum Allergy Rhinol. 2018;8(6):707–12. https://doi.org/10.1002/alr.22097.

7. Janda P, Sroka R, Baumgartner R, Grevers G, Leunig A. Laser treatment of hyperplastic inferior nasal turbinates: a review. Lasers Surg Med. 2001;28(5):404–13. https://doi.org/10.1002/lsm.1068.
8. Abdullah B, Singh S. Surgical interventions for inferior turbinate hypertrophy: a comprehensive review of current techniques and technologies. Int J Environ Res Public Health. 2021;18(7):3441. https://doi.org/10.3390/ijerph18073441.
9. Hol M, Huizing E. Treatment of inferior turbinate pathology: a review and critical evaluation of the different techniques. Rhinology. 2001;38:157–66.
10. Bielamowicz S, Hawrych A, Gupta A. Endoscopic inferior turbinate reduction: a new technique. Laryngoscope. 1999;109(6):1007–9. https://doi.org/10.1097/00005537-199906000-00030.
11. Friedman M, Tanyeri H, Lim J, Landsberg R, Caldarelli D. A safe, alternative technique for inferior turbinate reduction. Laryngoscope. 1999;109(11):1834–7. https://doi.org/10.1097/00005537-199911000-00021.
12. Nease CJ, Krempl GA. Radiofrequency treatment of turbinate hypertrophy: a randomized, blinded, placebo-controlled clinical trial. Otolaryngol—Head Neck Surg. 2004;130(3):291–9. https://doi.org/10.1016/j.otohns.2003.11.003.
13. Utley DS, Goode RL, Hakim I. Radiofrequency energy tissue ablation for the treatment of nasal obstruction secondary to turbinate hypertrophy. Laryngoscope. 1999;109(5):683–6. https://doi.org/10.1097/00005537-199905000-00001.
14. Gindros G, Kantas I, Balatsouras DG, Kaidoglou A, Kandiloros D. Comparison of ultrasound turbinate reduction, radiofrequency tissue ablation and submucosal cauterization in inferior turbinate hypertrophy. Eur Arch Otorrinolaringol. 2010;267(11):1727–33. https://doi.org/10.1007/s00405-010-1260-9.

Radiofrequency and Bioabsorbable Nasal Implantation for Treatment of Nasal Valve Obstruction

19

Greg E. Davis and Craig Miller

Key Points

- The nasal valve is a major component of nasal airway obstruction in many patients.
- Multiple devices are available on the market that surgically treat narrowing of the nasal valves, bypassing the need for patients to undergo reconstructive rhinoplasty.
- With recent advances, nasal valve compromise can be treated either in the operating room or in the office setting under local anesthesia.
- Patient selection and method of local anesthetic control are critical to performing a successful procedure.

Background

The internal nasal valve is an anatomically dynamic and complex area of the nasal cavity. This area is the narrowest region in the upper airway that can account for up to 70% of nasal respiratory resistance [1]. Anatomically, it is composed of the dorsal septum, upper lateral cartilage, and head of the inferior turbinate (Fig. 19.1). Both static (fixed) and dynamic (motion) challenges lead to nasal airway resistance.

Supplementary Information The online version contains supplementary material available at https://doi.org/10.1007/978-3-031-89191-5_19.

G. E. Davis (✉)
Otolaryngology, Proliance Surgeons, Seattle and Puyallup, WA, USA

C. Miller
Otolaryngology, Virginia Mason Franciscan Health, Seattle, WA, USA

J. T. Lee et al. (eds.), *Advances in Surgical and Medical Interventions for Recalcitrant Chronic Rhinosinusitis*,
https://doi.org/10.1007/978-3-031-89191-5_19

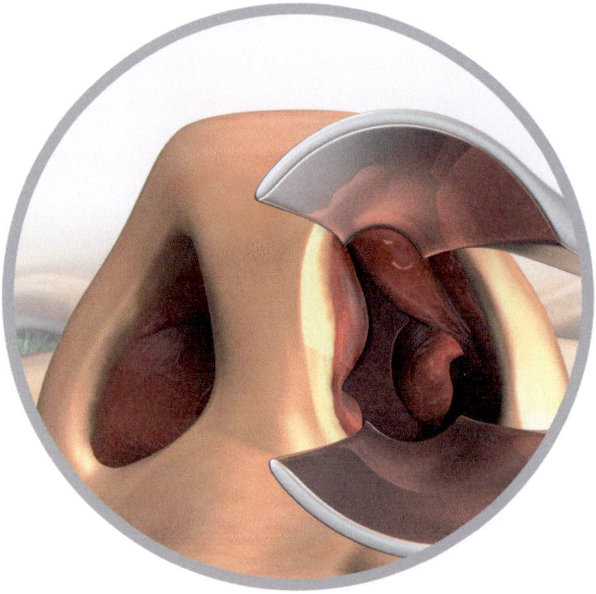

Fig. 19.1 Base view of the nose showing the internal nasal valve. Image courtesy of Aerin Medical

Static abnormalities include deviated nasal septum, inferior turbinate hypertrophy, and malpositioned (narrow) upper lateral cartilage. Dynamic abnormalities impact nasal resistance during active nasal inspiration when the sidewalls of the nose collapse due to weak upper lateral cartilages. This condition highlights Bernoulli's principle describing that as fluid velocity increases in a tube due to narrowing, the pressure in that tube must decrease. This decrease in pressure is akin to a vacuum effect and pulls in the surrounding inadequately supported tissue of the lateral nasal wall. The pathology of this event is called Nasal Valve Compromise (NVC), also called nasal valve collapse, and primarily relates to the internal nasal valve [2].

Dynamic nasal valve collapse attributed to weakness of the upper lateral cartilages can be managed via surgical and non-surgical techniques. Non-surgical techniques are typically temporary and consist of external nasal splints to support the cartilage collapse, such as breathe-right strips, or insertable devices to help stent open the nasal valve, such as nosecones or nasal dilators. Historically, invasive management of nasal valve collapse has consisted of surgical procedures to strengthen the upper lateral cartilages such as batten grafts and lateral crural strut grafts. These complex surgeries are predominantly performed by surgeons who obtained additional training in facial plastics or cosmetic fellowship programs [3]. Implanted nonabsorbable alloplastic grafts have been used; however these have increased risks of infection, extrusion, and high rates of revision surgery [4].

More recently, the development of two novel techniques to improve NVC has created simplified and effective options to treat NVC and lateral wall insufficiency that are available for the general otolaryngologist and rhinologist. The LATERA® (Stryker, Inc., Kalamazoo, MI) implant, a lateral nasal sidewall implant and the Vivaer® (Aerin Medical, Mountainview, CA) radio frequency (RF) device for nasal valve remodeling are currently readily available, low-morbidity treatment options for patients with NVC.

Surgical Technique

Bioabsorbable Nasal Sidewall Implant (LATERA)

LATERA is a bioabsorbable nasal implant used to support both the upper and lower lateral cartilages during inspiration. The implant is a 70:30 blend of poly(L-lactide) and poly(D-lactide) (Fig. 19.2). It is produced in two sizes, 24 and 20 mm. It is introduced via an endonasal insertion technique using a delivery device. This implant targets the caudal lateral region of the lateral crus of the lower lateral cartilage, a critical region for maintaining strength of the lateral nasal wall.

The implant consists of a forked end, which is positioned on the frontal process of the maxilla, and a body with a balled end, which extends caudally toward the alar region (Fig. 19.3). The implant conforms to the natural curvature of the lateral wall against the upper and lower lateral cartilages to provide support and strength to the lateral wall without change to the nasal aesthetic. Early prospective trials using the device found that 30 patients with dynamic NVC had improvement in their Nasal Obstruction Symptom Evaluation (NOSE) scores by an average of 42 points, improving from a mean pretreatment NOSE score of 65 to a 12-month post-treatment average of 23 points [4]. Additionally, there were no reports of significant change to cosmesis, implant migration, or associated infection. A recent systematic review and meta-analysis, reviewing five studies assessing NOSE scores and quality of life metrics following LATERA placement, concluded similar effectiveness and improvement in nasal breathing scores compared to sham surgery [5]. Histological analysis of LATERA at 24 months after implantation showed that the implant provides long-term structural support as it is replaced by fibrous tissue [6]. Long-term studies with 2-year follow-up demonstrated long-term stability [7, 8].

This procedure can be performed in the operating room either as an isolated procedure or in conjunction with septoplasty and inferior turbinate reduction. The minimally invasive technique and delivery system does allow for this to also be performed in the office setting under local anesthesia. Appropriate patient selection

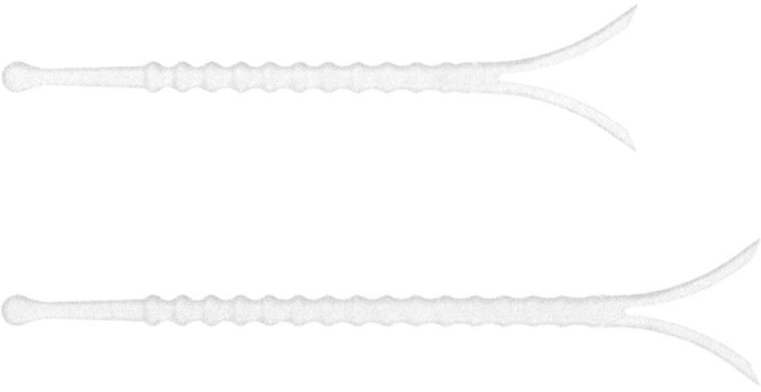

Fig. 19.2 Latera implant (permission to use image from Stryker)

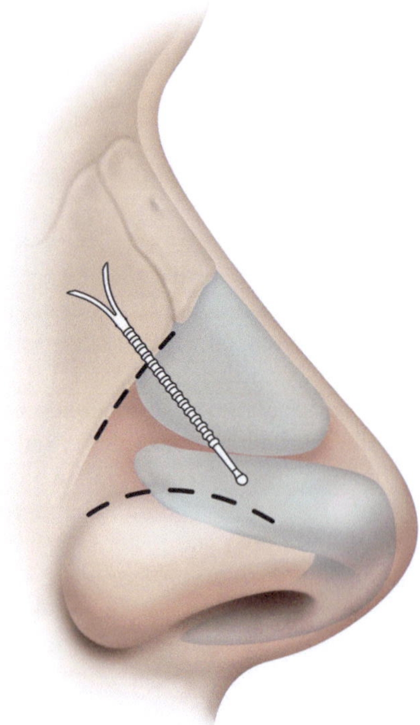

Fig. 19.3 Placement of Latera implant (permission granted to use image from Stryker)

and optimizing local anesthetic techniques improve patient experience and satisfaction.

Patient Selection

The ideal candidate for the LATERA procedure has mild to moderate dynamic nasal valve collapse with inspiration, a positive Cottle maneuver (improved breathing), mild to moderate inferior turbinate hypertrophy, and none or mild nasal septal deviation. A patient with severe septal deviation likely needs a septoplasty performed in conjunction with the LATERA procedure. Similarly, an inferior turbinate that is completely blocking the nasal space may benefit from a turbinate reduction either in addition to LATERA placement or in a separate procedure. An additional consideration should include the surgeon's perception of a patient's tolerance for an in-office versus an in-operating room procedure as this can significantly impact satisfaction during the procedure.

Local Anesthesia

Both topical and local anesthesia are necessary to provide optimal patient comfort. Local anesthesia injection, specifically lidocaine with epinephrine, can serve to decrease bleeding during the procedure, improve patient tolerance, and provide a hydro-dissected plane to improve device placement. The addition of 10% volume of

8.4% sodium bicarbonate to the local anesthetic can decrease the irritation caused by the acidic solution. Injection should proceed from the planned mucosal insertion and then in the tissue plane superficial to the upper and lower lateral cartilages along the planned trajectory of the device.

Surgical Technique

Apply a nasal decongestant, such as oxymetazoline spray, one hour before the procedure or as soon as is feasible prior to the procedure. This will aid in pain management and improve the visualization of the surgical field. Apply topical anesthesia with pledgets to numb the nasal ala. Use caution with direct infiltration of local anesthetic in the area as this may impair visualization due to local edema effects of the anesthetic.

Begin by marking the point of maximal lateral wall collapse with a skin marker during dynamic inspiration. This point will be the caudal aspect of the device. This point should not sit caudal to the alar crease, as this skin is thin and can lead to cosmetic concerns or device extrusion. Using the measuring tool, place a mark at the cephalad portion of the device. This must sit over the nasal bones. Lateral displacement of the forked end towards the medial canthus in patients who wear glasses can provide improved comfort during the healing process. Leaving the measuring tool in place, place a mark at the nasal rim corresponding to the vertical line of the planned device placement. This will provide a visual point in which to make the vestibular puncture.

Following an acceptable amount of time (usually 10–15 min), inject local anesthetic with a 27 g needle. Consider using 1% lidocaine with 1:200,000 epinephrine to minimize the cardiovascular and anxiety-inducing effect of epinephrine. Warning the patient of the potential brief tachycardia and anxiety associated with epinephrine administration can greatly reduce patient discomfort. Additionally, adding 10% volume of 8.4% sodium bicarbonate solution to the anesthetic mixture will decrease the sting of the solution. The local anesthetic agent should be injected into the nasal rim in the area of the planned insertion and then along the trajectory of the implant.

Using a sharp double prong skin hook, pull the ala laterally and place the delivery device at the caudal aspect of the lower lateral cartilage corresponding to the area where one would place a marginal incision. Directing the device towards the septum, pierce the mucosa. Once the cannula has pierced the nasal mucosa, direct this laterally to follow a superficial plane over the upper and lower lateral cartilages. Continue to follow the planned trajectory until the cannula reaches the cephalic mark at the nasal bones. Deploy the device by pressing the large green button in the center of the cannula and advancing the delivery component into the cannula component. It is important not to advance the cannula while doing this. Place a finger gently at the region where the device was deployed to anchor this in place and gently withdraw the cannula. Confirm that there is no aspect of the device that has extruded through the mucosal puncture point (Video 19.1).

Inform patients that it can take up to 3 months for the full effect of the procedure to be noticeable. Patients need to avoid manipulating the lateral nasal wall for the first 2 weeks so as not to dislodge the implant. Patients should be counseled that complications have been reported, including extrusion/need for retrieval of the device (4%, 22/543 implants), implant show or palpable on nasal surface (1%, 7/543 implants), and infection (1% 7/543 implants) [8].

Tips and Pearls

- Optimize the procedure room environment with distractions for the patient including playing music or a video monitor playing non-surgical images.
- A surgical headlight is helpful for visualization.
- Lateral displacement of the forked end towards the medial canthus in patients who wear glasses can provide improved comfort during the healing process.
- If there is bleeding from the mucosal penetration site, place gentle pressure along the nasal dorsum for a few minutes until the bleeding abates.

Radiofrequency Remodelling of the Lower Lateral Cartilage (Vivaer)

The Vivaer device became commercially available in the United States in 2018. This device uses RF energy at low temperature (60 °C) deployed by a temperature controlled bipolar device to reshape the cartilage of the lower lateral cartilage. It can also be used on soft tissue such as turbinate tissue or the septal swell body to superficially decrease the size of these structures. The initial research study reported on 50 patients who had nasal valve treatment and improved their NOSE scale scores by 69%; improving from a baseline average of 79.9 to a 26-week post-treatment average of 24.7 [9]. A two-year follow-up study on 39 of those subjects showed longevity of improvement with an average NOSE score of 26.5 (66.5% improvement from baseline) [10]. Finally, a long-term study of 29 subjects in the initial cohort who continued in the study reported their 48-month post-treatment NOSE score to be 25.7 (68.3% improvement compared to baseline) [11]. Perhaps the most interesting report was a prospective multi-center randomized controlled sham trial involving 117 subjects, 77 who received RF energy during the procedure compared to 40 who received the procedure without the deployment of RF energy [12]. The primary outcome measure was improvement in NOSE score > 20% or improvement in greater than or equal to 1 category of NOSE score severity compared to baseline. In the active treatment cohort, 88.3% responded favorably versus 42.5% in the sham treatment arm ($p < 0.001$).

The Vivaer procedure is effective in treating NVC. In addition, patient satisfaction was reported to be quite high on five questions queried in the initial study, ranging from 7.3 to 8.7 out of 10 [9]. Given that this procedure can be done under local anesthesia or also under general anesthesia, there are some techniques to be implemented to aid in patient satisfaction.

Patient Selection

The ideal candidate for the Vivaer procedure has mild to moderate dynamic nasal valve collapse with inspiration, a positive Cottle maneuver (improved breathing), mild to moderate inferior turbinate hypertrophy and none or mild nasal septal deviation. A patient with severe septal deviation likely needs a septoplasty performed in conjunction with the Vivaer procedure. Similarly, an inferior turbinate that is completely blocking the nasal space may benefit from a more aggressive turbinate reduction procedure rather than the superficial procedure that the Vivaer provides. An additional consideration should include the surgeon's perception of a patient's tolerance for an in-office versus an in-operating room procedure as this can significantly impact satisfaction during the procedure.

Local Anesthesia

The anterior nasal cavity, including the internal nasal valve, receives innervation from both the first and second branches of the trigeminal nerves. The first branch innervates the nasal skin and ala whereas the second branch innervates the internal lining of the nose. A combination of topical and locally injected anesthetic agents is often adequate to obtain exceptional anesthesia.

Surgical Technique

Similar to the Latera, patients can apply a nasal decongestant (such as oxymetazoline spray) an hour before the procedure or as soon as is feasible prior to the procedure to aid in pain management and improve the surgical field. A topical anesthetic, typically 4% lidocaine-soaked cotton or a 10% tetracaine gel can also be applied to the caudal nares. Following an acceptable amount of time (usually 10–15 min), inject local anesthetic with a 27 g needle. Consider using 1% lidocaine with 1:200,000 epinephrine and 10% volume of 8.4% sodium bicarbonate to minimize the cardiovascular and anxiety-inducing effect of epinephrine and to minimize the sting from the anesthetic. Some surgeons find it less painful to the patient if they apply a tapping motion to the ipsilateral infraorbital region during these injections.

The local anesthetic agent should be injected into the inferior turbinate head, septal swell body (if being treated) and then into the nasal side of the ala and lateral nasal wall junction targeting the lower lateral cartilage (Fig. 19.4). This last injection is the most pain inducing and is best done last after giving the turbinate injection 30–60 s to take effect. Additional anesthesia can be obtained by performing an infraorbital block. If this is going to be performed, prior to the injection, place viscous lidocaine-soaked cotton in the maxillary gingival sulcus to help minimize the pain of the injection.

Use the Vivaer device as indicated in non-overlapping areas. When applying the device to the internal nasal valve, use your contralateral hand to apply gentle pressure with a finger on the outside of the nasal sidewall to help straighten out any inward bowing cartilage. Several non-overlapping treatments can be applied to the length of the inferior turbinate and the septal swell body.

Post-operatively, we recommend patients use nasal gel or antibiotic ointment applied to the nostrils 2–3 times daily for the first 2 weeks to help minimize

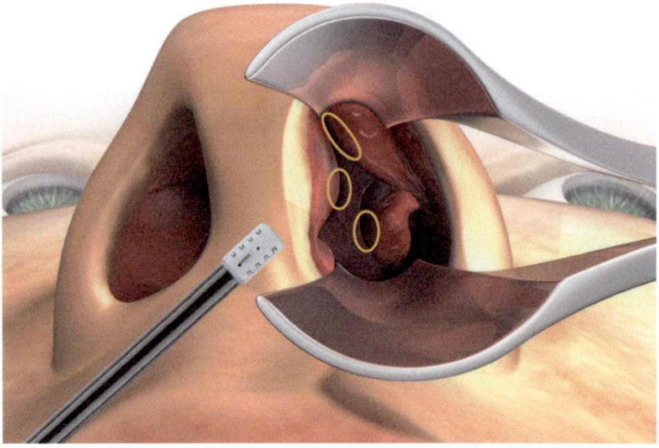

Fig. 19.4 Base view of the nasal cavity with yellow circles showing sites for local anesthetic injections and treatment sites. Image courtesy of Aerin Medical

crusting. Inform patients they will have a congested nose for 1–2 weeks before the congestion starts to improve and that it can take up to 3 months for the full effect of the procedure to be noticeable. Saline spray or irrigation can be helpful to help alleviate the congestion caused by the temporary swelling of the manipulated tissue (Video 19.2).

Tips and Pearls

- Optimize the procedure room environment with distractions for the patient including playing music or a video monitor playing non-surgical images.
- The procedure can be used with a surgical headlight or an endoscope.
- Following an acceptable amount of time (usually 10–15 min) inject local anesthetic with a 27 g needle. Consider using 1% lidocaine with 1:200,000 epinephrine and 10% volume of 8.4% sodium bicarbonate to minimize the cardiovascular and anxiety-inducing effect of epinephrine and to minimize the sting from the anesthetic. Some surgeons find it less painful to the patient if they apply a tapping motion to the ipsilateral infraorbital region during these injections.

References

1. Uddstromer M. Nasal respiration. Acta Otolaryngol Suppl. 1940;42
2. Cottle MH, Loring RM. Corrective surgery of the external nasal pyramid and the nasal septum for restoration of normal physiology. Ill Med J. 1946;90:119–35.
3. Rhee JS, Weaver EM, Park SS, Baker SR, Hilger PA, Kriet JD, et al. Clinical consensus statement: diagnosis and management of nasal valve compromise. Otolaryngol Head Neck Surg. 2010;143(1):48–59.
4. San Nicolo M, Stelter K, Sadick H, Bas M, Berghaus A. Absorbable implant to treat nasal valve collapse. Facial Plast Surg. 2017;33(2):233–40.
5. Kim DH, Lee HH, Kim SH, Hwang SH. Effectiveness of using a bioabsorbable implant (Latera) to treat nasal valve collapse in patients with nasal obstruction: systemic review and meta-analysis. Int Forum Allergy Rhinol. 2020;10(6):719–25.

6. Sanan A, Most SP. A bioabsorbable lateral nasal wall stent for dynamic nasal valve collapse: a review. Facial Plast Surg Clin North Am. 2019;27(3):367–71.
7. San Nicolo M, Berghaus A. Two-year sustained benefit of an absorbable implant for the treatment of NVC. OTO Open. 2017;1(3):2473974X17722982.
8. Sidle DM, Stolovitzky P, O'Malley EM, Ow RA, Nachlas NE, Silvers S. Bioabsorbable implant for treatment of nasal valve collapse with or without concomitant procedures. Facial Plast Surg. 2021;37(5):673–80.
9. Jacobowitz O, Driver M, Ephrat M. In-office treatment of nasal valve obstruction using a novel, bipolar radiofrequency device. Laryngoscope Investig Otolaryngol. 2019;4(2):211–7.
10. Ephrat M, Jacobowitz O, Driver M. Quality-of-life impact after in-office treatment of nasal valve obstruction with a radiofrequency device: 2-year results from a multicenter, prospective clinical trial. Int Forum Allergy Rhinol. 2021;11(4):755–65.
11. Jacobowitz O, Ehmer D, Lanier B, Scurry W, Davis B. Long-term outcomes following repair of nasal valve collapse with temperature-controlled radiofrequency treatment for patients with nasal obstruction. Int Forum Allergy Rhinol. 2022;
12. Silvers SL, Rosenthal JN, McDuffie CM, Yen DM, Han JK. Temperature-controlled radiofrequency device treatment of the nasal valve for nasal airway obstruction: a randomized controlled trial. Int Forum Allergy Rhinol. 2021;11(12):1676–84.

Part IV

Medical Interventions for Recalcitrant Chronic Rhinosinusitis

20 Topical Antibiotics in Treatment of Recalcitrant Chronic Rhinosinusitis

Keonho Albert Kong and Scott P. Stringer

Key Points

- The pathogenesis of chronic rhinosinusitis (CRS) is complex and multifactorial. Bacterial biofilms, microbiome dysbiosis, bacterial superantigens, antimicrobial resistance, and fungal antigens have all been suggested as contributors to CRS.
- Topical antimicrobial therapy theoretically delivers therapeutic medication directly to the affected sinuses of patients having undergone endoscopic sinus surgery with a low risk of systemic absorption.
- Despite this, evidence in support of topical antimicrobial therapy remains limited and the International Consensus Statement on Allergy and Rhinology does not recommend topical antimicrobial treatment for the routine management of CRS.
- There may be unrealized benefit in recalcitrant cases for topical antimicrobial therapy, or even in cases where CRS is due to manifestation of systemic conditions such as cystic fibrosis, vasculitis, or primary ciliary dyskinesia.

Background

The pathogenesis of chronic rhinosinusitis (CRS) is complex and multifactorial. The role of microorganisms in CRS has not yet been fully defined. However, biofilms, microbiome dysbiosis, bacterial superantigens, antimicrobial resistance, and

K. A. Kong
Department of Otolaryngology-Head and Neck Surgery, University of Mississippi Medical Center, Jackson, MS, USA
e-mail: kkong@umc.edu

S. P. Stringer
Department of Otolaryngology-Head and Neck Surgery, Virginia Commonwealth University School of Medicine, Richmond, VA, USA
e-mail: Scott.Stringer@vcuhealth.org

J. T. Lee et al. (eds.), *Advances in Surgical and Medical Interventions for Recalcitrant Chronic Rhinosinusitis*,
https://doi.org/10.1007/978-3-031-89191-5_20

fungal antigens have all been suggested as contributors. The complexity of its pathogenesis can make treatment of recalcitrant CRS especially challenging. Topical antibiotic therapy provides direct delivery of the therapeutic agent in high concentrations to the sinonasal mucosa. Systemic absorption from topical therapy is low, allowing side effects of systemic antimicrobial therapy to be minimized. There is the potential for mucociliary injury which may be associated with local adverse effects such as nasal congestion, epistaxis, irritation, and cough [1–3].

Based on current available evidence, the International Consensus Statement on Allergy and Rhinology does not recommend topical antimicrobial therapy (bacterial or fungal) for routine treatment of CRS with or without polyps [4]. There is substantial heterogeneity between studies, and insufficient trials have investigated specific subgroups of CRS. However, there may be utility for topical antimicrobials in recalcitrant CRS after endoscopic sinus surgery and in cases related to sinonasal manifestations of systemic conditions such as vasculitis, cystic fibrosis, primary ciliary dyskinesia, and other disorders.

In this chapter, we review current literature covering topical antibacterial and antifungal therapy for the treatment of chronic rhinosinusitis. We will also discuss the senior author's experience and recommendations with topical antimicrobial therapy.

Topical Antibacterial Therapy

Microbial dysbiosis and colonization of *Staphylococcus aureus* have been implicated in pathophysiology of CRS. Topical antibiotics are used in CRS in hopes that it would eliminate pathogenic bacteria and reset the patient's sinonasal flora. One prospective study evaluating the applicability of topical antibiotics, performed by Ezzat, et al. examined patients with biofilms and found that topical application of 0.3% ofloxacin TID for 12 weeks reduced biofilm burden via scanning electron microscopy by 80% [5]. Participants also reported a statistically significant reduction in RSI (Rhinosinusitis Symptom Inventory), nasal endoscopic, and CT-based CRSseverity scores.

Mupirocin is a carboxylic acid antibiotic that inhibits bacterial protein and RNA synthesis by reversibly binding isoleucyl-transfer RNA that is commonly used to decolonize methicillin resistant *S. aureus* (MRSA) and to treat skin/soft tissue MRSA infections. MRSA has been found in higher ratios in patients with CRS and its presence has been linked to poorer prognosis [6, 7]. A retrospective study by Solares et al. suggested that mupirocin nasal irrigations could be of benefit in MRSA-related CRS exacerbations [8]. However, only 7/42 cultures (16.7%) were treated with mupirocin irrigations alone, and most were treated with concurrent oral antibiotics. Jervis-Bardy et al. performed a prospective, double-blinded, placebo-controlled study comparing mupirocin rinses to saline rinses in *S. aureus* positive cultures after ESS [9]. Statistically significant benefit was noted at 1 month with *S. aureus* negative cultures in the mupirocin rinse group; however, the benefit did not persist to the 2–6 month follow-up visit. A meta-analysis by Kim et al., which included the two previously mentioned studies, studied the effect of mupirocin irrigations in *S. aureus* infection in the setting of CRS [10]. They showed a relative risk of 0.13 of residual infection through a random effects model meta-analysis of the pooled data. However, the proportion of residual staphylococcal infections was 0.53 at 6 months. Therefore, the authors concluded that short-term use of mupirocin irrigations was effective for recalcitrant staphylococcal CRS.

There may be a role for topical antibiotics in patients with cystic fibrosis (CF). Moss et al. performed a study of CF patients that underwent instillation of tobramycin irrigations via a secured catheter within the maxillary sinus placed intraoperatively. They found that the regular use of postoperative tobramycin irrigations reduced the need for revision surgery in CF by up to 2 years compared to those not using tobramycin irrigations [11]. Di Cicco et al. performed a double-blind controlled study of 27 patients with a diagnosis of CF and documented infection with *Pseudomonas aeruginosa* and/or *S. aureus* [12]. The patients were randomized to receive either a nasal spray formulation containing 0.2% sodium hyaluronate and 3% tobramycin or 0.2% sodium hyaluronate alone for 14 days. The hyaluronate-tobramycin group had a significant improvement in their hyposmia/anosmia and headache/facial pain with additional reductions in mucopurulent secretions at the ostiomeatal complex compared to the control group.

The utility of tobramycin irrigations has also been studied in CRS patients without cystic fibrosis with mixed conclusions. Derosiers et al., in a double-blind randomized controlled trial of patients with CRS refractory to medical and surgical treatment, found that the addition of tobramycin to large-particle nebulized aerosol therapy did not improve symptomatology or objective parameters of sinonasal inflammation [1]. Lee et al. retrospectively studied SNOT-20 outcomes of patients with high-volume topical antibiotic irrigations in CRS patients with previous sinus surgery [13]. A variety of antibiotics were included in the study including tobramycin, vancomycin, levofloxacin, mupirocin, gentamicin, ceftriaxone, and ceftazidime. There was no significant improvement in SNOT-20 scores in either CF and non-CF patients, but there was statistically significant improvement in Lund-Kennedy endoscopic scores in the non-CF group with 72% negative culture results for the targeted pathogen. Two systematic reviews by Rudmik et al. recommended against topical antibacterial therapy, yet the heterogeneity of the studies and their relatively small sample sizes were acknowledged as limitations for this recommendation [14, 15].

There are potential systemic and local side effects for topical antibacterial irrigations. These can be extrapolated from the known adverse side effects seen with enteral or parenteral administration of antibiotics. Smaller studies have shown increased levels of serum gentamicin without any clinically significant negative effect [16, 17]. Increased nasal congestion, sore throat, and cough have been reported in literature with topical administration of antibiotics [1, 3]. Workman et al. demonstrated that certain topical antibiotics can affect ciliary beat frequency [18]. Specifically, azithromycin and neomycin were cilio-stimulatory, and levofloxacin and tobramycin were cilio-inhibitory. The clinical implications of these ciliary changes are uncertain. A summary of the studies examining the role of topical antibacterial can be found in Table 20.1.

Table 20.1 Summary of topical antibacterial studies

Study	Level of evidence	Medical intervention	Number of patients	Reported outcomes
Kim et al. [10]	Meta-analysis	Mupirocin irrigation	101 (3 studies)	0.13 relative risk reduction of residual infection at 1 month after treatment (95% CI: 0.06–0.26, $p < 0.01$).
Ezzat et al. [5]	Prospective controlled	Topical ofloxacin (0.3%) intranasal 3 drops every 8 h × 12 weeks	37 (27 control)	Post-treatment reduction in RSI scoring, nasal endoscopic scoring, CT scan PNS score ($p < 0.001$), 80% biofilm disruption on SEM
Mainz et al. [28]	Double blind RCT	Inhalation with tobramycin (80 mg/2 mL) daily × 28 days using PARI sinus™ nebulizer	9 (6 treatment; 3 control)	6.67 point decrease in SNOT 20 in subject compared to 3.34 point increase in control ($p = 0.033$). No changes in endoscopy findings. Decrease in numbers of P. Aeruginosa colonies in 67% of treatment group.
Jervis-Bardy et al. [9]	Double blind RCT	Mupirocin irrigation twice daily	22 (13 treatment; 9 control)	Negative S aureus cultures in 8/9 mupirocin patients compared to 0/13 placebo control ($p < 0.01$). Improved LK endoscopic ($p < 0.01$) and SNOT 20 scores ($p = 0.06$)
Di Cicco et al. [12]	Double blind RCT	3%tobramycin and 0.2% sodium hyaluronate nasal spray for 14 days. Control group received hyaluronate only nasal spray	27 (14 treatment; 13 control)	There was improvement in mucopurulence at the OMC, and symptoms (hyposmia/anosmia, facial pain/headache) in treatment group compared to control

RSI rhinosinusitis symptom inventory, *SEM* scanning electron microscopy, *OMC* ostiomeatal complex

Overall, there is paucity of literature investigating the role and effect of topical antibiotics in recalcitrant CRS with mixed results in existing literature. Further studies specifically investigating the role of biofilms in recalcitrant CRS and the role of topical antibiotic therapy on its reduction are needed.

Topical Antifungal Therapy

Fungi are ubiquitous in the nasal cavities and sinuses of both individuals with and without CRS [19, 20]. They have been hypothesized to contribute to CRS pathogenesis due to stimulation of the host immune response [21]. Fungi have a role in the pathogenesis of two CRS phenotypes: allergic fungal sinusitis (AFS) and fungal ball/mycetoma. However, the role of fungi in the pathogenesis of other CRS subtypes is unclear. Amphotericin B binds to ergosterol in the fungal cell membrane

Table 20.2 Summary of topical antifungal studies

Study	Level of evidence	Medical intervention	Number of patients	Reported outcomes
Isaacs et al. [25]	Meta-analysis	Topical amphotericin B	284 (6 studies)	There were no statistically significant symptom, endoscopy, or radiologic outcomes between topical amphotericin B vs placebo
Sacks et al. [2]	Meta-analysis	Topical amphotericin B	327 patients (5 studies)	No improvement in QoL or endoscopy scores with topical amphotericin compared to placebo
Wang et al. [26]	Meta-analysis	Topical amphotericin B	300 patients (5 studies)	There was no difference between placebo and topical amphotericin B groups in QoL or endoscopy scores

and increases permeability, leading to cell death. Potential adverse effects of nasal burning, epistaxis, pruritus, and exacerbation of CRS have been reported with topical antifungal use [2]. Several randomized control trials have shown that there was no significant improvement in symptoms, radiographic findings, endoscopic staging with topical amphotericin B compared to placebo in CRS [22–24]. Additionally, three meta-analyses have demonstrated no benefit with topical amphotericin B in CRS with nasal polyps [2, 25, 26]. There are no significant studies investigating the role of topical amphotericin B in AFS so further studies are necessary [27]. A summary of the studies examining the role of topical antifungals in the treatment of CRS can be found in Table 20.2.

With both topical antibiotics and topical antifungal medications, it is important to note that most of these medications are prescribed through compounding pharmacies and are not covered by most insurance plans. This may inflict a financial burden on patients and should be discussed with them prior to prescription.

Senior Author's Practice

The senior author (SS) agrees with the consensus statements that topical antimicrobials should not be routinely used for treatment of CRS with or without polyps. However, we have seen anecdotal utility for topical antimicrobials in select cases. One such group of patients are those with recalcitrant type I chronic rhinosinusitis with chronic colonization of *S. aureus* that have undergone endoscopic sinus surgery. High-volume isotonic saline irrigations impregnated with mupirocin does seem to help in some of these patients with improvement in symptoms and endoscopic findings consistent with the previously referenced literature. Other antibiotics that have been useful include aminoglycosides, cephalosporins, and quinolones depending on cultures, treatment response, and patient allergies. Patients with sinonasal manifestation of various autoimmune mediated diseases and subsequent atrophic rhinosinusitis may also benefit. Mupirocin irrigations seem to help with the chronic crusting in these patient populations. In patients with cystic fibrosis or primary ciliary dyskinesia, culture-directed irrigations may help treat persistent chronic sinonasal disease.

Conclusions

Topical antimicrobial irrigations deliver medications directly to affected sinuses in patients who have had sinus surgery. Use of topical antimicrobial irrigations is not recommended for treatment of routine CRS. There may be a role for it in recalcitrant cases and in cases with manifestations from a systemic disease. Further studies that have bigger sample sizes and those that target specific patient subtypes are needed to determine presence and magnitude of benefit. Providers should consider its use on a case-by-case basis with thoughtful discussion with the patient.

References

1. Derosiers MY, Salas-Prato M. Treatment of chronic rhinosinusitis refractory to other treatments with topical antibiotic therapy delivered by means of a large-particle nebulizer: results of a controlled trial. Otolaryngol Head Neck Surg. 2001;125(3):265–9.
2. Sacks PL, Harve RJ, Rimmer J, et al. Topical and systemic antifungal therapy for the symptomatic treatment of chronic rhinosinusitis. Cochrane Database Syst Rev. 2011;8:CD008263.
3. Vaughan WC, Carvalho G. Use of nebulized antibiotics for acute infections in chronic sinusitis. Otolaryngol Head Neck Surg. 2002;127:558–68.
4. Orlandi RR, Kingdom TT, Smith TL, et al. International consensus statement on allergy and rhinology: rhinosinusitis 2021. Int Forum Allergy Rhinol. 2021;11(3):213–739.
5. Ezzat WF, Fawaz SA, Rabie H, et al. Effect of topical ofloxacin on bacterial biofilms in refractory post-sinus surgery rhino-sinusitis. Eur Arch Otorrinolaringol. 2015;272(9):2355–61.
6. Kim YC, Won HK, Lee JW, et al. Staphylococcus aureus nasal colonization and asthma in adults: systemic review and meta-analysis. J Allergy Clin Immunol Pract. 2019;7(2):606–15.e9
7. Feazel LM, Robertson CE, Ramakrishnan VR, et al. Microbiome complexity and Staphylococcus aureus in chronic rhinosinusitis. Laryngoscope. 2012;122:467–72.
8. Solares CA, Batra PS, Hall GS, et al. Treatment of chronic sinusitis exacerbations due to methicillin-resistant Staphylococcus aureus with mupirocin irritations. Am J Otolaryngol. 2006;27(3):161–5.
9. Jervis-Bardy J, Boase S, Psaltis A, et al. A randomized trial of mupirocin sinonasal rinses versus saline in surgically recalcitrant staphylococcal chronic rhinosinusitis. Laryngoscope. 2012;122(10):2148–53.
10. Kim JS, Kwon SH. Mupirocin in the treatment of staphylococcal infections in chronic rhinosinusitis: a meta-analysis. PLoS One. 2016;11:e0167369.
11. Moss RB, King VV. Management of sinusitis in cystic fibrosis by endoscopic surgery and serial antimicrobial lavage. Reduction in recurrence requiring surgery. Arch Otolaryngol Head Neck Surg. 1995;121(5):566–72.
12. Di Cicco M, Alicandro G, Claut L, et al. Efficacy and tolerability of a new nasal spray formulation containing hyaluronate and tobramycin in cystic fibrosis patients with bacterial rhinosinusitis. J Cyst Fibros. 2014;13(4):455–60.
13. Lee VS, Davis GE. Culture-directed topical antibiotic treatment for chronic rhinosinusitis. Am J Rhinol Allergy. 2016;30(6):414–7.
14. Rudmik L, Soler ZM. Medical therapies for adult chronic sinusitis: a systematic review. JAMA. 2015;314(9):926–39.
15. Rudmik L, Hoy M, Schlosser RJ, et al. Topical therapies in the management of chronic rhinosinusitis: an evidence-based review with recommendations. Int Forum Allergy Rhinol. 2013;3(4):281–98.
16. Whatley WS, Chandra RK, MacDonald CB. Systemic absorption of gentamicin nasal irrigations. Am J Rhinol. 2006;20:251–4.

17. Wong KK, Marglani O, Westerberg BD, et al. Systemic absorption of topical gentamicin sinus irrigation. J Otolaryngol Head Neck Surg. 2008;37:395–8.
18. Workman AD, Carey RM, Kohanski MA, Adappa ND, Palmer JN, Cohen NA. Effects of ophthalmologic solutions on sinonasal ciliated epithelium. Int Forum Allergy Rhinol. 2017;7:801–8.
19. Braun H, Buzina W, Freudenschuss K, et al. 'Eosinophilic fungal rhinosinusitis': a common disorder in Europe? Laryngoscope. 2003;113(2):264–9.
20. Lawrence LA, Mulligan JK, Roach C, et al. Superoxide dismutase reduces the inflammatory response to Aspergillus and Alternaria in human sinonasal epithelial cells derived from patients with chronic rhinosinusitis. Am J Rhinol Allergy. 2015;29(2):89–93.
21. Fokkens WJ, Lund VJ, Hopkins C, et al. European position paper on rhinosinusitis and nasal polyps 2020. Rhinology. 2020;58(Suppl S29):1–464.
22. Ebbens FA, Scadding GK, Badia L, et al. Amphotericin B nasal lavages: not a solution for patients with chronic rhinosinusitis. J Allergy Clin Immunol. 2006;118:1149–56.
23. Weschta M, Rimek D, Formanek M, et al. Topical antifungal treatment of chronic rhinosinusitis with nasal polyps: a randomized, double-blind clinical trial. J Allergy Clin Immunol. 2004;113:1122–8.
24. Jian RS, Twu CW, Liang KL. Efficacy of nasal irrigation with 200mug/mL amphotericin B after functional endoscopic sinus surgery: a randomized, placebo-controlled, double-blind study. Int Forum Allergy Rhinol. 2018;8:41–8.
25. Isaacs S, Fakhri S, Luong A, et al. A meta-analysis of topical amphotericin B for the treatment of chronic rhinosinusitis. Int Forum Allergy Rhinol. 2011;1(4):250–4.
26. Wang T, Su J, Feng T. The effectiveness of topical amphotericin B in the management of chronic rhinosinusitis: a meta-analysis. Eur Arch Otorrinolaringol. 2015;272(8):1923–9.
27. Tan CW, Psaltis AJ. Latest development on topical therapies in chronic rhinosinusitis. Curr Opin Otolaryngol Head Neck Surg. 2020;28(1):25–30.
28. Mainz JG, Schadlich K, Schien C, et al. Sinonasal inhalation of tobramycin vibrating aerosol in cystic fibrosis patients with upper airway Pseudomonas aeruginosa colonization: results of a randomized, double-blind, placebo-controlled pilot study. Drug Des Devel Ther. 2014;8:209–17.

Intravenous Antimicrobial Therapy

21

Amy V. Dora and Matthew Bidwell Goetz

Abbreviations

ESBL	Extended-spectrum beta-lactamases
HIV	Human immunodeficiency virus
IV	Intravenous
MRSA	Methicillin-resistant *Staphylococcus aureus*
MSSA	Methicillin-sensitive *Staphylococcus aureus*
NGS	Next-generation sequencing
PO	Per os

Key Points

- Recalcitrant chronic rhinosinusitis (CRS) is a notoriously difficult-to-treat inflammatory disease of noninfectious origin; most individuals with this disease have had persistent or relapsing symptoms despite surgical and medical therapies, typically inclusive of prior antibiotic therapy.
- Colonization of the sinuses, in addition to host risk factors such as immune compromise, anatomic disruption, and environmental exposures, causes patients with CRS to be susceptible to acute and potentially recurrent bacterial, fungal, and mycobacterial infections.

A. V. Dora
Infectious Diseases, VA Greater Los Angeles Healthcare System, Los Angeles, CA, USA
e-mail: amy.dora@va.gov

M. B. Goetz (✉)
Infectious Diseases, VA Greater Los Angeles Healthcare System, Los Angeles, CA, USA

Clinical Medicine, David Geffen School of Medicine at UCLA, Los Angeles, CA, USA
e-mail: matthew.goetz@va.gov

J. T. Lee et al. (eds.), *Advances in Surgical and Medical Interventions for Recalcitrant Chronic Rhinosinusitis*,
https://doi.org/10.1007/978-3-031-89191-5_21

- CRS patients with severe infection may warrant systemic antibiotic therapy, including intravenous, pathogen-directed therapy. However, stewardship regarding the use of systemic antimicrobials is necessary to prevent the emergence of resistance and the adverse effects of long-term intravenous antibiotic therapy.

Background

Chronic rhinosinusitis is defined by symptoms of nasal discharge or obstruction for at least 12 weeks, accompanied either by facial pain, facial pressure, or by hyposmia [1–3]. Diagnostic confirmation is provided by documentation of nasal polyps, mucopurulent discharge, edema, or mucosal changes within the osteomeatal complex or sinuses by endoscopy or computed tomography imaging.

The manifestations of chronic rhinosinusitis are due to inflammation of the sinuses, which is often accompanied by chronic colonization and biofilm formation by a variety of bacteria and fungi not normally found in the sinuses (i.e., dysbiosis of the sinuses). Although fluctuations in these microbial populations may cause symptom flares that merit antibiotic therapy, chronic rhinosinusitis per se is not mediated by infection and may not benefit from chronic antibiotic therapy [3–5].

This chapter will discuss the diagnosis and management of those cases of serious infection which do warrant systemic antibiotic therapy, with particular attention to recalcitrant chronic rhinosinusitis, i.e., those cases of chronic rhinosinusitis that fail to respond to adequate surgery, intranasal corticosteroid treatment, and up to two short courses of antibiotics or systemic corticosteroids in the prior year; importantly, this definition does not specify receipt of previous culture-directed therapy [1].

When Is Recalcitrant Chronic Rhinosinusitis Infectious?

When considering further antibiotic therapy for persons with recalcitrant chronic rhinosinusitis, it is important to consider the reasons for failure of prior antibiotic therapy and whether symptom flares are due to infectious or noninfectious causes. Failure of antimicrobial therapy in an infection may be due to (1) failure to identify the pathogenic organism, (2) pathogen resistance to antimicrobial therapy, (3) anatomic complications of infections (e.g., osteomyelitis), (4) inadequate source control, (5) suboptimal antimicrobial bioavailability or dosing, or (6) insufficient duration of therapy. Notably, despite microbial colonization of the sinuses, recalcitrant disease need not be due to infection, rendering any antimicrobial therapy ineffective in symptom abatement [5]. The overlap between chronic rhinosinusitis, chronic recalcitrant rhinosinusitis, and chronic infectious rhinosinusitis is shown in Fig. 21.1.

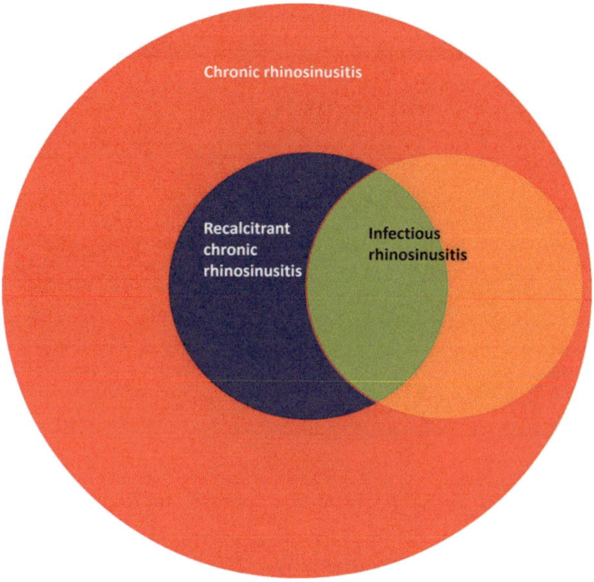

Fig. 21.1 Infectious rhinosinusitis and the overlap between chronic and recalcitrant disease. Chronic rhinosinusitis is described as the waxing and waning presence of symptoms; ongoing inadequate control of symptoms despite multimodal interventions (steroids, antibiotics, surgery) has led to the description of recalcitrant disease. Acute worsening of symptoms (described as flares) can result from either acute infection (infectious rhinosinusitis) or other noninfectious triggers

Before committing a patient with recalcitrant chronic rhinosinusitis to additional antibiotic therapy, it is important to confirm the infectious etiology of a flare by verifying the presence of both a compatible clinical syndrome and causative pathogen. However, determining whether antibiotic therapy is warranted is often difficult. First, the symptoms of infectious chronic rhinosinusitis and noninfectious flares of chronic rhinosinusitis, e.g., rhinorrhea, mucopurulence, altered sense of smell, facial pain, and nasal obstruction, overlap. Additionally, identification of the responsible infectious pathogen(s) may be challenging due to the indistinct boundaries between colonization and infection and the presence of polymicrobial biofilms [6] in the setting of dysbiosis of the sinuses [4, 5]. Both the clinical context and pathogen identification are essential for determining if an organism is a true cause of infection or an innocent bystander. Although making a precise clinical and microbiological diagnosis is difficult, this is of great clinical importance, as unnecessary or prolonged antimicrobial therapy carries the risks of side effects and promotes colonization of the sinus by resistant pathogens.

If the patient is clinically stable, the differential diagnoses listed in Table 21.1 should be evaluated prior to initiating antimicrobial therapy for infectious rhinosinusitis flare. As this chapter will focus on the indications for usage of intravenous antibiotic therapy, we will not cover noninfectious causes for flares of chronic rhinosinusitis in depth.

Table 21.1 Chronic rhinosinusitis symptoms and the infectious differential diagnosis

Infectious differential of chronic rhinosinusitis flares
Viral rhinosinusitis
– Coronaviruses including *SARS-CoV-2*
– *Rhinovirus*
– *Influenza*
– *Adenovirus*
– *Parainfluenza*
Bacterial rhinosinusitis
– *Streptococcus pneumoniae*
– Oral S*treptococcus* spp.
– *Haemophilus influenzae*
– *Moraxella catarrhalis*
– *Staphylococcus aureus*
– *Enterobacterales*
– *Pseudomonas aeruginosa*
– *Burkholderia cepacia complex*
– Mixed aerobic and anaerobic infection
Fungal rhinosinusitis
– Invasive: *Zygomycetes*, *Aspergillus*, *Fusarium*
– Allergic: *Aspergillus*, *Alternaria*
Uncommon pathogens
– *Klebsiella ozaenae*
– Atypical mycobacteria

Chronic rhinosinusitis symptoms can represent a wide range of diagnostic possibilities. Although this list focuses on microbiological causes, it is important to also consider the noninfectious differential of these symptoms. This is inclusive of diagnoses such as nonallergic rhinitis, allergic rhinitis, allergic fungal rhinosinusitis, structural abnormalities (septal perforation, nasal valve dysfunction, septal deviation, adenoidal hypertrophy), neuralgia, vascular etiology, trauma, neoplasm, congenital causes, and temporal arteritis [51]

Predisposing Risk Factors in Infectious Chronic Rhinosinusitis

Chronic rhinosinusitis is characterized by disruption of epithelial barriers, disturbances in the normal sinus flora (dysbiosis), and chronic inflammation, all of which increase the risk of acute infectious exacerbations [7]. Tissue disruption in the sinuses, incited by viral infections, atrophic rhinitis, and anatomic disruption (nasal cavity deformation, neoplasms, nasal polyposis, trauma, surgery) further increase susceptibility to biofilm formation, fluctuating polymicrobial colonization of the sinuses, and progression to complicated infection by organisms not typically seen in acute bacterial rhinosinusitis, especially in the setting of a recurrent course of antibiotic therapy [4]. A similar sequence of events occurs in patients with mechanical dysfunction of mucociliary clearance e.g., primary ciliary dyskinesia and cystic fibrosis.

Specific immunologic defects also predispose to recurrent infections. Patients with a primary immunodeficiency, such as complement deficiencies, immunoglobulin G deficiency, immunoglobulin A deficiency, or common variable immunodeficiency (CVID), have a high risk of frequent, recurrent infections, including rhinosinusitis [8], with more severe disease presentations. More severe and/or unusual infections can also be seen in persons receiving immunosuppressant therapy, such as patients with organ transplantation, those on therapy with agents such as rituximab or chronic steroid therapy, or those with bone marrow suppression due to cytotoxic therapy for malignancies, poorly controlled diabetes, or advanced HIV infection.

Altogether, compromised host defenses, whether due to tissue disruption, immunologic factors, or impaired mucociliary clearance, increase the risk of recurrent infections, progression to complicated infection, and repeated antimicrobial therapy exposure, accompanied by sinus colonization with resistant organisms and subsequent difficult-to-treat infections.

The Ecology and Microbiology of Infectious Chronic Rhinosinusitis

The organisms comprising the normal sinonasal microbiome are highly diverse. In comparison with chronic rhinosinusitis, there is replacement of this normal flora with a more restricted range of organisms. A growing body of evidence indicates that replacement of the normal diverse microbiome is both a consequence of chronic inflammation and prior antibiotic use and a risk factor for recurrent disease flares [5, 9]. Although acute bacterial rhinosinusitis is typically caused by *Streptococcus pneumonia*, *Haemophilus influenzae*, or *Moraxella catarrhalis* [9], the microbiology of chronic rhinosinusitis infection more often involves methicillin-sensitive and methicillin-resistant *Staphylococcus aureus* (MSSA and MRSA), gram-negative organisms including *Pseudomonas aeruginosa*, and anaerobes [4]. Anatomic disruption also affects the sinus flora, for example, exposure to bisphosphonate therapy can result in oroantral fistula from osteonecrosis of the maxilla [10], with subsequent polymicrobial infection due to oral flora. A careful history of the insults and exposures to the sinonasal environment can broaden the microbial differential for the infectious etiology of a rhinosinusitis exacerbation.

Underlying chronic diseases also impact the microbial composition of the sinus flora. In cystic fibrosis, the upper airways can be colonized with MRSA, *P. aeruginosa*, or *Burkholderia* species, which can lead to infection [11]. Patients with poorly controlled diabetes, chronic steroid use, or malignancy not only have frequent, recurrent bacterial infections but are also at risk for more rare invasive fungal diseases of the sinuses, similar to patients with hematopoietic stem cell transplants [12]. A high index of suspicion for *Mucorales* infection is important, as it is extremely destructive and rapidly progressive, and aggressive treatment can be lifesaving. Rarely, atypical mycobacteria [13, 14], *Nocardia* spp. [15], or even protozoa [16] can be the responsible pathogens and require specialized microbiological processing and cultures. Concern for infection by these pathogens should prompt consultation with infectious disease pharmacists to guide antibiotic selection, given the potential for breeding further resistance.

Finally, specific environmental exposures can increase the risk of more atypical infections. Both freshwater swimming and contaminated nasal irrigation can predispose individuals to amoebic disease, with a risk of developing amoebic meningoencephalitis [16]. Occupational exposures such as exposure to work in soil, hay, and freshwater sources can increase the risk of fungal rhinosinusitis with *Scedosporium* spp. [17] Additionally, substance use can provide an opportunity for organisms not intrinsic to the nasal passages to infect the sinuses, either by direct introduction or disruption of anatomy (e.g., smoking marijuana and *Aspergillus* sinus disease; cocaine resulting in septal perforation; tobacco resulting in increased inflammation and risk for neoplasms).

Anatomically Complicated Infections

Inadequate source control can lead to ongoing infection, secondary complications, and antibiotic resistance. Identifying and controlling the source of infection is especially important in complicated infections that originate outside the sinuses or extend from the sinuses into other tissues. For example, pathogen-directed therapy based on cultures from direct aspiration of the maxillary sinus may still result in treatment failure if an odontogenic infection, such as a periapical abscess with sinus extension, is not addressed with adequate drainage. Alternatively, infection can be complicated by bacteremia, extension from the sinuses into the orbits, abscess development, erosion into the bone (osteomyelitis), or extension into the brain, leading to meningitis, intracranial abscess, or cavernous sinus thrombosis. Diagnosis of these secondary complications requires a high level of clinical suspicion. Clinical symptoms and exam findings should be reviewed for alarm signs (Table 21.2), including headaches, loss of vision, and meningismus. Infectious disease consultation is recommended to guide antimicrobial therapy in these populations.

Imaging is essential in defining the anatomic involvement of infection, guiding surgical intervention, and selecting antimicrobial therapy effective within the infected space. Comprehensive computed tomography including imaging of the brain in addition to the sinuses or orbits should be considered [18]. Contrast media may be helpful in evaluating for complications such as cavernous sinus thrombosis or abscess. Magnetic resonance imaging can be very useful in identifying complications such as intracranial abscess, orbital complications, or invasive fungal sinusitis [18]. Further specialist consultation can be helpful in determining appropriate diagnostics and therapeutics.

Table 21.2 Alarm symptoms in chronic rhinosinusitis and associated infectious complications

Alarm signs and symptoms	Complications of rhinosinusitis
Neurologic deficits Severe headache	Intracranial abscess Bacterial meningitis/encephalitis Superior sagittal and cavernous sinus thrombosis Subperiosteal abscess Epidural empyema Subdural empyema
Periorbital edema Diplopia/blindness	Pre-septal cellulitis Orbital cellulitis Orbital abscess
Neck pain/stiffness	Bacterial meningitis Lemierre's syndrome (septic thrombophlebitis)
Nasal/palatal eschar	Mucormycosis Necrosis
qSOFA[a] or SIRS[b] criteria: – Fever >38.0 °C or hypothermia <36.0 °C – Tachycardia >90 beats/min – Tachypnea >20 breaths/min – Leukocytosis $>12 \times 10^9$/l or leukopenia $<4 \times 10^9$/l – Altered mentation	Two or more signs indicate the presence of sepsis, complicating one of the above infections (e.g., sepsis)
Hypotension End-organ system dysfunction	Septic shock Toxic shock syndrome (group A *Streptococcus* infection)

Alarm signs or the documented presence of a complication from infectious rhinosinusitis should prompt an infectious disease consultation to assist with treatment
[a]SIRS: systemic inflammatory response syndrome
[b]qSOFA: quick sequential organ failure assessment

Identifying the Pathogen and Susceptibility

Pathogen identification and susceptibility testing are necessary to guide antibiotic treatment especially in the context of prior antibiotic therapy. Direct sampling for culture from the sites of infection provides the most relevant information. Superficial cultures of the nasal passages are not recommended, as they recover clinically irrelevant contaminants or commensal organisms; at a minimum, either endoscopic cultures of the middle meatus or direct aspiration of the sinuses via antral puncture should be obtained [19]. If there is concern for secondary complications, such as an abscess or osteomyelitis, attempts should be made to obtain cultures from these sources, e.g., cultures of abscess contents or bone biopsy to obtain bone cultures, if safe and feasible.

Obtaining multiple cultures allows for adequate material to be sent for specialized aerobic, anaerobic, fungal, mycobacterial, or nocardial cultures. Specifics on optimal specimen, method of collection, and specimen transport details are enumerated in the Guide to Utilization of the Microbiology Laboratory for Diagnosis of Infectious Diseases: 2018 Update by the Infectious Diseases Society of America and the American Society for Microbiology [19]. Although fresh tissue or fluid is necessary for culturing organisms for definitive identification and susceptibility testing, histologic examination of formalin-fixed tissues using specialized stains (e.g., Grocott's Methenamine Silver stain for fungi) can still aid in diagnosis [20].

Traditional cultures may demonstrate aerobic and anaerobic bacterial organism growth in days, whereas fungi and mycobacteria may require weeks of incubation for growth [21, 22]. If tissue availability is limited, both specialist consultation with infectious disease and the microbiology laboratory can help prioritize testing based on clinical likelihood. Apart from traditional culture media, rapid and advanced diagnostics have greatly assisted the identification and susceptibility testing of pathogens; many of these tests are now widely available. If no organism is identified by such means, frozen tissue can be sent to specialized referral laboratories for next-generation sequencing (NGS), wherein genetic material from the sample is amplified and sequenced to determine pathogen identification, virulence markers, and genes conferring antimicrobial resistance [23].

The identification of the pathogen responsible for a flare of recalcitrant rhinosinusitis is often challenging even when appropriate cultures are obtained. Not only are there issues related to potential sampling error, but also recalcitrant chronic rhinosinusitis is characterized by chronic dysbiosis, wherein the sinus flora has been shaped by prior antimicrobial therapy and polymicrobial biofilm formation [4]. Dysbiosis complicates the assessment of the contribution of any single organism to infectious syndromes, as the presence of symptoms may be due to the synergistic effects of multiple organisms and as symptomatic flares may reflect fluctuations in the relative density of organisms and associated inflammation [7, 24]. As is the case with other polymicrobial infections (e.g., aspiration pneumonia, intra-abdominal foot infections, bacterial vaginosis), therapeutic success does not necessarily require treatment of all identified microorganisms.

The Role of Intravenous Antimicrobial Therapy

There are no specific infectious disease guidelines for the use of empiric intravenous antimicrobial therapy in chronic rhinosinusitis. There is a dearth of high-quality studies examining the utility of intravenous antibiotics for chronic rhinosinusitis [5]; the literature is limited to small uncontrolled cohort studies with variable short-term success and high relapse rates [25–27]. A Cochrane review published in 2016 was not able to identify any randomized controlled trials of intravenous antibiotic therapy [28]. Reviews of the available cohort studies have concluded that in light of the reported complications of intravenous antibiotics agents for chronic rhinosinusitis, such as deep vein thrombosis, drug reactions, and other adverse effects [29], intravenous antibiotics should not be routinely used in chronic rhinosinusitis, with exceptions for acute infectious complications, such as intracranial or intra-orbital infections [25, 30]. As discussed earlier in Fig. 21.1, intravenous antibiotics are only beneficial in patients with rhinosinusitis flares that are caused by infection, and the risk-benefit profile of intravenous therapy supports its use only in documented, complicated, or invasive infections, where adequate tissue concentrations of effective antibiotics cannot be achieved by oral administration.

When to Start Empiric Intravenous Antimicrobial Therapy

Due to the variability of host factors and presentation of disease, our belief is that the best approach in treatment includes careful identification of anatomic involvement and causative organism by obtaining the results of cultures prior to initiating therapy. If the patient with suspected infection is clinically stable, it is appropriate to defer antimicrobial treatment and to expedite obtaining cultures for true culture-directed therapy.

The severity of illness; the likelihood of infectious complications, e.g., intracranial infection; and the presence of impaired host defenses that may predispose patients to rapid clinical progression should be the main considerations in deciding when and whether to start empiric antimicrobial therapy in chronic rhinosinusitis. Empiric antibiotic therapy is necessary in patients who have severe presentations (i.e., symptoms noted in Table 21.2) or life-threatening or complicated infections, such as meningoencephalitis, orbital involvement, epidural or subdural empyema, brain abscess, or bacteremia. Notably, individuals meeting at least two of the systemic inflammatory reaction syndrome criteria (fever >38.0 °C or hypothermia <36.0 °C, tachycardia >90 beats/minute, tachypnea >20 breaths/minute, leukocytosis $>12 \times 10^9$/l, or leukopenia $<4 \times 10^9$/l) may have developed sepsis, complicating one of the above infections [31]. When accompanied by hypotension or end-organ system dysfunction, these findings indicate the presence of septic shock and should prompt urgent initiation of antibiotics; consultation with infectious disease is highly recommended. Host risk factors may lower the threshold for treatment given the potential risk for complications. Special populations such as those with cystic fibrosis, those with primary ciliary dyskinesia, and those who are profoundly immunosuppressed (e.g., organ transplantation, poorly controlled diabetes, and primary immunodeficiency) have an increased risk for severe, extensive infection with risk for progression with secondary complications and catastrophic consequences including hospitalization, transplant organ loss, or death. The prevention of these outcomes is essential.

If sepsis is present or the infection is complicated, e.g., osteomyelitis of surrounding bone or concern for necrosis and decreased blood supply, preference should be given to initiating intravenous antimicrobial therapy to ensure rapid antimicrobial activity and adequate concentrations of effective antibiotics at the site of infection. When considering severe complications of infectious rhinosinusitis such as intraocular infection or intracranial penetration, infectious disease specialist involvement is recommended.

Prior to starting empiric intravenous therapy, it is essential to draw two sets of blood cultures; sinus cultures should be obtained as soon as possible. The use of intravenous antibiotics with activity against gram-positive (*Staphylococcus* spp. and *Streptococcus* spp.) and gram-negative (*Enterobacterales* and *P. aeruginosa*) bacteria is often appropriate, given the risk of resistant organisms due to the frequent prior use of antibiotics in this patient population; however, the risk of emerging antimicrobial resistance must be weighed, as there may be few options to treat a future infection with a highly resistant organism.

By definition, patients with recalcitrant disease have been exposed to prior antimicrobial therapy. Consequently, presentation of an acute infectious flare inevitably leads to concern about infection by organisms resistant to narrow-spectrum antibiotics. However, consideration needs to be given to the particulars of the patient. The best predictor of infection by resistant organisms is prior infection or colonization by that organism [32]. Other considerations include repeated exposures to specific antibiotics. Examples include the selection of fluoroquinolone-resistant flora (and, for complex reasons, MRSA) due to prior fluoroquinolone exposure [33] and the selection of extended-spectrum beta-lactamase (ESBL)-producing organisms, such as *Klebsiella* or *E. coli*, by frequent use of penicillins and cephalosporins, which then require therapy with a carbapenem [34]. In addition to antimicrobial susceptibilities on the individual level, community-level susceptibilities and nosocomial exposures should be considered when choosing empiric treatment. Local hospital antibiograms that report the prevalence of resistant organisms in various settings (inpatient versus outpatient clinics) can guide empiric antibiotic selection.

Finally, the severity of infection does not correlate with antimicrobial resistance. Pathogens such as fully susceptible *Staphylococcus* spp. and *Streptococcus* spp. can cause life-threatening infections in persons with normal host defenses and even more so in select populations, such as patients with primary immunodeficiencies, including complement deficiencies, immunoglobulin G deficiency, immunoglobulin A deficiency, or common variable immunodeficiency (CVID), or those with poorly controlled HIV infection. Options for empiric intravenous antimicrobial therapy for adequate coverage are provided in Table 21.3.

Table 21.3 Empiric intravenous and oral antimicrobial therapy

Suspected pathogens	Intravenous therapy	Oral therapy
MRSA	Vancomycin 15 mg/kg IV loading dose* Daptomycin 8 mg/kg IV q24h Linezolid 600 mg IV q12h Ceftaroline 600 mg IV q12h*	Doxycycline 100 mg PO q12h Minocycline 100 mg PO q12h Trimethoprim/sulfamethoxazole 160 mg/800 mg PO q12h* Linezolid 600 mg PO q12h
MSSA	Oxacillin 2 g IV q6h Cefazolin 1 g IV q8h* Also covered by MRSA agents	Cefadroxil 500 g PO q12h Cephalexin 500 mg PO q6h Amoxicillin/clavulanate * 875 mg/125 mg PO q12h Also covered by MRSA agents

(continued)

Table 21.3 (continued)

Suspected pathogens	Intravenous therapy	Oral therapy
Oral streptococci *Streptococcus pneumoniae* *Haemophilus influenzae* *Moraxella catarrhalis*	Cefuroxime 750 mg IV q8h* Ceftriaxone 1 g IV q24h Ampicillin/sulbactam 3 g IV q6h* Levofloxacin 500 mg IV q12h* Moxifloxacin 400 mg IV q24h	Amoxicillin/clavulanate* 875 mg/125 mg PO q12h Cefuroxime 250 mg PO q12h Cefpodoxime 200 mg PO q12h* Levofloxacin 500 mg PO daily* Moxifloxacin 400 mg PO q24h
Enterobacterales (if resistance is not suspected)	Ceftriaxone 1 g IV q24h	Cefpodoxime 200 mg PO q12h Trimethoprim/sulfamethoxazole 160 mg/800 mg PO q12h Ciprofloxacin 500 mg PO q12h
Enterobacterales (if resistance IS suspected, e.g., extended-spectrum beta-lactamase	Ertapenem* 1 g IV q24h Meropenem* 1 g IV q8h	Trimethoprim/sulfamethoxazole 160 mg/800 mg PO q12h* Ciprofloxacin 500 mg PO q12h*
P. aeruginosa	Ciprofloxacin 400 mg IV q8h* Levofloxacin 750 mg IV q12h* Cefepime 2 g IV q8h* Ceftazidime 2 g IV q8h* Piperacillin/tazobactam 3.375 g IV q12h* Meropenem 1 g IV q8h* Aztreonam 2gm IV q8h* (if true penicillin/cephalosporin allergy is present)	Ciprofloxacin 750 mg PO q12h* Levofloxacin 750 mg PO q12h*
**Mucorales/Zygomycetes	Liposomal amphotericin 5–10 mg/kg IV q24h	Posaconazole Isavuconazole

In the setting of increased severity of disease or highly complicated infections (e.g., intra-orbital infections, empiric intravenous therapy should be initiated to ensure adequate tissue concentrations of effective antibiotics. Intravenous antibiotic therapy should target suspected pathogens based on individual host risk factors, prior cultures, and local antibiograms, which can indicate risk for resistance. In the presence of invasive fungal disease, an infectious disease specialist should be consulted to guide dose and duration, in conjunction with prompt surgical management. Patients with ongoing symptoms indicating infection and pending microbiologic culture data may benefit from the initiation of empiric oral therapy if clinically stable in the outpatient setting. Again, the selection of empiric therapy should be guided by prior culture data if available, as well as local antibiograms. Clindamycin is not favored as empiric therapy due to inducible resistance in *S. aureus* and potential difficulties with tolerability. For critically ill patients, dosing adjustment should be determined in consultation with pharmacists and infectious disease specialists.

*Renal dosing adjustments needed

**Infectious disease consultation strongly recommended. Oral agents for mucorales/zygomycetes should not be used for acute, uncontrolled disease prior to surgical intervention.

Empiric Oral Antimicrobial Therapy

Whereas empiric intravenous therapy is justifiable for persons with severe disease, culture-directed therapy is strongly preferred in persons with non-severe disease for whom, when there is an indication for antibiotics, oral antimicrobial therapy is usually appropriate. In the occasional circumstances that warrant empiric oral antimicrobial therapy without waiting for culture and susceptibility results, we recommend following the choices listed in Table 21.3 while taking into consideration prior culture results and historical risk factors as discussed in the previous section on intravenous antibiotic therapy. A synopsis of international guideline recommendations for oral antibiotics in persons with chronic rhinosinusitis has been recently published [5].

Oral Versus Intravenous Therapy

Antimicrobial therapy, when tailored to the pathogen and anatomic location to ensure tissue penetration, can be efficacious as either oral or intravenous therapy. For example, recent studies have shown that oral antimicrobial therapy, when selected on the basis of oral bioavailability and activity in the infected space, is non-inferior to intravenous therapy in the treatment of endocarditis and osteomyelitis [35, 36]. Thus, while appropriate for uncomplicated cases of infection, oral therapy is also an important therapeutic option for patients with chronic rhinosinusitis complicated by osteomyelitis and other severe disease manifestations, who have achieved clinical stability after an initial course of intravenous antibiotics and any necessary surgical interventions.

Therapeutic Considerations for Specific Pathogens

Staphylococcus

S. aureus is a commonly found pathogen in chronic rhinosinusitis that may form biofilms and cause recurrent infections [4, 37]. MRSA is a concern, especially in patients with prior MRSA colonization or infection, repeated prior antimicrobial use, or nosocomial infections. Active intravenous antimicrobials against MRSA include vancomycin and daptomycin; decreased activity or resistance to either of these agents is unusual and, when found, should prompt infectious disease consultation. Methicillin-susceptible *S. aureus* (MSSA) is best treated with either oxacillin or a first-generation cephalosporin such as cefazolin, though oxacillin is superior if there is concern for intracranial infection.

Coagulase-negative staphylococci, e.g., *Staphylococcus epidermidis*, are common commensal organisms or "skin contaminants." Recovery of these organisms can represent sampling error or colonization. However, heavy growth of coagulase-negative staphylococci in multiple, appropriately obtained cultures may represent true infection and warrant treatment. Methicillin resistance among different coagulase-negative *Staphylococcus* spp. has become more prevalent over time, making vancomycin or daptomycin appropriate treatment choices while awaiting definitive susceptibility test results [38].

Streptococcus

Streptococcus pneumoniae is a common pathogen in acute bacterial sinusitis and contributes to acute bacterial exacerbations of chronic rhinosinusitis as well. Invasive disease is particularly a concern in persons with defects in antibody or complement production (e.g., common variable hypogammaglobulinemia or complement deficiency states), who are at an increased risk of meningitis and bacteremia. Fully vaccinated individuals have good protection against severe infection with this organism. Resistance to penicillin as well as ceftriaxone is increasing, but in most parts of the world, it is a concern primarily in intracranial infections [39]; although both vancomycin and linezolid remain active against *S. pneumoniae*, infectious disease consultation should be obtained to assure appropriate dosing in these complex infections.

Streptococcus pyogenes (i.e., group A streptococci) is part of the beta-hemolytic streptococcus group. It is commonly a cause of pharyngitis, and its presence in the oral flora can be a risk factor for sinus infection. Though it is reliably sensitive to penicillin and cephalosporins, when complicated by necrotizing fasciitis or toxic shock syndrome, the addition of clindamycin to halt toxin production is strongly recommended.

Although often grouped with viridans streptococci, *Streptococcus anginosus* and its similar counterparts, *Streptococcus intermedius* and *Streptococcus constellatus*, are particularly virulent and invasive, with a tendency to metastasize to various organ systems (typically the brain, lungs, and liver) and form abscesses should it become a bloodstream infection [40]. The presence of these organisms on culture should prompt a more thorough evaluation to confirm whether infection is localized or complicated, as source control will impact treatment. *S. anginosus* is adequately treated by penicillins or cephalosporins; most microbiology labs will not perform susceptibility testing due to the reliability of antibiotic activity.

Other viridans group streptococci bacteria are associated with the oropharynx and are a common cause of odontogenic infections and can be either commensals or true pathogens [41]. These are sensitive to penicillins and cephalosporins.

Enterococcus

Although *Enterococcus faecalis* and *E. faecium* are rarely the root cause of flares of chronic rhinosinusitis, they have the potential to result in invasive infection in immunocompromised hosts. Susceptibility testing is essential for appropriate treatment, as vancomycin resistance is becoming increasingly common, particularly in

E. faecium. *E. faecalis* is more reliably sensitive to ampicillin; in penicillin-allergic patients, vancomycin, daptomycin, and linezolid are alternative agents. When vancomycin resistance is detected, antimicrobials should be selected based on susceptibility data; generally, daptomycin and linezolid (available in both intravenous and oral forms) are reliable options. Of note, the susceptibility to daptomycin can be dose-dependent and may require very high doses (10–12 mg/kg) in life-threatening infections.

Enterobacterales

Enterobacterales is a family of enteric organisms that includes *Enterobacter* spp., *Citrobacter* spp., *Klebsiella* spp., and *Escherichia coli*. Although uncommonly seen in healthy sinus flora, these organisms are more common colonizers in chronic rhinosinusitis and have the propensity to cause infection [42]. Importantly, these organisms along with *Serratia marcescens* and *Acinetobacter baumannii* can develop inducible resistance by producing extended-spectrum beta-lactamases, leading to cephalosporin resistance and necessitating treatment with broader-spectrum antibiotics, such as carbapenems [34].

Pseudomonas

P. aeruginosa is a gram-negative organism with diverse drug resistance mechanisms including inducible resistance gene expression (beta-lactamases), efflux pumps, and altered permeability to antimicrobials [43]. The effectiveness of antibiotic therapy is further adversely affected by biofilm formation particularly in persons with mucociliary disorders and/or multiple courses of prior antibiotic therapy. Due to the frequency of resistance, the selection of therapy should be susceptibility-dependent. Although piperacillin/tazobactam, cefepime, aztreonam, and meropenem can often be used for *P. aeruginosa*, more resistant isolates may require consideration of aminoglycosides (e.g., tobramycin), colistin, or newer agents, as discussed below.

Other Gram-Negative Organisms

Haemophilus influenzae and *Moraxella catarrhalis* are commonly implicated in acute bacterial rhinosinusitis but can also cause acute exacerbations of chronic rhinosinusitis [42]. Although vaccination has reduced the incidence of *H. influenzae* type B, type A and other nontypeable strains are increasingly causes of invasive infection [44]. For both *H. influenzae* and *M. catarrhalis*, beta-lactamase presence (indicating penicillin resistance) is common [45]. Beta-lactam/beta-lactamase inhibitor combinations such as ampicillin/sulbactam or third-generation cephalosporins can be especially efficacious when susceptibility is unknown.

Eikenella corrodens is present in the human oral flora and can be a source of periodontal infections. In cases of odontogenic sources of rhinosinusitis flares, it is important to consider this organism, as clindamycin resistance is frequently seen [46]. *Eikenella* is usually seen in polymicrobial infections; therefore, third-generation cephalosporins such as ceftriaxone and beta-lactam/beta-lactamase inhibitor combinations (e.g., amoxicillin/clavulanate or ampicillin/sulbactam) can be helpful here as well, as they are active against oral anaerobes.

Anaerobes

The altered microbiota in chronic rhinosinusitis includes diverse anaerobes such as *Prevotella*, *Porphyromonas*, *Peptostreptococcus*, and *Fusobacterium* [7]. However, when recovered on appropriately obtained (i.e., anaerobic) cultures, specific antibiotic therapy is usually not necessary, unless there is abscess formation or tissue necrosis. Although penicillin, ceftriaxone, and clindamycin are suitable for some mixed aerobic-anaerobic infections, the addition of metronidazole or the use of a beta-lactam/beta-lactamase inhibitor combination (such as ampicillin/sulbactam and piperacillin/tazobactam) or, much less often, a carbapenem (e.g., ertapenem) is warranted in severe, complex infections. Monotherapy with metronidazole, an agent which has activity against only anaerobes, is not appropriate, as anaerobes are invariably part of a polymicrobial infection that requires antimicrobial coverage beyond the anaerobic spectrum.

Multidrug-Resistant Organisms

The emergence of highly resistant organisms is an increasing societal problem [47–49]. Some of these phenotypes are still rare, such as vancomycin-resistant *S. aureus*; however, others are increasingly more prevalent, such as meropenem-resistant *Acinetobacter baumannii*, *Burkholderia cepacia* complex (especially in persons with cystic fibrosis), and carbapenemase-producing carbapenem-resistant *Enterobacterales* (e.g., carbapenem-resistant *K. pneumoniae*). Recently developed antibiotics, such as ceftolozane-tazobactam, meropenem-vaborbactam, ceftazidime-avibactam, eravacycline, and cefiderocol can be lifesaving, but resistance to these antimicrobials has also occurred. The presence of multidrug-resistant organisms on cultures necessitates infectious disease consultation, as patients with true infection may require combination therapy for treatment.

Candida and Other Fungal Pathogens

Often, in patients with a history of recent broad-spectrum antibiotics, or those with specific immunodeficiencies, bacterial cultures may yield growth of *Candida* species, even though *Candida* is a fungus. In the absence of oral candidiasis (thrush), or another complication (such as an abscess) where *Candida* may also be cultured, it should be regarded as a colonizer or contaminate and not treated unless tissue invasion is demonstrated by histopathology.

While fungal rhinosinusitis will not be discussed in detail, it is important to recognize when the clinical picture, cultures, or imaging studies indicate the presence of other fungal organisms, such as *Aspergillus* and zygomycetes. When mycobacteria are isolated, infectious disease consultation can aid in determining if these results are contaminant, local infection, allergy-mediated disease, or invasive infection and if therapy should be initiated.

Treatment Duration and Other Complicating Factors

For a bacterial flare of chronic rhinosinusitis without complications such as abscess, osteomyelitis or other disease extending beyond the sinuses, a reasonable treatment duration is 7–10 days, especially if adequate drainage of the sinuses is achieved and an appropriate clinical response to antibiotics is demonstrated. Complicating factors such as osteomyelitis, abscess formation, or invasive disease such as bacteremia, ocular/orbital involvement, or extension to the brain may require further imaging, surgical debridement, and/or source control prior to determining the antibiotic course duration. Any concern for possible prolongation of therapy may warrant further discussion with an infectious disease consultant for guidance.

The role of extended antimicrobial therapy duration to decrease inflammation by altering the composition of the sinus microbiota in chronic rhinosinusitis remains to be fully defined. Macrolides, typically administered orally, are considered to have an anti-inflammatory effect. There may be a role for these antibiotics for this anti-inflammatory effect rather than for pathogen-directed therapy [5].

Antimicrobial Stewardship

Antimicrobial stewardship is of utmost importance given that antibiotic overuse drives the emergence of drug-resistant organisms and can greatly limit treatment choices that require the use of less convenient and/or more toxic antibiotics; in worst case scenarios, there is no effective therapy. The first step in stewardship is to ensure the accuracy of the diagnosis of infection and the identity of the responsible microorganism(s). Next is the prudent selection of empiric antibiotic therapy to avoid unnecessarily broad-spectrum therapy. When the pathogen is identified, prompt de-escalation of broad-spectrum antimicrobial therapy in favor of pathogen-directed therapy is strongly recommended. These measures, combined with limiting the duration of therapy to decrease perturbation of the normal sinus microbiome, can mitigate the emergence of resistant organisms and the risk of individual treatment side effects (such as eosinophilic pneumonia from daptomycin or tendinopathy with fluoroquinolone usage) or the emergence of *Clostridium difficile*-associated diarrheal illness [50].

Although long-term therapy is needed in complex cases such as osteomyelitis, prescribing long-term intravenous antibiotic therapy is fraught with its own complications. Administration of intravenous therapy often requires prolonged hospitalizations, with prolonged length of stay due to either coordination for home health delivery of antibiotics or due to potential delays in obtaining a peripherally inserted central catheter for home administration. Peripherally inserted central catheters carry their own risk of complications such as associated thrombosis, line infection, or cellulitis. Home intravenous antibiotic administration also requires consideration of antimicrobial cold storage, patient education and health literacy, coordination of durable medical equipment, and home health nursing for laboratory monitoring of drug levels and safety, as well as possible administration of antimicrobial therapy if the patient or caregivers are unable to do so. Intravenous antibiotics administered at home should always be monitored by a physician, and ideally a pharmacist and nursing staff to assist in coordination of care delivery and safety monitoring, as the potential longer-term complications of home intravenous antibiotics include eosinophilia, acute kidney injury, transaminase elevation, or other medication-specific complications. When appropriate, oral therapy should be used to avoid many of these complications.

References

1. Fokkens WJ, Lund VJ, Hopkins C, Hellings PW, Kern R, Reitsma S, et al. European position paper on rhinosinusitis and nasal polyps 2020. Rhinology. 2020;58(Suppl S29):1–464.
2. Desrosiers M, Evans GA, Keith PK, Wright ED, Kaplan A, Bouchard J, et al. Canadian clinical practice guidelines for acute and chronic rhinosinusitis. Allergy Asthma Clin Immunol. 2011;7(1):2.
3. Rosenfeld RM, Piccirillo JF, Chandrasekhar SS, Brook I, Ashok Kumar K, Kramper M, et al. Clinical practice guideline (update): adult sinusitis. Otolaryngol Head Neck Surg. 2015;152(2 Suppl):S1–S39.
4. Brook I. Microbiology of chronic rhinosinusitis. Eur J Clin Microbiol Infect Dis. 2016;35(7):1059–68.
5. Smith SS, Kim R, Douglas R. Is there a role for antibiotics in the treatment of chronic rhinosinusitis? J Allergy Clin Immunol. 2022;149(5):1504–12.
6. Al-Mutairi D, Kilty SJ. Bacterial biofilms and the pathophysiology of chronic rhinosinusitis. Curr Opin Allergy Clin Immunol. 2011;11(1):18–23.
7. Wu D, Bleier BS, Wei Y. Current understanding of the acute exacerbation of chronic rhinosinusitis. Front Cell Infect Microbiol. 2019;9:415.
8. Sedaghat AR, Kuan EC, Scadding GK. Epidemiology of chronic rhinosinusitis: prevalence and risk factors. J Allergy Clin Immunol Pract. 2022;10(6):1395–403.
9. Biswas K, Hoggard M, Jain R, Taylor MW, Douglas RG. The nasal microbiota in health and disease: variation within and between subjects. Front Microbiol. 2015;9:134.
10. Hwang CS, Lee C, Chae HS, Han C, Yang HW, Lee YS, et al. Characteristics of chronic maxillary sinusitis in patients with a history of long-term bisphosphonate use. Am J Rhinol Allergy. 2019;33(5):500–6.
11. Chaaban MR, Kejner A, Rowe SM, Woodworth BA. Cystic fibrosis chronic rhinosinusitis: a comprehensive review. Am J Rhinol Allergy. 2013;27(5):387–95.

12. Marty FM, Cosimi LA, Baden LR. Breakthrough zygomycosis after voriconazole treatment in recipients of hematopoietic stem-cell transplants. N Engl J Med. 2004;350(9):950–2.
13. Hicks MD, Karempelis PS, Janus SC. Mycobacterium chelonae sinusitis in an immunocompetent adult. JAMA Otolaryngol Head Neck Surg. 2016;142(8):805–6.
14. Tichenor WS, Thurlow J, McNulty S, Brown-Elliott BA, Wallace RJ Jr, Falkinham JO 3rd. Nontuberculous Mycobacteria in household plumbing as possible cause of chronic rhinosinusitis. Emerg Infect Dis. 2012;18(10):1612–7.
15. Katz P, Fauci AS. Nocardia asteroides sinusitis. Presentation as a trimethoprim-sulfamethoxazole responsive fever of unknown origin. JAMA. 1977;238(22):2397–8.
16. Kofman A, Guarner J. Infections caused by free-living amoebae. J Clin Microbiol. 2022;60(1):e0022821.
17. Naik PP, Bhatt K, Richards EC, Bates T, Jahshan F, Chavda SV, et al. A rare case of fungal rhinosinusitis caused by Scedosporium apiopermum. Head Neck Pathol. 2021;15(3):1059–63.
18. Mafee MF, Tran BH, Chapa AR. Imaging of rhinosinusitis and its complications: plain film, CT, and MRI. Clin Rev Allergy Immunol. 2006;30(3):165–86.
19. Miller JM, Binnicker MJ, Campbell S, Carroll KC, Chapin KC, Gilligan PH, et al. A guide to utilization of the microbiology laboratory for diagnosis of infectious diseases: 2018 update by the Infectious Diseases Society of America and the American Society for Microbiology. Clin Infect Dis. 2018;67(6):e1–e94.
20. Guarner J, Brandt ME. Histopathologic diagnosis of fungal infections in the 21st century. Clin Microbiol Rev. 2011;24(2):247–80.
21. Bosshard PP. Incubation of fungal cultures: how long is long enough? Mycoses. 2011;54(5):e539–45.
22. Pfyffer GE, Wittwer F. Incubation time of mycobacterial cultures: how long is long enough to issue a final negative report to the clinician? J Clin Microbiol. 2012;50(12):4188–9.
23. Gautam SS, Kc R, Leong KW, Mac Aogáin M, O'Toole RF. A step-by-step beginner's protocol for whole genome sequencing of human bacterial pathogens. J Biol Methods. 2019;6(1):e110.
24. Cho DY, Hunter RC, Ramakrishnan VR. The microbiome and chronic rhinosinusitis. Immunol Allergy Clin N Am. 2020;40(2):251–63.
25. Tanner SB, Fowler KC. Intravenous antibiotics for chronic rhinosinusitis: are they effective? Curr Opin Otolaryngol Head Neck Surg. 2004;12(1):3–8.
26. Anand V, Levine H, Friedman M, Krespi Y, Panje W, Schettino R, et al. Intravenous antibiotics for refractory rhinosinusitis in nonsurgical patients: preliminary findings of a prospective study. Am J Rhinol. 2003;17(6):363–8.
27. Fowler KC, Duncavage JA, Murray JJ, Tanner S. Chronic sinusitis and intravenous antibiotic therapy: resolution, recurrence, and adverse events. J Allergy Clin Immunol. 2003;111(2):S85.
28. Head K, Chong LY, Piromchai P, Hopkins C, Philpott C, Schilder AG, et al. Systemic and topical antibiotics for chronic rhinosinusitis. Cochrane Database Syst Rev. 2016;4(4):CD011994.
29. Lin JW, Kacker A, Anand VK, Levine H. Catheter- and antibiotic-related complications of ambulatory intravenous antibiotic therapy for chronic refractory rhinosinusitis. Am J Rhinol. 2005;19(4):365–9.
30. Soler ZM, Oyer SL, Kern RC, Senior BA, Kountakis SE, Marple BF, et al. Antimicrobials and chronic rhinosinusitis with or without polyposis in adults: an evidenced-based review with recommendations. Int Forum Allergy Rhinol. 2013;3(1):31–47.
31. Comstedt P, Storgaard M, Lassen AT. The systemic inflammatory response syndrome (SIRS) in acutely hospitalised medical patients: a cohort study. Scand J Trauma Resusc Emerg Med. 2009;17:67.
32. Jones BE, Brown KA, Jones MM, Huttner BD, Greene T, Sauer BC, et al. Variation in empiric coverage versus detection of methicillin-resistant Staphylococcus aureus and Pseudomonas aeruginosa in hospitalizations for community-onset pneumonia across 128 US veterans affairs medical centers. Infect Control Hosp Epidemiol. 2017;38(8):937–44.
33. Couderc C, Jolivet S, Thiebaut AC, Ligier C, Remy L, Alvarez AS, et al. Fluoroquinolone use is a risk factor for methicillin-resistant Staphylococcus aureus acquisition in long-term care facilities: a nested case-case-control study. Clin Infect Dis. 2014;59(2):206–15.

34. Harris PNA, Tambyah PA, Lye DC, Mo Y, Lee TH, Yilmaz M, et al. Effect of Piperacillin-Tazobactam vs Meropenem on 30-day mortality for patients with E coli or Klebsiella pneumoniae bloodstream infection and ceftriaxone resistance: a randomized clinical trial. JAMA. 2018;320(10):984–94.
35. Li HK, Rombach I, Zambellas R, Walker AS, McNally MA, Atkins BL, et al. Oral versus intravenous antibiotics for bone and joint infection. N Engl J Med. 2019;380(5):425–36.
36. Iversen K, Ihlemann N, Gill SU, Madsen T, Elming H, Jensen KT, et al. Partial oral versus intravenous antibiotic treatment of endocarditis. N Engl J Med. 2019;380(5):415–24.
37. Prince AA, Steiger JD, Khalid AN, Dogrhamji L, Reger C, Eau Claire S, et al. Prevalence of biofilm-forming bacteria in chronic rhinosinusitis. Am J Rhinol. 2008;22(3):239–45.
38. Becker K, Heilmann C, Peters G. Coagulase-negative staphylococci. Clin Microbiol Rev. 2014;27(4):870–926.
39. Kim L, McGee L, Tomczyk S, Beall B. Biological and epidemiological features of antibiotic-resistant Streptococcus pneumoniae in pre- and post-conjugate vaccine eras: a United States perspective. Clin Microbiol Rev. 2016;29(3):525–52.
40. Claridge JE 3rd, Attorri S, Musher DM, Hebert J, Dunbar S. Streptococcus intermedius, Streptococcus constellatus, and Streptococcus anginosus ("Streptococcus milleri group") are of different clinical importance and are not equally associated with abscess. Clin Infect Dis. 2001;32(10):1511–5.
41. Doern CD, Burnham CA. It's not easy being green: the viridans group streptococci, with a focus on pediatric clinical manifestations. J Clin Microbiol. 2010;48(11):3829–35.
42. Brook I. Microbiology of sinusitis. Proc Am Thorac Soc. 2011;8(1):90–100.
43. Lister PD, Wolter DJ, Hanson ND. Antibacterial-resistant Pseudomonas aeruginosa: clinical impact and complex regulation of chromosomally encoded resistance mechanisms. Clin Microbiol Rev. 2009;22(4):582–610.
44. Soeters HM, Blain A, Pondo T, Doman B, Farley MM, Harrison LH, et al. Current epidemiology and trends in invasive haemophilus influenzae disease-United States, 2009-2015. Clin Infect Dis. 2018;67(6):881–9.
45. Beekmann SE, Heilmann KP, Richter SS, Garcia-de-Lomas J, Doern GV, Group GS. Antimicrobial resistance in Streptococcus pneumoniae, Haemophilus influenzae, Moraxella catarrhalis and group A beta-haemolytic streptococci in 2002-2003. Results of the multinational GRASP Surveillance Program. Int J Antimicrob Agents. 2005;25(2):148–56.
46. Udaka T, Hiraki N, Shiomori T, Miyamoto H, Fujimura T, Inaba T, et al. Eikenella corrodens in head and neck infections. J Infect. 2007;54(4):343–8.
47. Jernigan JA, Hatfield KM, Wolford H, Nelson RE, Olubajo B, Reddy SC, et al. Multidrug-resistant bacterial infections in U.S. hospitalized patients, 2012–2017. N Engl J Med. 2020;382(14):1309–19.
48. Global burden of bacterial antimicrobial resistance in 2019: a systematic analysis. Lancet. 2022;399(10325):629–55.
49. CDC. COVID-19: U.S. Impact on Antimicrobial Resistance, Special Report 2022. Atlanta, GA: U.S. Department of Health and Human Services, CDC; 2022. [Available from: https://www.cdc.gov/drugresistance/covid19.html]
50. Curran J, Lo J, Leung V, Brown K, Schwartz KL, Daneman N, et al. Estimating daily antibiotic harms: an umbrella review with individual study meta-analysis. Clin Microbiol Infect. 2022;28(4):479–90.
51. Bachert C, Pawankar R, Zhang L, Bunnag C, Fokkens WJ, Hamilos DL, et al. ICON: chronic rhinosinusitis. World Allergy Organ J. 2014;7(1):25.

Topical Corticosteroid Therapy in Recalcitrant Chronic Rhinosinusitis

22

Daniel R. Romano, Daniel P. Lander, and John S. Schneider

Key Points

- Glucocorticoids have long been a cornerstone of therapy in the treatment of chronic rhinosinusitis (CRS), and nasal steroid sprays remain a first-line treatment in many consensus statements.
- A number of CRS patients will experience continued or recurrent symptoms despite appropriate surgical management and medical maintenance therapy with intranasal saline irrigations and simple nasal steroid sprays.
- While short courses of oral steroids may lead to temporary symptom control in these patients, the numerous side effects of systemic steroids make this an unattractive option for long-term CRS management.
- Alternative delivery mechanisms for topical steroid therapy, including intranasal steroid irrigations and the exhalation delivery system with fluticasone propionate (EDS-FLU), have demonstrated improved paranasal sinus medication distribution in the treatment of CRS.
- Though local factors, systemic conditions, and/or steroid resistance may contribute to refractory CRS, studies have shown that improved outcomes are often possible in these patients with improved topical steroid delivery.

D. R. Romano · D. P. Lander · J. S. Schneider (✉)
Department of Otolaryngology-Head & Neck Surgery, Washington University School of Medicine, St. Louis, MO, USA
e-mail: d.r.romano@wustl.edu; daniel.lander@wustl.edu; jsschnei@wustl.edu

J. T. Lee et al. (eds.), *Advances in Surgical and Medical Interventions for Recalcitrant Chronic Rhinosinusitis*,
https://doi.org/10.1007/978-3-031-89191-5_22

Background

Glucocorticoids are a cornerstone in the treatment of chronic rhinosinusitis (CRS). Intranasal corticosteroid sprays are consistently recommended as a first-line treatment for CRS in published clinical practice guidelines, evidence-based reviews, and multidisciplinary and international consensus statements; and short courses of oral steroids can be a useful adjunct for symptomatic CRS refractory to topical steroids and saline rinses [1–8]. Daily nasal steroid sprays are also a standard part of long-term, postoperative medical maintenance regimens that are designed to prevent or delay the relapse of sinus disease after surgery. Meta-analyses have shown that intranasal corticosteroids administered via a breath actuated dry-powder inhaler device, nasal spray, or drop can decrease symptom severity and reduce polyp burden in CRS [9–11]. However, nasal steroid sprays alone may be inadequate for symptom control in the treatment of CRS. Up to half of patients may not achieve adequate symptom control with an appropriate medical therapy protocol involving a 3-month, twice-daily regimen of nasal steroid sprays and saline rinses, a $\geq$ 3-week course of systemic antibiotics, and a 21-day oral steroid taper [12]. Medically refractory CRS veritably represents a major health issue, with patients failing medical therapy reporting a similar health-related quality of life to those with end-stage renal disease requiring dialysis [13] and experiencing mean annual productivity costs greater than patients with diabetes, severe asthma, and chronic migraine [14].

Surgery is often indicated in cases of failed medical therapy and has been shown to result in clinically and statistically significant improvement in average health-related quality of life [13]. However, a segment of patients will experience continued or recurrent symptoms despite appropriate surgical management and medical maintenance therapy. Refractory, recalcitrant, and treatment-resistant are terms that are often used to describe these patients, and difficult-to-treat CRS is defined in the 2020 European Position Paper on Rhinosinusitis and Nasal Polyps (EPOS 2020) as continued CRS symptoms despite adequate surgery, an appropriate regimen of topical corticosteroids, and up to two short courses of oral steroids or antibiotics in a one-year period [2]. Several small studies have shown that short courses of oral steroids can reduce polyp burden in even surgically refractory CRS [15, 16]. However, this effect is often transient, with polyps returning to baseline 8–10 weeks after discontinuation of oral corticosteroids [15, 16]. Additionally, chronic oral steroid use is not recommended for CRS management due to the side effects of oral steroids, which include delayed wound healing, glaucoma, cataracts, osteoporosis, hyperglycemia, psychiatric disturbance, and suppression of the hypothalamic-pituitary-adrenal axis (HPA axis) [17].

As a result, patients with refractory CRS commonly end up undergoing multiple surgical interventions and repeated courses of systemic steroids and antibiotics. Unfortunately, antibiotic usage is a primary driver of antibiotic resistance, and even short-term oral steroid therapy (i.e., $<$ 14–30 days) has been associated with an increased incidence of serious if rare adverse events such as sepsis, cardiac failure, pathologic fractures, venous thromboembolism, and gastrointestinal bleeding [18, 19]. Nevertheless, the efficacy of oral steroids in treating even surgically refractory CRS suggests that some patients' poor response to nasal steroid sprays may be due to limited drug delivery to sinus tissue, rather than a true insensitivity to glucocorticoid action. Supporting this, multiple imaging studies in adult patients have revealed that contrast material and radionuclide agents administered via nasal spray are primarily deposited in the anterior and inferior regions of the nasal cavity (e.g., nasal floor, anterior septum, and inferior meatus) and in the nasopharynx, without measurable delivery to the frontal recess or paranasal sinuses regardless of previous sinus surgery [20–22]. In contrast, other steroid delivery methods such as large volume nasal saline irrigation and exhalation delivery systems facilitate greater deposition in the upper posterior region of the nasal cavity, frontal recess, middle meatus, olfactory cleft, and maxillary sinuses [21, 23–25]. Meanwhile, steroid-eluting sinus stents allow for sustained release of steroid compounds directly at the site of disease. These alternative means of topical glucocorticoid delivery and their respective roles in the management of recalcitrant CRS are the primary focus of the present review.

Sinusitis and Steroids: A Brief Review of Physiology

Chronic Rhinosinusitis

CRS is not a single disease entity but rather a syndrome characterized by persistent, symptomatic mucosal inflammation of the nasal cavity and sinuses, defined by 12 weeks of at least two of the four cardinal symptoms: (1) nasal congestion or obstruction; (2) purulent nasal drainage; (3) facial pressure, pain, or fullness; and (4) hyposmia [2, 4, 5, 8]. A formal diagnosis requires evidence of mucosal inflammation on radiographic studies (e.g., computed tomography [CT] imaging) or sinonasal endoscopy. CRS is classically subdivided into CRS with (CRSwNP) and without nasal polyposis (CRSsNP). CRSwNP is often considered a type 2 inflammatory disease and CRSsNP a type 1 or type 3 inflammatory disease. However, a recently growing body of evidence has upended the paradigm that the absence or presence of nasal polyps is necessarily indicative of the underlying inflammatory environment in CRS [26, 27], and EPOS 2020 has recommended differentiating the management of type 2 and non-type 2 disease (i.e., endotype) rather than basing it on CRSwNP or CRSsNP (i.e., phenotype) [2]. With that said, information regarding the inflammatory endotype of a patient's sinonasal disease is not commonly available, and research inclusion and exclusion criteria and regulatory approvals still often reference the CRSw/sNP classification paradigm. With this, a major current benefit of steroid drugs is their ability to target both common and distinct inflammatory pathways, including those involved in type 1, 2, and 3 inflammation.

Glucocorticoids

The human glucocorticoid receptor (GR) is a member of the nuclear transcription factor receptor superfamily. GR binds to its ligand (glucocorticoids) in the cell's cytoplasm, and the ligand-bound GR is translocated from the cytosol to the nucleus, regulating gene expression by (1) directly binding glucocorticoid response elements (GREs) in the enhancers and promoters of target genes, (2) physically interacting with (an)other transcription factor(s) ("tethering"), or (3) composite binding of the GR to a GRE and (an)other transcription factor(s) [28, 29]. Genomic activity of the GR modulates the expression of up to 20% of the genes in the human genome [30]. Glucocorticoids can also exert more rapid (i.e., in seconds to minutes) but poorly understood, nongenomic effects [28, 29]. Glucocorticoids are involved in a number of important physiological processes, including glucose metabolism, growth, development, reproduction, and immune response. The anti-inflammatory actions of glucocorticoids are multifaceted and include the downregulation of proinflammatory cytokines (e.g., IL-1, IL-6, TNF), decreased expression of adhesion molecules (e.g., SELE, VLA4) on the vascular endothelium and circulating leukocytes, and decreased chemokine production [28]. The specific mechanisms regarding glucocorticoids in CRS treatment remain incompletely characterized. However, studies have shown that glucocorticoid treatment is significantly associated with the reduced expression of the mucin gene MUC4 [31], the eosinophil chemokine eotaxin-2 [32], and the endothelial adhesion molecule P-selectin [33], as well as reduced numbers of eosinophils, $CD4^+$ T cells, and cells expressing the type 2 cytokines IL-4 and IL-13 [33] in nasal polyp tissue.

Delivery of steroids to sinonasal tissue is achieved either by (1) systemic administration of oral or intravenous steroids, (2) topical application of steroid preparations, or (3) intra-polyp glucocorticoid injections. Topical delivery is the main administration route for steroid therapy in CRS, as this allows administration of a higher concentration of glucocorticoid directly to sites of sinonasal inflammation, with minimal systemic exposure. Improved delivery methods for topical steroid therapy are an important source of innovation in the medical treatment of CRS. However, local factors such as microbiome composition, cytokine profile, biofilms, and osteitis may influence the efficacy of steroids regardless of delivery mechanism. Some systemic disorders such as asthma, diabetes mellitus, or a primary immunodeficiency disease might also affect a patient's responsiveness to glucocorticoid therapies. When discussing the important role of improved topical steroid delivery methods in the management of refractory CRS, these variables must be carefully considered as inherent limitations of steroid therapy and potential confounders in current studies.

Intranasal Steroid Irrigations

Rationale

The primary rationale for the use of large-volume, low-pressure nasal irrigations for topical steroid therapy in CRS derives from drug distribution studies that demonstrated greater drug delivery to the sphenoethmoidal and frontal recesses, middle meatus, and maxillary sinus with nasal irrigation when compared to topical nasal sprays [21, 25]. Nasal irrigation also provides the benefit of mechanical lavage with improved mucociliary clearance, removal of biofilms, mucus, bacteria, and secreted inflammatory mediators. Available approaches for nasal irrigations range from syringes with nasal adapters to powered irrigation devices. The most common method used for intranasal steroid irrigation (in studies and in clinical experience) involves low-pressure, large-volume irrigations with a nasal squeeze bottle with steroid drops, creams, capsules, or respules added off-label to the saline irrigation solution.

Evidence

There are several blinded, randomized, placebo-controlled studies examining the impact of steroid irrigations on symptom severity (Table 22.1) [34–40]. Some of these studies are limited by smaller patient populations with heterogeneity among the presenting symptoms. However, most of these studies demonstrate a statistically significant improvement in subjective and objective outcomes with regard to CRS treatment. The most recent RCT examined adult patients with budesonide irrigations (n = 33) versus isotonic saline irrigations (n = 22) in the postoperative period twice daily for 3 months and found that the SNOT-22 at 2 weeks was significantly lower in the budesonide irrigation group at 2 weeks and 3 months postoperatively with a significant difference in the Lund-Kennedy Endoscopic Score [34]. In contrast, studies by Rawal et al. and Rotenberg et al. have found no significant differences in outcomes between budesonide and saline irrigation [39, 40].

Multiple uncontrolled prospective studies have demonstrated similar reductions in SNOT-22 [41–45], symptom severity [45], Lund-Kennedy Endoscopic Score [42, 43, 45], and oral steroid use [43] in CRS patients following treatment with steroid irrigations. In these studies, 63–75% of patients saw at least a minimal clinically important difference (MCID) in SNOT score [41, 43, 44]. However, due to the uncontrolled nature of these studies, it is challenging to separate the actual effect of intranasal steroid irrigations from the natural course of disease; the mechanical action of large-volume, low-pressure rinses; the beneficial effect of functional endoscopic sinus surgery (ESS) or adjuvant nonsurgical therapies (e.g., saline rinses, post-op steroid tapers), when used; and, in the case of patient-reported outcomes, a placebo effect. And even the more objective measures, such as Lund-Kennedy Endoscopic Score, were subject to bias, as scorers were not clearly blinded to whether the patient was pre- or post-irrigation [42, 43].

Placebo effects are a major challenge in clinical studies of CRS treatment, with nasal saline irrigations often used as the placebo, although this treatment is also standard in the postoperative management of CRS. As a result, the placebo arm of many studies has also shown a statistically significant improvement in not only subjective but also some objective CRS outcomes in a newly published systematic review and meta-analysis [46]. Steroid irrigations are at a special disadvantage in

Table 22.1 Summary of the current highest-quality studies of intranasal steroid irrigations for chronic rhinosinusitis (CRS)

Study	Design	Primary inclusion/exclusion criteria	Intervention/ comparison (n^a)	Additional study procedures	Results[b]
Ahamed, et al. (2024) [34]	Single-center, double-blind randomized controlled trial	Adult patients undergoing endoscopic sinus surgery for CRS No tumors or secondary sinusitis No oral steroid use No previous closure of a CSF leak	Post-operative nasal budesonide (1 mg budesonide in 400-mL normal saline; $n = 33$) *vs* isotonic saline irrigation ($n = 22$), 100 mL per nostril *via* sinus rinse bottle, twice daily for 3 months	Post-operative care included a nasal steroid spray, a 7-day antibiotic course (amoxicillin-clavulanate 875–125 mg), and endoscopic debridement at 1 week, 2 weeks, and 3 months	*Subjective Outcome Measures*: Significant difference in mean SNOT-22 score at 2 weeks (26.69 *vs* 30.54, $p < 0.01$) and 3 months (11.34 *vs* 17.27, $p < 0.01$) *Objective Outcome Measures*: Significant difference in mean LKES at 2 weeks (4.06 *vs* 4.50, $p = 0.031$) and 3 months (1.45 *vs* 2.68, $p < 0.01$) *Safety Results/Adverse Events*: No related adverse events in either one of the groups
Megow, et al. (2024) [35]	Single-center, double-blind randomized controlled trial	Adult patients status post bilateral full-house endoscopic sinus surgery for CRSwNP or CRSsNP No oral steroid use or antibiotics	Intranasal budesonide irrigation (1 mg budesonide, once daily) + isotonic saline irrigation (once daily) + Isotonic saline nebulizer (once daily) ($n = 16$) *vs* isotonic saline irrigation (twice daily) + intranasal budesonide nebulizer (500 μg budesonide, once daily) ($n = 12$), for a period of 6 weeks		*Subjective Outcome Measures*: No significant difference in mean SNOT-22 score at 6 weeks ($p > 0.05$) No significant difference in mean VAS score at 6 weeks ($p > 0.05$) *Objective Outcome Measures*: No significant difference in mean discharge/ inflammation/polyp score at 6 weeks ($p > 0.05$) *Safety Results/Adverse Events*: No adverse events in either one of the groups

Jiramongkolchai, et al. (2020) [36]	Single-center, double-blind randomized controlled trial	Adult patients with a CRS diagnosis SNOT-22 > 9 No nasal polyps No previous sinus surgery No comorbid mucociliary disorder or medical condition requiring prolonged steroid treatment No sinusitis associated with an autoimmune condition or vasculitis No steroid nasal sprays, intranasal irrigations, or systemic antibiotics in the past 2 weeks	Intranasal mometasone irrigation (1.2 mg per capsule, 2 capsules per irrigation *via* sinus rinse bottle + nasal saline spray (n = 23) *vs* intranasal saline irrigation + nasal mometasone spray (50 μg per spray, 2 sprays per nostril) (n = 24), once daily for 8 weeks	No other steroid nasal sprays or intranasal irrigations were permitted during the treatment period A segment of subjects (n = 10 per group) was randomly selected to complete cosyntropin (ACTH) stimulation testing at enrollment and completion	*Subjective Outcome Measures*: No significant least square mean difference in SNOT-22 score change at 8 weeks (95% CI −17.7 to 0.58) No significant difference in the percentage of participants with a clinically meaningful improvement in SNOT-22 at 8 weeks (81 *vs* 64%, 95% CI −9% to 44%) *Objective Outcome Measures*: No significant least square mean difference in LKES change at 8 weeks (95% CI −0.84 to 1.15) *Safety Results/Adverse Events*: No significant difference in ACTH stimulation test results after 8 weeks of intranasal mometasone irrigation (24.22 *vs* 24.18 μg/dL cortisol, 95% CI −3.83 to 3.75 μg/dL cortisol) or nasal mometasone spray (23.91 *vs* 23.19 μg/dL cortisol, 95% CI −3.41 to 1.97 μg/dL cortisol) No related serious adverse events in either one of the groups

(continued)

Table 22.1 (continued)

Study	Design	Primary inclusion/exclusion criteria	Intervention/ comparison (n^a)	Additional study procedures	Results[b]
Harvey, et al. (2018) [37]	Multi-center, double-blind randomized controlled trial	Adult patients undergoing endoscopic sinus surgery for CRSwNP or CRSsNP after failure of ≥6 weeks of standard medical therapy (which included saline irrigations, a nasal steroid spray, a ≥3-week course of prednisone [for CRSwNP], and antibiotics [for purulent nasal secretions or positive microbiology cultures]) No previous sinus surgery No unilateral sinus pathology (e.g., odontogenic or allergic fungal sinusitis, etc.) or sinusitis associated with systemic conditions (e.g., autoimmune or vasculitic disorders, immunodeficiency, etc.) Not using immunosuppressive agents; other systemic drugs were permitted during the treatment period No clinically significant deviation of the anterior or caudal nasal septum	Post-operative mometasone nasal irrigation (2 mg mometasone in 240-mL normal saline, 240 mL per irrigation *via* sinus rinse bottle) + nasal placebo spray ($n = 21$) *vs* intranasal placebo irrigation + nasal mometasone spray (1 mg per side) ($n = 23$), once daily for 12 months	No systemic steroids or antibiotics were permitted in the 4-week period before surgery Surgery involved a wide maxillary antrostomy, a complete sphenoethmoidectomy, a Draf3 or Draf2a frontal sinusotomy, and septoplasty if a deviation was impairing sinus cavity access Post-operative care included a 10-day antibiotic course (amoxicillin-clavulanate 875–125 mg; adapted to operative cultures as needed) and a 3-week prednisone taper (25 mg × 1 week, 12.5 mg × 1 week, 5 mg × 1 week); patients were allowed to perform additional saline irrigations	*Subjective Outcome Measures*: Significantly greater improvement in mean nasal blockage VAS score at 12 months (−69.91 *vs* −36.12, $p = 0.029$); no significant difference in average total VAS symptom score change at 12 months (−28.67 *vs* − 21.14, $p = 0.213$) Significant difference in average drainage and fever VAS score at 12 months (7.31 *vs* 34.22, $p < 0.01$; 1.13 *vs* 5.73, $p = 0.03$); no significant differences in the other average VAS symptom scores at 12 months No significant difference in mean SNOT-22 score change at 12 months (−29.26 *vs* − 31.62, $p = 0.725$) No significant difference in average global sinonasal function score change at 12 months (+7.31 *vs* + 6.07, $p = 0.347$) *Objective Outcome Measures*: Significantly greater improvement in mean LM score at 12 months (−12.07 *vs* −7.39, $p = 0.031$) Significant difference in average mLKES at 12 months (7.33 *vs* 21.78, $p = 0.018$) *Safety Results/Adverse Events*: No related adverse events in either one of the groups

Tait, et al. (2018) [38]	Single-center, double-blind randomized controlled trial	Adult patients with a CRS diagnosis SNOT-22 > 9 No antibiotics in the past 2 weeks No sinus surgery within the past 6 weeks No comorbid mucociliary disorder, CSF leak, ocular herpes, pulmonary tuberculosis infection, or medical condition requiring prolonged steroid treatment	Intranasal budesonide irrigation (1 mg budesonide in 1-bottle normal saline; $n = 29$) *vs* intranasal lactose irrigation ($n = 32$) with one half of sinus rinse bottle, once daily for 30 days		Subjective *Outcome Measures*: No significant difference in mean SNOT-22 score change at 30 days (20.7 *vs* 13.6, 95% CI −2 to 16) No significant difference in the percentage of participants with a clinically meaningful improvement in SNOT-22 at 30 days (79 *vs* 59%, 95% CI −2.5 to 42.5%) No significant difference in the percentage of participants reporting improvement on the clinical global impressions scale at 30 days (83 *vs* 67%, 95% CI −6 to 38%) *Objective Outcome Measures*: No significant difference in average LKES change at 30 days (3.4 *vs* 2.7, 95% CI −0.6 to 2.0) *Safety Results/Adverse Events*: No related adverse events in either one of the groups
Rawal, et al. (2015) [39]	Single-center, single-blind randomized controlled trial	English-speaking, adult patients undergoing endoscopic sinus surgery for CRSwNP after failure of conservative management	Post-operative nasal budesonide (2 mL of 0.5 mg/2 mL budesonide in 1-quart normal saline; $n = 24$) *vs* isotonic saline irrigation ($n = 18$), 60 mL per nostril *via* sinus rinse bottle, twice daily for 3–6 months	Peri-operative care included a 12-day prednisone taper (40 mg × 3 days, 30 mg × 3 days, 20 mg × 3 days, 10 mg × 3 days)	*Subjective Outcome Measures*: No significant difference in RSOM-31 at 0–2 weeks ($p = 0.64$), 3–8 weeks ($p = 0.84$), or 3–6 months ($p = 0.79$) No significant difference in RSDI at 0–2 weeks ($p = 0.93$), 3–8 weeks ($p = 0.60$), or 3–6 months ($p = 0.78$) No significant difference in SNOT-22 at 0–2 weeks ($p = 0.48$), 3–8 weeks ($p > 0.05$), or 3–6 months ($p = 0.40$) *Objective Outcome Measures*: No significant difference in UPSIT score change at 3–8 weeks ($p = 0.55$) or 3–6 months ($p = 0.99$) No significant difference in the proportion of "improved," "same," and "worsened" PEA threshold test scores at 3–8 weeks ($p = 0.78$) or 3–6 months ($p = 0.99$)

(continued)

Table 22.1 (continued)

Study	Design	Primary inclusion/exclusion criteria	Intervention/ comparison (n[a])	Additional study procedures	Results[b]
Rotenberg, et al. (2011) [40]	Single-center, double-blind randomized controlled trial	Adult patients undergoing endoscopic sinus surgery for CRSwNP after failure of ≥6 months of standard medical therapy (which included nasal steroids, intranasal saline irrigations, systemic steroids and/or antibiotics as indicated, and appropriate allergy management if applicable) Severe chronic sinus disease, with a LKES ≥8 A Samter's triad phenotype Nonsmoking No previous sinus surgery No other corticosteroid usage	Post-operative budesonide nasal irrigation (2 mL of 0.5 mg/mL budesonide in 1-bottle normal saline, 60 mL per nostril *via* sinus rinse bottle; $n = 20$) *vs* isotonic saline irrigation + nasal budesonide spray (64 µg per nostril) ($n = 19$) *vs* isotonic saline irrigation alone ($n = 21$), twice daily for 12 months	Extent of surgery was tailored to the patient, but included at minimum a polypectomy, maxillary antrostomy, and ethmoidectomy Post-operative care included a 3-week prednisone taper	*Subjective Outcome Measures*: No significant difference in mean SNOT-21 score at 6 (28.2 *vs* 27.4 *vs* 29.7, $p > 0.05$) or 12 (42.2 *vs* 47.9 *vs* 42.5, $p > 0.05$) months *Objective Outcome Measures*: No significant difference in mean LKES at 6 (1.2 *vs* 1.5 *vs* 1.5, $p > 0.05$) or 12 (4.4 *vs* 4.1 *vs* 3.7, $p > 0.05$) months No significant difference in mean LM score at 12 months (13.4 *vs* 12.7 *vs* 11.8, $p > 0.05$) *Safety Results/Adverse Events*: No significant difference in average intraocular pressure at 6 (13.9 *vs* 12.9 *vs* 12.4, $p > 0.05$) or 12 (12.9 *vs* 13.4 *vs* 13.1, $p > 0.05$) months All patients had normal ACTH levels at 6 and 12 months

CI confidence interval, *CRSwNP/sNP* CRS with and without nasal polyposis, *DIP* discharge, inflammation, and polyps/edema, *LKES* Lund-Kennedy Endoscopic Score, *LM* Lund-Mackay, *mLKES* Modified Lund-Kennedy Endoscopic Score, *PEA* phenyl ethyl alcohol, *RSDI* Rhinosinusitis Disability Index, *RSOM-31* 31-Item Rhinosinusitis Outcome Measure, *SNOT-21* 21-Item Sino-Nasal Outcome Test, *SNOT-22* 22-Item Sino-Nasal Outcome Test, *UPSIT* University of Pennsylvania Smell Identification Test, *VAS* visual analog scale

[a]included in the analysis

[b]of intergroup comparisons, unless otherwise stated

placebo-controlled randomized studies, as saline irrigations (the vehicle for placebo) are an active intervention (e.g., by removal of biofilms) and an important part of CRS management [1, 2, 4–8, 47]. Variability in surgical extent, irrigation technique, and/or perioperative management is another common problem in examining the literature on steroid irrigations, potentially contributing to the many negative studies. Ultimately, the randomized controlled literature on intranasal steroid irrigations in CRS treatment is challenging to interpret due to the wide variability in study population, steroid type and dose, and irrigation device, frequency, volume, and duration.

Recently, some randomized controlled literature examining the impact of steroid irrigations have conducted blinded comparisons to traditional first-line therapies (i.e., intranasal saline irrigations and nasal steroid sprays) [36, 37]. These studies suggest that intranasal steroid irrigations are at least no worse than the consensus first-line treatment of nasal steroid spray and saline lavage. Harvey et al. (2018) reported significantly greater improvements in average nasal blockage visual analog scale (VAS) score (−69.91 vs − 36.12, $p = 0.029$) and mean Lund-Mackay score (−12.07 vs −7.39, $p = 0.031$) at 12 months in patients who underwent treatment with mometasone irrigation and a nasal placebo spray, versus intranasal placebo irrigation and a nasal mometasone spray, after primary sinus surgery [37]. However, it was unclear from the article text whether the authors corrected for multiple testing. A second study reported a nonsignificant least square mean difference in SNOT-22 improvement, favoring mometasone irrigation with nasal saline spray over intranasal saline irrigation with nasal mometasone spray (95% CI −17.7–0.58) in patients without previous surgery [36]. Similarly, a single-center double-blinded RCT comparing budesonide irrigations to nebulized intranasal budesonide found no significant difference in SNOT-22, VAS scores, or discharge/inflammation/polyp score [35].

Steroid irrigations remain an off-label treatment for CRSwNP and are often not covered by patient insurance. Filling prescriptions for steroid irrigations may additionally require preparation by specialized compounding pharmacies. Nonetheless, many otolaryngology practitioners view glucocorticoid irrigations as a potentially beneficial, generally well-tolerated, and safe option for CRS patients who experience continued or recurrent symptoms despite using a nasal steroid spray. In the International Consensus Statement on Allergy and Rhinology: Rhinosinusitis 2021 (ICAR-RS-2021), steroid irrigations received a Grade A recommendation for postoperative patients with a CRSsNP diagnosis and a strong recommendation for CRSwNP that is uncontrolled by nasal steroid sprays [4]. However, published clinical practice guidelines have largely relegated steroid irrigation to an option [6, 47], or otherwise provided no official recommendation for glucocorticoid lavage [1, 2, 7], in CRS.

Patient adherence with steroid irrigation is 90–100% in blinded randomized controlled studies [36–40]. However, tolerance of and adherence to intranasal irrigations is a major issue in clinical practice. Gutierrez et al. (2024) reported that patients undergoing treatment with intranasal steroid irrigations showed a mean medication possession ratio (MPR) of 0.44 (i.e., patients possessed steroid irrigations on only 44% of treatment days), with 15.5% and 12.7% of patients reporting problems with medication cost and irrigation use, respectively [48]. Adverse events related to steroid irrigation are rare, mild, and mostly localized (e.g., nasal pain, irritation, or epistaxis), and blinded RCTs reported no significant HPA axis suppression or intraocular pressure elevations after a year of twice-daily steroid irrigations [36, 40]. However, citing concerns about the unregulated nature of steroid irrigations (e.g., no high-quality safety data, no aftermarket surveillance, no standardization of dosing or administration, potential variability in compounded medication), some experts have urged doctors to consider screening patients for HPA suppression and other complications of chronic glucocorticoid exposure [49].

Although off-label nasal steroid irrigation is a common clinical practice in contemporary CRS management, there continues to be little consensus on the appropriate indications and optimal irrigation regimen, delivery device (e.g., neti pot vs a nasal squeeze bottle), and steroid choice (type and dose). Patient positioning during irrigations is an important factor that is often overlooked. Cadaveric studies have demonstrated significant differences in irrigation distribution with variable head positioning [50–54], with optimal irrigation of the paranasal sinuses in the "vertex" (i.e., with nose down) or "vertex to floor" position (i.e., with Frankfort horizontal line angled >90° to the ground). The authors typically instruct patients to perform nasal rinses while leaning over a sink or basin, as this position is well tolerated by most patients. Cadaveric studies have also demonstrated significant differences in irrigation distribution depending on the extent of surgery [50, 52, 53, 55–57]. No well-designed, randomized controlled study has demonstrated statistically significant improvement in subjective or objective CRS outcomes for intranasal steroid over placebo irrigations in CRS patients in the absence of previous sinus surgery.

The Exhalation Delivery System

Rationale

The exhalation delivery system with fluticasone propionate (EDS-FLU) is a breath-actuated device composed of a nosepiece and a mouthpiece. Exhalation through the mouthpiece causes the administration of steroid into the nasal cavity via the nosepiece and closes the soft palate, causing the air and steroid to turn 180° into the opposite nasal passage at the nasopharynx (so-called bidirectional delivery) rather than escape the nasal cavity and paranasal sinuses. Positive pressure delivery to the nostril also stents open the nasal valve, facilitating the deposition of fluticasone propionate in the deeper areas of the nasal cavity. Scintigraphy studies have demonstrated greater distribution of Tc-labeled material to the upper posterior region of the nasal cavity and paranasal sinuses with the EDS-FLU compared to standard nasal delivery devices [23, 24]. Another major benefit of EDS-FLU is a decreased dependence on patient and device positioning, with more reproducible nasal deposition than a standard nasal aerosol spray [23, 24].

Evidence

EDS-FLU has had demonstrable efficacy and has been well tolerated by patients in multiple studies. Reported adherence rates with EDS-FLU are as high as 97–99% during the study period [58, 59], and most patients reported that the delivery system was somewhat or very comfortable (74–82% at 1–12 months) and easy to administer (85–90% at 1–12 months) [60–62]. Large, double-blind, randomized placebo-controlled studies have demonstrated statistically significant advantages of EDS-FLU over placebo in multiple objective and subjective measures in patients with CRSwNP and CRSsNP (Table 22.2) [58–60, 63, 64]. Adverse events related to EDS-FLU were generally local and of mild severity and included headache, nasopharyngitis, and septal erythema or ulceration. Epistaxis occurred in a dose-dependent rate in EDS-FLU groups across studies (1.4% [5/348] in placebo groups, 4.3% [7/161] in 93-μg EDS-FLU groups, 8.1% [28/344] in 186-μg EDS-FLU groups, and 10.5% [36/344] in 372-μg EDS-FLU groups) [60, 63, 64].

EDS-FLU was approved for the treatment of CRSwNP in patients ≥18 years by the US Food and Drug Administration (FDA) in 2017 and, more recently, for the treatment of adult patients with CRSsNP in 2024. Expansion of indications to CRSsNP was a result of ReOpen1 and 2 trials, a pair of RCTs that demonstrated significant improvement in mean paranasal sinus opacification, nasal symptom scores, and SNOT-22 with EDS-FLU in patients with CRSsNP, versus placebo [63]. Notably, EDS-FLU is the only medication that is currently FDA approved for CRSsNP. However, EDS-FLU is more expensive than standard first-line therapies; therefore, it is usually reserved for patients who do not respond to nasal steroid sprays or irrigations. Han et al. (2021) recommended the consideration of EDS-FLU in patients with CRSwNP and continued objective and subjective evidence of CRS after a 1-month trial of a nasal steroid spray [3].

Currently available formulations of EDS-FLU deliver 93 μg of fluticasone propionate per spray, with a recommended dose by the manufacturer of one to two sprays per nostril (186–372 μg) twice daily. Multiple dose-response studies have been published and have demonstrated no statistically significant differences in evaluated outcomes for 372-μg versus 186-μg dosing [63, 64]. A phase 1 randomized crossover study revealed greater systemic steroid exposure with 372 μg of EDS-FLU compared to 400 μg delivered via traditional fluticasone propionate delivery devices [65]. However, average systemic exposure remains much lower than that of inhaled corticosteroids used for pulmonary disease (440 μg) [65], and other studies have shown no significant HPA axis suppression, intraocular pressure elevations, or increased cataract diagnoses, with 12 months of twice-daily 372-μg EDS-FLU treatment [58–62, 64]. These studies together suggest that systemic absorption of EDS-FLU at maximum labeled dosages does not have a significant clinical impact.

The randomized controlled literature on EDS-FLU demonstrates several notable shortcomings. Currently, each RCT examining EDS-FLU compares results to placebo only. No studies have compared EDS-FLU treatment directly to standard steroid spray applications or intranasal steroid or saline irrigations. Therefore, the

Table 22.2 Summary of the current highest-quality studies of the exhalation delivery system with fluticasone propionate (EDS-FLU) for chronic rhinosinusitis (CRS)

Study	Design	Primary inclusion/ exclusion criteria	Intervention/ comparison (n^a)	Additional study procedures	Results[b]
ReOpen2 [63]	Multi-center, double-blind randomized controlled trial	≥ 18 years of age Bilateral CRSsNP diagnosis ≥ 25% opacification of ethmoid sinuses and ≥ 1 maxillary sinus on pre-treatment CT scan No sinus surgery within 6 months of screening	Fluticasone propionate (372 µg, *n* = 73; or 186 µg, *n* = 72) *vs* placebo (*n* = 75) EDS, twice daily for 24 weeks	7- to 21-day placebo run-in Randomization was stratified according to previous sinus surgery (yes/no) After 4 weeks, a non-sedating antihistamine was permitted as rescue therapy	*Subjective Outcome Measures*: Significantly greater improvement in morning combined symptom score in the 372-µg (−1.74 *vs* −0.81 LSMC, $p = 0.001$) and 186-µg EDS-FLU groups (−1.54 *vs* − 0.81 LSMC, $p = 0.011$) at 4 weeks Significantly greater improvement in several of the cardinal nasal symptom scores in the 372-µg and 186-µg EDS-FLU groups at 4, 8, and 12 weeks Significantly greater improvement in SNOT-22 in the 372-µg (−15.54 *vs* − 8.72 LSMC, $p = 0.029$) and 186-µg EDS-FLU groups (−19.45 *vs* − 8.72 LSMC, $p < 0.001$) at 24 weeks Significantly greater percentage of participants reporting improvement on the PGIC scale in the 372-µg (91.3 *vs* 60.9%, $p < 0.001$) and 186-µg EDS-FLU groups (84.3 *vs* 60.9%, $p = 0.004$) at 24 weeks Significantly greater percentage of subjects who reported a global rating of "much improved" or "very much improved" in the 372-µg (56.5 *vs* 24.6%, $p < 0.001$) and 186-µg EDS-FLU groups (62.9 *vs* 24.6%, $p < 0.001$) at 24 weeks *Objective Outcome Measures*: Significantly greater improvement in mean paranasal sinus opacification in the 372-µg (−5.14 *vs* +1.19 LSMC, $p = 0.009$) and 186-µg EDS-FLU groups (−7.00 *vs* + 1.19 LSMC, $p < 0.001$) at 24 weeks
ReOpen1 [63]	Multi-center, double-blind randomized controlled trial	≥18 years of age Bilateral CRSwNP or CRSsNP diagnosis ≥ 25% opacification of ethmoid sinuses and ≥1 maxillary sinus on pre-treatment CT scan No polyps extending beyond attachment of inferior turbinate No sinus surgery within 6 months of screening	Fluticasone propionate (372 µg, *n* = 107; or 186 µg, *n* = 110) *vs* placebo (*n* = 110) EDS, twice daily for 24 weeks	7- to 21-day placebo run-in Randomization was stratified according to the presence of nasal polyps (yes/no) and prior history of sinus surgery (yes/no) After 4 weeks, a non-sedating antihistamine was permitted as rescue therapy	*Subjective Outcome Measures*: Significantly greater improvement in morning combined symptom score in the 372-µg (−1.60 *vs* − 0.62 LSMC, $p < 0.001$) and 186-µg EDS-FLU groups (−1.58 *vs* − 0.62 LSMC, $p < 0.001$) at 4 weeks Significantly greater improvement in several of the cardinal nasal symptom scores in the 372-µg and 186-µg EDS-FLU groups at 4, 8, and 12 weeks Significantly greater improvement in SNOT-22 in the 372-µg (−22.77 *vs* − 10.16 LSMC, $p < 0.001$) and 186-µg EDS-FLU groups (−18.05 *vs* −10.16 LSMC, $p = 0.001$) at 24 weeks Significantly greater percentage of participants reporting improvement on the PGIC scale in the 372-µg (81.6 *vs* 59.6%, $p < 0.001$) and 186-µg EDS-FLU groups (78.8 *vs* 59.6%, $p = 0.004$) at 24 weeks Significantly greater percentage of subjects who reported a global rating of "much improved" or "very much improved" in the 372-µg (54.1 *vs* 25.5%, $p < 0.001$) and 186-µg EDS-FLU groups (44.4 *vs* 25.5%, $p = 0.006$) at 24 weeks *Objective Outcome Measures*: Significantly greater improvement in mean paranasal sinus opacification in the 372-µg (−6.20 *vs* −1.60 LSMC, $p = 0.018$) and 186-µg EDS-FLU groups (−5.58 *vs* −1.60 LSMC, $p = 0.045$) at 24 weeks

NAVIGATE II [60]	Multi-center, double-blind randomized controlled trial	≥18 years of age Bilateral nasal polyposis with ≥ moderate nasal congestion (i.e., morning nasal congestion/obstruction score of ≥2 for ≥5 of the past 7 days) ≤ 5 lifetime sinus surgeries No sinus surgery within 6 months of screening ≤ 1 episode of epistaxis in the past 1 month Patients with asthma or COPD were included if (1) no exacerbations in the past 3 months and (2) inhaled corticosteroids ≤1000 µg beclomethasone (or equivalent) daily with a stable dose for ≥3 months	Fluticasone propionate (372 µg, $n = 82$; 186 µg, $n = 80$; or 93 µg, $n = 80$) vs placebo ($n = 79$) EDS, twice daily for 16 weeks	7- to 14-day placebo run-in After 4 weeks, a non-sedating antihistamine was permitted as rescue therapy Subjects who completed the 16-week double-blind period were enrolled in an 8-week open-label phase, consisting of treatment with 372-µg EDS-FLU twice daily (see citation for results)	*Subjective Outcome Measures*: Significantly greater improvement in morning nasal congestion/obstruction symptom score in the 372-µg (−0.62 *vs* − 0.24 LSMC, $p < 0.001$), 186-µg (−0.68 *vs* − 0.24 LSMC, $p < 0.001$), and 93-µg EDS-FLU groups (−0.59 *vs* − 0.24 LSMC, $p < 0.001$) at 4 weeks; no significant differences among EDS-FLU groups Significantly greater improvement in multiple other morning and evening nasal symptom scores in the 372-µg, 186-µg, and 93-µg EDS-FLU groups at 4, 8, and 16 weeks Significantly greater improvement in SNOT-22 in the 372-µg (−21.05 *vs* − 11.70 LSMC, $p < 0.001$), 186-µg (−21.43 *vs* − 11.70 LSMC, $p < 0.001$), and 93-µg EDS-FLU groups (−21.14 *vs* − 11.70 LSMC, $p < 0.001$) at 16 weeks Significantly greater percentage of subjects who reported a global rating of "much improved" or "very much improved" in the 372-µg (67.9 *vs* 31.5%, $p < 0.001$), 186-µg (68.0 *vs* 31.5%, $p < 0.001$), and 93-µg EDS-FLU groups (68.0 *vs* 31.5%, $p < 0.001$) at 16 weeks Significantly greater improvement in MOS sleep-R sleep disturbance score in the 372-µg (+14.30 *vs* + 10.03 LSMC, $p < 0.05$), 186-µg (+15.78 *vs* + 10.03 LSMC, $p < 0.05$), and 93-µg EDS-FLU groups (+14.26 *vs* + 10.03 LSMC, $p < 0.05$) at 16 weeks Significantly greater improvement in RSDI in the 372-µg (−16.69 *vs* − 7.80 LSMC, $p < 0.001$), 186-µg (−15.37 *vs* − 7.80 LSMC, $p < 0.05$), and 93-µg EDS-FLU groups (−15.54 *vs* − 7.80 LSMC, $p < 0.05$) at 16 weeks Significantly greater improvement in SF-36 mental score in the 372-µg (+3.53 *vs* + 1.42 LSMC, $p < 0.05$) and 93-µg EDS-FLU groups (+3.76 *vs* + 1.42 LSMC, $p < 0.05$) at 16 weeks; no significant difference in the 186-µg EDS-FLU group (+3.44 *vs* + 1.42 LSMC, $p > 0.05$) Significantly greater improvement in SF-36 physical score in the 372-µg (+5.09 *vs* + 2.89 LSMC, $p < 0.05$) and 93-µg EDS-FLU groups (+4.40 *vs* + 2.89 LSMC, $p < 0.05$) at 16 weeks; no significant difference in the 186-µg EDS-FLU group (+4.62 *vs* + 2.89 LSMC, $p > 0.05$) Statistical reduction in the percent of patients who were considered eligible for surgical evaluation in the 372-µg (21.0 *vs* 54.9%, $p = 0.034$), 186-µg (17.8 *vs* 52.5%, $p = 0.014$), and 93-µg EDS-FLU groups (16.7 *vs* 50.0%, $p = 0.006$) after 16 weeks *Objective Outcome Measures*: Significantly greater improvement in total polyp grade[c] in the 372-µg (−1.41 *vs* − 0.61 LSMC, $p < 0.001$), 186-µg (−1.22 *vs* − 0.61 LSMC, $p < 0.001$), and 93-µg EDS-FLU groups (−1.31 *vs* − 0.61 LSMC, $p < 0.001$) at 16 weeks Significantly greater percentage of patients experiencing ≥1-point improvement in total polyp grade[c] in the 372-µg (69.1 *vs* 43.5%, $p < 0.05$), 186-µg (63.0 *vs* 43.5%, $p < 0.05$), and 93-µg EDS-FLU groups (68.4 *vs* 43.5%, $p < 0.05$) at 16 weeks No significant difference in the percent of patients who experienced polyp elimination in ≥1 side of the nose in the 372-µg (13.6 *vs* 4.3%, $p > 0.05$), 186-µg (8.2 *vs* 4.3%, $p > 0.05$), or 93-µg EDS-FLU groups (12.7 *vs* 4.3%, $p > 0.05$) at 16 weeks *Safety Results/Adverse Events*: No significant difference in average intraocular pressure change or new diagnosis of lens cataracts Adverse events reported more often with EDS-FLU therapy and in ≥2% of patients included headache, epistaxis, nasal erythema and septal ulceration

(continued)

Table 22.2 (continued)

Study	Design	Primary inclusion/ exclusion criteria	Intervention/ comparison (n^a)	Additional study procedures	Results[b]
NAVIGATE I [64]	Multi-center, double-blind randomized controlled trial	≥ 18 years of age Bilateral nasal polyposis with ≥ moderate nasal congestion (i.e., morning nasal congestion/obstruction score of ≥2 for ≥5 of the past 7 days) Bilateral nasal patency ≤ 5 lifetime sinus surgeries No sinus surgery within 6 months of screening No COPD or asthma exacerbations within 3 months of screening No allergic rhinitis with a seasonality coinciding with the first 4 weeks of randomization	Fluticasone propionate (372 µg, $n = 79$; 186 µg, $n = 80$; or 93 µg, $n = 81$) *vs* placebo ($n = 82$) EDS, twice daily for 16 weeks	7- to 14-day placebo run-in After 4 weeks, a non-sedating antihistamine was permitted as rescue therapy; no other medication for nasal congestion was permitted during the treatment period Subjects who completed the 16-week double-blind period were enrolled in an 8-week open-label phase, consisting of treatment with 372-µg EDS-FLU twice daily (see citation for results)	*Subjective Outcome Measures*: Significantly greater improvement in morning nasal congestion/obstruction symptom score in the 372-µg (−0.62 *vs* − 0.24 LSMC, $p < 0.001$), 186-µg (−0.54 *vs* − 0.24 LSMC, $p = 0.002$), and 93-µg EDS-FLU groups (−0.49 *vs* − 0.24 LSMC, $p = 0.010$) at 4 weeks; no significant differences among EDS-FLU groups Significantly greater improvement in multiple other morning and evening nasal symptom scores in the 372-µg, 186-µg, and 93-µg EDS-FLU groups at 4, 8, and 16 weeks Significantly greater improvement in SNOT-22 in the 372-µg (−19.80 *vs* − 10.96 LSMC, $p < 0.001$), 186-µg (−19.56 *vs* − 10.96 LSMC, $p < 0.001$), and 93-µg EDS-FLU groups (−18.32 *vs* − 10.96 LSMC, $p < 0.001$) at 16 weeks Significantly greater improvement in MOS sleep-R sleep disturbance score in the 186-µg EDS-FLU group (−14.24 *vs* − 8.53 LSMC, $p < 0.05$) at 16 weeks; no significant difference in the 372-µg (−10.66 *vs* − 8.53 LSMC, $p > 0.05$) or 93-µg EDS-FLU group (−10.69 *vs* − 8.53 LSMC, $p > 0.05$) Significantly greater percentage of subjects who reported a global rating of "much improved" or "very much improved" in the 372-µg (66.7 *vs* 41.2%, $p < 0.001$), 186-µg (67.1 *vs* 41.2%, $p < 0.001$), and 93-µg EDS-FLU groups (61.6 *vs* 41.2%, $p < 0.05$) at 16 weeks Significantly greater improvement in RSDI in the 372-µg (−16.37 *vs* − 10.71 LSMC, $p < 0.05$), 186-µg (−16.44 *vs* − 10.71 LSMC, $p < 0.05$), and 93-µg EDS-FLU groups (−17.08 *vs* − 10.71 LSMC, $p < 0.05$) at 16 weeks Significantly greater improvement in SF-36 mental score in the 186-µg (+4.03 *vs* + 0.70 LSMC, $p < 0.05$) and 93-µg EDS-FLU groups (+3.19 *vs* + 0.70 LSMC, $p < 0.05$) at 16 weeks; no significant difference in the 372-µg EDS-FLU group (+1.83 *vs* + 0.70 LSMC, $p > 0.05$) Significantly greater improvement in SF-36 physical score in the 93-µg EDS-FLU group at 16 weeks (+4.12 *vs* + 2.67 LSMC, $p < 0.05$); no significant difference in the 372-µg (+3.58 *vs* + 2.67 LSMC, $p > 0.05$) or 186-µg EDS-FLU group (+5.19 *vs* + 2.67 LSMC, $p > 0.05$) Statistical reduction in the percentage of patients who were considered eligible for surgical evaluation in the 372-µg (25.3 *vs* 60.3%, $p < 0.05$) and 93-µg EDS-FLU groups (23.0 *vs* 55.6%, $p < 0.05$) after 16 weeks; no significant difference in the 186-µg (30.4 *vs* 55.0%, $p > 0.05$) or placebo groups (39.7 *vs* 64.6%, $p > 0.05$) *Objective Outcome Measures*: Significantly greater improvement in total polyp grade[c] in the 372-µg (−1.06 *vs* − 0.45 LSMC, $p < 0.001$), 186-µg (−1.03 *vs* − 0.45 LSMC, $p < 0.001$), and 93-µg EDS-FLU groups (−0.96 *vs* − 0.45 LSMC, $p = 0.004$) at 16 weeks; no significant differences among EDS-FLU groups Significantly greater percentage of patients experiencing ≥1-point improvement in total polyp grade[c] in the 372-µg (72.0 *vs* 41.2%, $p < 0.001$) and 186-µg EDS-FLU groups (66.2 *vs* 41.2%, $p < 0.05$) at 16 weeks; no significant difference in the 93-µg EDS-FLU group (56.0 *vs* 41.2%, $p > 0.05$) No significant difference in the percentage of patients who experienced polyp elimination in ≥1 side of the nose in the 372-µg (18.7 *vs* 13.2%, $p > 0.05$), 186-µg (17.6 *vs* 13.2%, $p > 0.05$), or 93-µg EDS-FLU groups (25.3 *vs* 13.2%, $p > 0.05$) at 16 weeks *Safety Results/Adverse Events*: No significant difference in average intraocular pressure change or new diagnosis of lens cataracts Adverse events reported more often with EDS-FLU therapy and in >5% of patients included epistaxis, mucosal erythema, acute sinusitis and septal ulceration

Hansen, et al. (2010) [58]	Single-center, double-blind randomized controlled trial	18–65 years of age CRS, with no visible nasal polyps on endoscopic evaluation Verified palate closure and bilateral nasal patency Ability to trigger the breath actuation device mechanism No cleft palate or cystic fibrosis No sinus surgery for nasal polyps in the past 3 months No systemic steroids in the past 2 months No other steroids except for inhaled corticosteroids ≤1000 μg beclomethasone (or equivalent) daily with a stable dose for ≥3 months for treatment of asthma No nostril dilation devices No treatment with ritonavir or other established CYP3A inhibitors	Fluticasone propionate (400 μg, $n = 10$) *vs* placebo ($n = 10$) EDS, twice daily for 12 weeks	14- to 16-day treatment-free run-in Investigators provided oxymetazoline and an antihistamine (a 10 mg loratadine tablet) as rescue therapies for severe symptoms; intranasal sodium cromoglycate and antimuscarinics, neuroleptics, decongestants, antihistamines, and leukotriene receptor antagonists were otherwise prohibited Subjects using saline rinses were allowed to continue	*Subjective Outcome Measures*: No significant difference in median total RSOM-31 score change at 12 weeks (−62.0 *vs* − 5.0, $p > 0.05$) Significantly greater median improvement in RSOM-31 nasal domain score at 4 (−11.0 *vs* + 6.0, $p = 0.009$), 8 (−21.0 *vs* + 3.0, $p = 0.016$), but not 12 (−18.0 *vs* − 1.0, $p > 0.05$) weeks Significantly greater median improvement in morning combined symptom scores at 8 (−2.00 *vs* − 0.16, $p = 0.030$) and 12 (−2.00 *vs* + 0.43, $p = 0.038$) weeks; no significant difference in median change in morning combined symptom score at 4 weeks (−1.78 *vs* − 0.10, $p > 0.05$) Significantly greater median improvement in evening combined symptom scores at 4 (−1.95 *vs* + 0.09, $p = 0.028$), 8 (−2.00 *vs* − 0.22, $p = 0.034$), and 12 (−2.00 *vs* + 0.68, $p = 0.034$) weeks Significantly greater median improvement in morning and evening nasal discomfort scores at 12 weeks (−0.67 *vs* + 0.00, $p = 0.027$; −0.90 *vs* + 0.00, $p = 0.027$), evening nasal discomfort score at 4 weeks (−0.51 *vs* − 0.03, $p = 0.044$), and evening olfactory symptom score at 12 weeks (−0.17 *vs* + 0.00, $p = 0.048$); no significant differences in other median nasal symptom score changes No significant difference in median change in CRS symptom VAS at 12 weeks (−13.0 *vs* + 2.0, $p > 0.05$) *Objective Outcome Measures*: Significantly greater improvement in median LMES edema at 4 ($p = 0.015$), 8 ($p = 0.017$), and 12 ($p = 0.015$) weeks; no significant difference in median change in nasal discharge LMES at 4 ($p > 0.05$), 8 ($p > 0.05$), or 12 ($p > 0.05$) weeks Significantly greater median improvement in PNIF at 4 (+35.0 *vs* − 2.5 L/min, $p = 0.006$), 8 (+50.0 *vs* + 10.0 L/min, $p = 0.030$), but not 12 (+40.0 *vs* + 25.0 L/min, $p > 0.05$) weeks No significant difference in nasal volume change No significant difference in median MRI score change at 12 weeks ($p = 0.11$) No significant difference in mean usage of antihistamine (4.3 *vs* 12.1% of days during the study period, $p > 0.05$) or oxymetazoline (1.2 *vs* 0.0% of days during the study period, $p > 0.05$) *Safety Results/Adverse Events*: No clinically apparent adrenal suppression on morning cortisol testing Adverse events reported by 90% of the EDS-FLU group and 90% of the control group No serious adverse events in either one of the groups

(continued)

Table 22.2 (continued)

Study	Design	Primary inclusion/ exclusion criteria	Intervention/ comparison (n[a])	Additional study procedures	Results[b]
Vlckova, et al. (2009) [59]	Multi-center, double-blind randomized controlled trial	18–65 years of age Bilateral nasal polyposis with a mild or moderate grade on the Lildholdt scale (i.e., 1 or 2) Verified palate closure and bilateral nasal patency Ability to trigger the breath actuation device mechanism No cleft palate, cystic fibrosis, allergic rhinitis, or purulent nasal infection No sinus surgery for nasal polyps or systemic steroids in the past 3 months No other steroids except for inhaled corticosteroids ≤1000 μg beclomethasone (or equivalent) daily with a stable dose for ≥3 months for treatment of asthma	Fluticasone propionate (400 μg, $n = 54$) *vs* placebo ($n = 55$) EDS, twice daily for 12 weeks	14- to 16-day treatment-free run-in No saline rinses or nostril dilation devices were permitted during the treatment period Investigators provided oxymetazoline and an antihistamine (a 10 mg loratadine tablet) as rescue therapies for severe symptoms; no other medication usage that would interfere with study evaluation (e.g., intranasal sodium cromoglycate or antimuscarinics, neuroleptics, decongestants, antihistamines, or leukotriene receptor antagonists, etc.) was permitted	*Subjective Outcome Measures*: Significantly greater improvement in average morning and evening combined symptom scores at 4 (−0.67 *vs* + 0.31, $p < 0.001$; −0.74 *vs* + 0.45, $p < 0.001$), 8 (−1.01 *vs* + 0.35, $p < 0.001$; −1.03 *vs* + 0.46, $p < 0.001$), and 12 (−1.11 *vs* + 0.31, $p < 0.001$; −1.09 *vs* + 0.44, $p < 0.001$) weeks Significantly greater improvement in average morning and evening nasal blockage scores at 4 (−0.25 *vs* − 0.02, $p < 0.05$; −0.26 *vs* + 0.06, $p < 0.01$), 8 (−0.33 *vs* + 0.00, $p < 0.05$; −0.31 *vs* + 0.06, $p < 0.01$), and 12 (−0.39 *vs* − 0.05, $p < 0.05$; −0.34 *vs* + 0.03, $p < 0.05$) weeks Significantly greater improvement in average morning and evening nasal discomfort scores at 4 (−0.18 *vs* + 0.16, $p < 0.001$; −0.24 *vs* + 0.13, $p < 0.001$), 8 (−0.20 *vs* + 0.12, $p < 0.01$; −0.24 *vs* + 0.09, $p < 0.001$), and 12 (−0.22 *vs* + 0.21, $p < 0.001$; −0.27 *vs* + 0.18, $p < 0.001$) weeks Significantly greater improvement in average morning and evening rhinitis symptom scores at 4 (−0.19 *vs* + 0.20, $p < 0.001$; −0.18 *vs* + 0.19, $p < 0.001$), 8 (−0.28 *vs* + 0.16, $p < 0.001$; −0.25 *vs* + 0.16, $p < 0.001$) and 12 (−0.27 *vs* + 0.11, $p < 0.01$; −0.21 *vs* + 0.08, $p < 0.05$) weeks Significantly greater improvement in average morning and evening olfactory symptom scores at 8 weeks (−0.19 *vs* + 0.06, $p < 0.05$; −0.22 *vs* + 0.15, $p < 0.01$) and evening olfactory symptom score at 12 weeks (−0.26 *vs* + 0.13, $p < 0.01$); no significant differences in other average olfactory symptom score changes Significantly greater percentage of subjects who reported a global rating of "improved" or "very much improved" at 12 weeks (76 *vs* 27%, $p < 0.001$) *Objective Outcome Measures*: Significantly greater improvement in mean Lildholdt score at 4 (−0.28 *vs* + 0.00, $p < 0.05$), 8 (−0.63 *vs* + 0.15, $p < 0.001$), and 12 (−0.98 *vs* + 0.23, $p < 0.001$) weeks Significantly greater percentage of subjects with a reduced score on the Lildholdt scale at 4 (22 *vs* 7%, $p = 0.011$), 8 (43 *vs* 7%, $p < 0.001$), and 12 (57 *vs* 9%, $p < 0.001$) weeks Significant difference in mean polyp size, expressed as a percent of the lateral wall of the nasal cavity, at 4 (13.86 *vs* 18.26%, $p < 0.001$), 8 (11.62 *vs* 18.73%, $p < 0.001$), and 12 (8.85 *vs* 19.18%, $p < 0.001$) weeks Significant difference in mean PNIF at 4 (106.8 *vs* 102.4 L/min, $p < 0.05$), 8 (113.8 *vs* 100.5 L/min, $p < 0.01$), and 12 (116.8 *vs* 96.0 L/min, $p < 0.001$) weeks Significantly greater improvement in mean PNIF at 12 weeks (+17.7 *vs* − 3.2 L/min, $p < 0.001$) Significantly lower utilization of antihistamine (3.1 *vs* 22.4% of days during the study period, $p < 0.001$) and oxymetazoline (0.0 *vs* 1.2% of days during the study period, $p = 0.025$) *Safety Results/Adverse Events*: No change in morning plasma cortisol levels at 12 weeks (−0.75 *vs* − 0.38 μg/dL) Epistaxis was the most common treatment-emergent adverse event (11.1 *vs* 0.0%) Treatment-emergent adverse events occurred in 24% of the EDS-FLU group and 20% of the control group No related serious adverse events in either one of the groups

CRSwNP/sNP CRS with and without nasal polyposis, *LMES* Lund-Mackay Endoscopic Score, *LSMC* least square mean change, *MOS Sleep-R* Medical Outcomes Study Sleep Scale-Revised, *PGIC* Patient Global Impression of Change, *PNIF* peak nasal inspiratory flow, *RSDI* Rhinosinusitis Disability Index, *RSOM-31* 31-Item Rhinosinusitis Outcome Measure, *SF-36* 36-Item Short-Form Health Survey, *SNOT-22* 22-Item Sino-Nasal Outcome Test, *VAS* visual analog scale

[a]included in the analysis

[b]of intergroup comparisons, unless otherwise stated

[c]on a 6-point modified Lildholdt scale

superiority of twice-daily EDS-FLU treatment over standard topical steroid therapies in the treatment of CRS has not been rigorously established. Nevertheless, a small prospective, uncontrolled study and one post hoc analysis of data pooled from the Navigate I and II studies both demonstrated statistically significant improvements in multiple objective and subjective measures with EDS-FLU in patients with continued CRSwNP symptoms on other topical nasal steroids, including steroid irrigation [66, 67]. Additional subgroup analyses of pooled data from high-quality, randomized controlled studies have shown that twice-daily EDS-FLU treatment also improves outcomes in CRSw/sNP patients with recurrent symptoms after previous sinus surgery [68, 69].

Steroid-Eluting Sinus Stents

Rationale

While nasal sprays, powders, and irrigations are rapidly cleared from the nasal cavity [23, 24], steroid-eluting sinus stents enable the sustained release of steroid compounds at the site of disease. Bioabsorbable, self-expanding, steroid-eluting sinus stents were originally developed to maintain sinus patency and reduce inflammation after endoscopic surgery [70]. The first FDA-approved drug-eluting sinus stents were designed for endoscopic placement in the ethmoid cavity during surgery to maintain patency and deliver steroids locally. These stents were composed of a polylactide-co-glycolide (PLGA) polymer impregnated with 370-μg mometasone furoate, a design that allows for the gradual, controlled release of steroid over a 30-day period. Animal studies with mometasone furoate-coated bioabsorbable stents demonstrated effective mucosal drug delivery, with negligible systemic absorption [70], and further studies in human subjects showed that the stents were generally well tolerated and entirely resorbed within 45–60 days [71, 72].

Rationale

Original FDA approval of steroid-eluting stents for ethmoid sinus surgery was based on blinded, randomized, placebo-controlled studies that demonstrated reduced postoperative ethmoid inflammation, polypoid changes, adhesions, and need for adhesion lysis and/or oral steroids on short-term (i.e., < 60-day) follow-up (Table 22.3) [72, 73]. Additional, smaller versions of the steroid-eluting implants have since been developed for frontal sinus application and have demonstrated improved postoperative outcomes after frontal sinus surgery [74, 75]. Steroid-eluting ethmoid sinus implants are currently indicated in patients ≥18 years to maintain patency following ethmoid surgery, and the newer stents are indicated for placement in the surgically opened maxillary os, ethmoid cavity, or frontal recess in adult patients. Two Chinese FDA-approved, bioabsorbable, steroid-eluting sinus stents (652-μg mometasone furoate on a PLGA polymer) have demonstrated improved

Table 22.3 Summary of the current highest-quality studies of steroid-eluting sinus stents for chronic rhinosinusitis (CRS)

Study	Design	Primary inclusion/exclusion criteria	Intervention/comparison (n^a)	Additional study procedures	Results[b]
LANTERN [91]	Multi-center, single-blind randomized controlled trial	Adult patients with a CRS diagnosis and continued symptoms (i.e., an average 4-cardinal symptom composite score ≥ 7 over the past 7 days) despite ≥2 trials of medical therapy, at least one of which was a ≥ 4-week course of nasal steroid spray Bilateral Zinreich MRI score ≥ 4 in the frontal sinuses, sphenoid sinuses, or posterior ethmoids No previous sinus surgery No systemic steroids in the past 1 month No invasive fungal sinusitis, immunodeficiency, severe asthma, mycetoma, or mucocele No allergic rhinitis with a seasonality coinciding with the first 4 weeks of randomization	A self-expanding, steroid-eluting matrix placed in the bilateral middle meatuses in a clinic setting (LYR-210; 7500-μg mometasone furoate, $n = 21$; or 2500-μg mometasone furoate, $n = 23$) *vs* bilateral sham insertion ($n = 23$)	Sham procedure involved delivery system insertion without stent placement; patients were blinded to group allocation using blindfolds during the procedure and subsequent endoscopic evaluations After 24 weeks, implants were removed; controls underwent sham removal procedures A daily intranasal saline irrigation was required during the follow-up period and 14-day washout Nasal steroid sprays, systemic steroids, monoclonal antibodies, and oral decongestants were not permitted except as rescue treatment during screening and follow-up periods; the study permitted stable regimens of inhaled corticosteroids for asthma pharmacotherapy and non-sedating antihistamines	*Subjective Outcome Measures*: Significantly greater improvement in average nasal blockage score in patients treated with 7500-µg LYR-210 at 16 ($p = 0.013$), 20 ($p = 0.007$), and 24 ($p = 0.005$) weeks Significantly greater improvement in mean facial pain score in patients treated with 7500-µg LYR-210 at 12 ($p = 0.048$), 16 ($p = 0.011$), 20 ($p = 0.005$), and 24 ($p = 0.007$) weeks, and patients treated with 2500-µg LYR-210 at 20 weeks ($p = 0.033$) Significantly greater improvement in average nasal discharge score in patients treated with 7500-µg LYR-210 at 16 ($p = 0.012$), 20 ($p = 0.017$), and 24 ($p = 0.007$) weeks, and patients treated with 2500-µg LYR-210 at 16 ($p = 0.023$) and 20 ($p = 0.037$) weeks Significantly greater improvement in mean 4-cardinal symptom composite score in patients treated with 7500-µg LYR-210 at 16 ($p = 0.021$), 20 ($p = 0.012$), and 24 ($p = 0.016$) weeks Significantly greater improvement in mean SNOT-22 score in patients treated with 7500-µg LYR-210 at 8 ($p = 0.039$), 16 ($p = 0.008$), 20 ($p = 0.001$), and 24 ($p = 0.001$) weeks, and patients treated with 2500-µg LYR-210 at 20 weeks ($p = 0.028$) *Objective Outcome Measures*: Significantly greater improvement in mean bilateral Zinreich MRI score for the ethmoid sinuses in patients treated with 7500-µg LYR-210 at 24 weeks ($p = 0.031$) Significantly lower utilization of rescue therapy in patients treated with 7500-ug LYR-210 (HR 0.1, $p < 0.05$) *Safety Results/Adverse Events*: No clinically significant increases in intraocular pressure or diagnosed cataract in either LYR-210 group No significant reductions in morning plasma cortisol levels at 4, 12, or 24 weeks No related serious adverse events

Kern, et al. (2018) [88]	Multi-center, double-blind randomized controlled trial	Patients ≥18 years with a CRS diagnosis who were candidates for revision sinus surgery (i.e., bilateral nasal polyposis [with a grade ≥ 2 on ≥1 side] with ≥ moderate nasal congestion [i.e., nasal congestion/obstruction score of ≥2 for ≥5 of the past 7 days] and ethmoid obstruction despite a prior bilateral total ethmoidectomy + daily nasal steroid spray usage for the past 14 days) Received or refused at least 1 course of high-dose steroid treatment in the past 1 year Polyp grade < 4 on each side No diabetes mellitus, invasive fungal sinusitis, or acute bacterial sinus infection No condition that requires oral steroids, chemotherapy, or immunotherapy No diagnosed subcapsular cataracts or glaucoma	A bioabsorbable, self-expanding, drug-eluting stent placed in the patient's bilateral ethmoid cavities in a clinic setting (Sinuva®, 1350-μg mometasone furoate in a polymer matrix, $n = 201$) *vs* bilateral sham insertion ($n = 99$)	Sham procedure involved delivery system insertion without stent placement Budesonide irrigations, nebulized steroids, and oral steroids were not permitted in the 14-day period before the procedure was performed; parenteral steroid injection was restricted for 30 days before A daily steroid spray (200-µg mometasone furoate, once daily) was required during the follow-up period Budesonide irrigations and nebulized and systemic steroids were prohibited during the follow-up period; oral inhaled corticosteroids were allowed for asthma control Implants were removed by day 60 to allow blinding of sinus surgeons (the blinded, 3-member, review panel) to group assignment in video recordings of nasal endoscopies	*Subjective Outcome Measures*: Significantly greater improvement in average nasal obstruction/congestion symptom score at 30 (−0.80 *vs* − 0.56, $p = 0.0074$), 60 ($p = 0.0129$), and 90 (−0.93 *vs* − 0.69, $p = 0.0248$) days A significantly greater percentage of participants experiencing clinically meaningful improvements in nasal obstruction/congestion score (i.e., ≥ 0.5-point or ≥ 1.0-point reduction) at 30 days (62.8 *vs* 50.5%, $p = 0.0440$; 44.2 *vs* 25.8%, $p = 0.0022$) Significantly greater improvement in mean olfactory symptom score at 90 days (−1.20 *vs* − 0.76, $p = 0.0470$) No significant difference in average facial pain score change at 90 days (−0.77 *vs* − 0.90, $p = 0.9130$) *Objective Outcome Measures*: Significantly greater improvement in mean bilateral polyp grade at 90 days, as determined by the blinded, 3-member, review panel (−0.56 *vs* − 0.15, $p = 0.0073$) and at 14 ($p < 0.0001$), 30 ($p < 0.0001$), 60 ($p < 0.0001$), and 90 ($p < 0.0001$) days, as determined by the study site investigators Significantly greater percentage of participants experiencing clinically meaningful improvements in polyp grade (i.e., ≥ 1.0-point or ≥ 2.0-point reduction) at 90 days, as per scores from the study site investigators (72.0 *vs* 36.7%, $p < 0.0001$; 47.5 *vs* 16.3%, $p < 0.0001$) Significantly greater improvement in mean VAS score for percentage ethmoid obstruction at 90 days, as determined by the blinded, 3-member, review panel (−11.3 *vs* − 1.9, $p = 0.0007$) and at 14 ($p < 0.0001$), 30 ($p < 0.0001$), 60 ($p < 0.0001$), and 90 ($p < 0.0001$) days, as determined by the study site investigators Significant difference in the percent of patients who remained candidates for revision sinus surgery, as determined by the study site investigators, at 90 days (39.0 *vs* 63.3%, $p = 0.0004$) *Safety Results/Adverse Events*: Device-related adverse events included nasal discomfort, parosmia, rhinalgia, as well as a single device-related serious adverse event (epistaxis necessitating surgical cauterization)

(continued)

Table 22.3 (continued)

Study	Design	Primary inclusion/exclusion criteria	Intervention/comparison (n^a)	Additional study procedures	Results[b]
RESOLVE [89, 90]	Multi-center, double-blind randomized controlled trial	Patients ≥18 years with a CRS diagnosis who were candidates for revision sinus surgery (i.e., recurrent CRS symptoms and bilateral nasal polyposis [with a grade ≥ 2 on ≥1 side] with ethmoid obstruction despite an uncomplicated bilateral ethmoidectomy performed >3 months ago + ongoing intranasal steroid irrigation or spray + at least 1 course of systemic steroids in the past 6 months) Polyp grade < 4 on each side No immunodeficiency, invasive fungal sinusitis, acute bacterial sinus infection, type 1 insulin-dependent diabetes, or oral steroid-dependent condition No diagnosis of glaucoma, nuclear sclerotic or cortical cataracts ≥ grade 3, or posterior subcapsular cataracts	A bioabsorbable, self-expanding, drug-eluting stent placed in the patient's bilateral ethmoid cavities in a clinic setting (Sinuva®, 1350-*μ*g mometasone furoate in a polymer matrix, $n = 53$) *vs* bilateral sham insertion ($n = 47$)	Sham procedure involved delivery system insertion without stent placement; patients were blinded to group assignment using a blindfold and noise-cancelling headphones during the procedure and subsequent endoscopic evaluations Intranasal steroid irrigations and oral steroids were not permitted in the 2-week period before the procedure was performed A daily steroid spray (100-μg mometasone furoate, each side, once daily) was required during the follow-up period Intranasal saline irrigation or spray was encouraged after the procedure Steroid nasal rinses were not allowed during the 90-day follow-up period; oral inhaled corticosteroids were allowed for asthma control Implants were removed on day 60 to allow blinding of sinus surgeons (the blinded, 3-member, review panel) to group assignment in video recordings of nasal endoscopies	*Subjective Outcome Measures*: No significant difference in average nasal obstruction/congestion score change at 90 days (−1.33 *vs* − 0.67, $p = 0.137$) or 6 months (−1.06 *vs* − 0.44, $p = 0.124$) Significantly greater improvement in mean NOSE score at 6 months (−25.6 *vs* − 12.2, $p = 0.021$) *Objective Outcome Measures*: Significantly greater improvement in mean bilateral polyp grade at 7 ($p < 0.05$), 14 ($p < 0.05$), 30 ($p < 0.05$), 45 ($p < 0.05$), 60 ($p < 0.05$), 90 (−1.0 *vs* − 0.1, $p = 0.016$), and 180 (−0.71 *vs* + 0.02, $p = 0.018$) days as determined by the study site investigators; no significant difference at 3 months as determined by the blinded, 3-member, review panel (−0.76 *vs* − 0.38, $p = 0.099$) Significantly greater improvement in mean VAS score for percentage ethmoid obstruction, as determined by either the study site investigators at 7 ($p < 0.05$), 14 ($p < 0.05$), 30 ($p < 0.05$), 45 ($p < 0.05$), 60 ($p < 0.05$), 90 (−21.5 *vs* + 1.3, $p = 0.001$), and 180 (−16.5 *vs* + 4.96, $p < 0.001$) days, or the blinded, 3-member, review panel at 3 months (−17.1 *vs* − 5.6, $p = 0.010$) *Safety Results/Adverse Events*: No clinically significant increases in intraocular pressure or diagnosed cataract in either one of the groups Adverse events were similar between groups and included sinusitis, asthma, headache, epistaxis, presyncope, nasopharyngitis, and upper respiratory tract infection

Luong, et al. (2018) [74]	Multi-center, single-blind randomized controlled trial	Adult patients undergoing endoscopic sinus surgery for CRSwNP or CRSsNP Evidence of bilateral frontal sinus disease on computed tomography imaging (i.e., LM score ≥ 1 per side) No immunodeficiency, invasive fungal sinusitis, acute bacterial sinus infection, type 1 insulin-dependent diabetes or oral steroid-dependent condition	A bioabsorbable, self-expanding, drug-eluting stent placed in the patient's left or right frontal sinus opening (Propel® contour, 370-μg mometasone furoate in polylactide-co-glycolide [PLGA], $n = 80$) *vs* surgery alone without stent on the other side ($n = 80$) (Intrapatient comparison, with treatment side randomized)	Extent of surgery included at least a bilateral frontal sinusotomy (Draf IIa or IIb, using traditional sinus instruments, a balloon, or both), with ≥5-mm frontal sinus opening Post-operative care included a 10-day antibiotic course; saline nasal sprays or irrigation were encouraged Oral inhaled corticosteroids were allowed for asthma control; after 14 days, steroid nasal sprays were permitted Implants were removed on day-21 to allow blinding of a sinus surgeon (the blinded independent reviewer) to group assignment in video recordings of nasal endoscopies	*Objective Outcome Measures*: Significantly lower percentage of sinuses having an endoscopic indication for postsurgical intervention (i.e., scar tissue debridement or oral steroid treatment), as determined by either the study site investigators at 30 (16.0 *vs* 33.3%, 95% CI −27.9 to −6.7%) and 90 (95% CI −21.0 to −2.4%) days, or a blinded independent reviewer at 30 days (11.5 *vs* 32.8%, 95% CI −35.1 to −7.6%) Significant difference in mean VAS score for inflammation at 30 (23.1 *vs* 35.6, 95% CI −18.3 to −6.4), but not 90 (26.0 *vs* 31.9, 95% CI −11.3 to 0.3) days Significantly lower prevalence of restenosed or occluded frontal sinuses (i.e., frontal sinus patency grade ≥ 1) at 30 (13.3 *vs* 36.0%, 95% CI −33.5 to −11.9%) and 90 (23.2 *vs* 40.6%, 95% CI −28.6 to −6.1%) days Significant difference in average frontal sinus opening diameter at 30 (6.3 *vs* 4.5 mm, 95% CI 1.3 to 2.5 mm) and 90 (5.7 *vs* 4.7 mm, 95% CI 0.2 to 1.7 mm) days Significant difference in mean frontal sinus LM score at 90 days (0.7 *vs* 0.9, 95% CI −0.3 to −0.1) *Safety Results/Adverse Events*: No device-related adverse events
Smith, et al. (2016) [75]	Multi-center, single-blind randomized controlled trial	Adult patients undergoing endoscopic sinus surgery for CRSwNP or CRSsNP Evidence of bilateral frontal sinus disease on computed tomography imaging (i.e., LM score ≥ 1 per side) No immunodeficiency, invasive fungal sinusitis, acute bacterial sinus infection, type 1 insulin-dependent diabetes, or oral steroid-dependent condition	A bioabsorbable, self-expanding, drug-eluting stent placed in the patient's left or right frontal sinus opening (Propel® mini, 370-μg mometasone furoate in polylactide-co-glycolide [PLGA], $n = 67$) *vs* surgery alone without stent on the other side ($n = 67$) (intrapatient comparison, with treatment side randomized)	Extent of surgery included at least a bilateral frontal sinusotomy (Draf IIa or IIb, using traditional sinus instruments, a balloon, or both), with ≥5-mm frontal sinus opening Post-operative care included a 10-day antibiotic course; saline nasal sprays or irrigation were encouraged Oral inhaled corticosteroids were allowed for asthma control; after 14 days, steroid nasal sprays were permitted Implants were removed on day-21 to allow blinding of a sinus surgeon (the blinded independent reviewer) to group assignment in video recordings of nasal endoscopies	*Objective Outcome Measures*: Significantly lower percentage of sinuses having an endoscopic indication for postsurgical intervention (i.e., scar tissue debridement or oral steroid treatment) at 30 days, as determined by either the study site investigators (16.5 *vs* 41.8%, $p < 0.0001$) or a blinded independent reviewer (38.8 *vs* 62.7%, $p = 0.0070$) Significant difference in mean VAS score for inflammation at 30 days (24.7 *vs* 41.3, $p < 0.0001$) Significantly lower prevalence of restenosed or occluded frontal sinuses at 30 days (21.1 *vs* 46.1%, $p = 0.0002$) Significant difference in average frontal sinus opening diameter at 30 days (5.9 *vs* 4.4 mm, $p < 0.0001$) *Safety Results/Adverse Events*: No device-related adverse events

(continued)

Table 22.3 (continued)

Study	Design	Primary inclusion/exclusion criteria	Intervention/comparison (n^a)	Additional study procedures	Results[b]
Wang, et al. (2023) [76]	Multi-center, single-blind randomized controlled trial	18 to 65-year-old patients undergoing a full house endoscopic sinus surgery, endoscopic middle turbinate resection, and polypectomy for bilateral eCRSwNP (defined as CRSwNP in which polyp tissue shows either (1) proportion of eosinophils >27% of total infiltrating cells or (2) > 55 eosinophils/hpf) No cataract, glaucoma, immunodeficiency, acute fungal sinus infection, acute bacterial sinus infection, an oral steroid-dependent condition, or severe diabetes or hypertension	A bioabsorbable, drug-eluting stent placed in the patient's left or right ethmoid sinus cavity ± a second stent in the frontal recess (Xiangtong®, 652-μg mometasone furoate in polylactide-co-glycolide [PLGA], $n = 95$) *vs* surgery alone without stent on the other side ($n = 95$) (intrapatient comparison, with treatment side randomized)	Septoplasty was permitted for severe nasal septal deviation A stent was placed in the frontal recess if the frontal sinus was well aerated with a frontal ostium diameter of ≥10 mm in the anterior–posterior direction Post-operative care included saline nasal sprays or irrigations, and mucolytics and leukotriene receptor antagonists if medically indicated Steroid nasal sprays were allowed after surgery; oral steroids were not permitted during the follow-up period	*Subjective Outcome Measures*: Significant difference in the average total nasal symptoms (5.47 *vs* 6.41, $p = 0.001$) and nasal obstruction scores (0.92 *vs* 1.35, $p < 0.01$) at 8 weeks; no significant differences in other average nasal symptom scores *Objective Outcome Measures*: Significant difference in mean LKES at 4 (3.21 *vs* 3.80, $p = 0.001$), 8 (1.96 *vs* 2.77, $p < 0.001$), and 12 (1.05 *vs* 2.05, $p < 0.001$) weeks; subscores for crusting at 2 (1.53 *vs* 0.98, $p < 0.001$) and 8 (0.20 *vs* 0.36, $p < 0.01$) weeks; scarring at 4 weeks (0.26 *vs* 0.41, $p < 0.05$); discharge at 12 weeks (0.30 *vs* 0.73, $p < 0.001$); and edema at 2 (1.35 *vs* 1.65, $p < 0.01$), 4 (0.95 *vs* 1.30, $p < 0.001$), 8 (0.74 *vs* 1.03, $p < 0.01$), and 12 (0.65 *vs* 1.00, $p < 0.01$) weeks; no significant differences in other endoscopic scores No significant difference in the total nasal volume or resistance, minimal cross-sectional area, or nasal nitric oxide levels at 2, 4, 8, or 12 weeks Significantly lower median disease volumetric score in the ethmoid (25.0 *vs* 30.0, $p = 0.011$) and frontal (31.0 *vs* 35.0, $p = 0.032$) sinuses at 8 weeks Significantly lower median eosinophil count in the ethmoid sinus mucosa at 4 weeks (30.0 *vs* 60.0, $p = 0.011$) *Safety Results/Adverse Events*: No significant difference in morning plasma cortisol levels at 4 or 12 weeks No device-related adverse events

Huang, et al. (2022) [77]	Multi-center, single-blind randomized controlled trial	CRS patients undergoing bilateral endoscopic sinus surgery 18–65 years of age Bilateral CRSwNP or CRSsNP diagnosis Not using immunosuppressive agents No diabetes, glaucoma, acute fungal sinus infection, acute bacterial sinus infection, ocular hypertension, or autoimmune disease	A bioabsorbable, drug-eluting stent placed in the patient's left or right ethmoid sinus cavity (BISORB®, 652-μg mometasone furoate in polylactide-co-glycolide [PLGA], $n = 181$) *vs* non-steroid impregnated, bioabsorbable packing on the other side (NasoPore®, $n = 181$) (intrapatient comparison, with treatment side randomized)	Post-operative care included a 7-day antibiotic course Saline nasal sprays and intranasal saline irrigations were allowed before and after surgery After 30 days, steroid nasal sprays were permitted	*Objective Outcome Measures*: Significantly lower percentage of sinuses meeting criteria for postsurgical intervention (i.e., endoscopic middle turbinate lateralization score ≥ 3, or adhesion or polyp score ≥ 2) at 30 days, as determined by either the study site investigators (33.7 *vs* 66.3%, $p < 0.0001$) or a blinded, 3-member, review panel (14.38 *vs* 75.00%, $p < 0.0001$) Lower frequency of polyp formation (i.e., polyp grade ≥ 2) at 14 (16.57 *vs* 44.75%, $p < 0.0001$), 30 (22.65 *vs* 54.14%, $p < 0.0001$), and 90 (6.78 *vs* 25.42%, $p < 0.0001$) days, as determined by the study site investigators No significant difference in the percent of sinuses with a lateralized middle turbinate at 14 (0.00 *vs* 0.00%), 30 (0.55 *vs* 0.55%, $p = 1.00$), or 90 (0.00 *vs* 0.00%) days, as determined by the study site investigators Significantly lower percentage of sinus cavities with severe adhesions at 90 (7.63 *vs* 25.42%, $p = 0.0003$), but not 14 (0.00 *vs* 0.00%) or 30 (0.55 *vs* 2.21%, $p = 0.0833$) days, as determined by the study site investigators *Safety Results/Adverse Events*: No significant difference in average intraocular pressure at 14 (15.54 *vs* 15.68, $p > 0.05$), 30 (15.09 *vs* 15.30, $p > 0.05$), or 90 (14.97 *vs* 14.87, $p > 0.05$) days No significant difference in apparent lens opacities at 14, 30, or 90 days No device-related adverse events occurred during the follow-up period
Rawl, et al. (2020) [114]	Single-center, single-blind randomized controlled trial	Adult patients undergoing endoscopic sinus surgery for CRSwNP or CRSsNP No previous sinus surgery No immunodeficiency, cystic fibrosis, or ciliary disorder	A bioabsorbable, self-expanding, drug-eluting stent placed in the bilateral middle meatuses (Propel®, 370-μg mometasone furoate in polylactide-co-glycolide [PLGA], $n = 22$) *vs* Merocel® packs wrapped in non-latex glove material ($n = 18$)	Extent of surgery included ≥ a total ethmoidectomy, maxillary antrostomy, and middle turbinate management Post-operative care included oral steroids, antibiotics, and budesonide irrigations Spacers were removed at 8–10 days to enable blinded review of nasal endoscopy video recordings	*Subjective Outcome Measures*: No significant difference in mean SNOT-22 scores at 8–10 days (29.9 *vs* 29.1, $p = 0.9248$), 20 days (21.6 *vs* 9.7, $p = 0.0528$), 1 month (10.6 *vs* 7.1, $p = 0.4871$), or 3 months (12.0 *vs* 13.3, $p = 0.8087$) *Objective Outcome Measures*: Significant difference in mean VAS score for right- and left-sided middle turbinate lateralization at 8–10 days (1.73 *vs* 0.38, $p = 0.0399$; 2.45 *vs* 0.43, $p = 0.0231$), but not at 20 days (2.00 *vs* 1.38, $p = 0.4187$; 2.10 *vs* 2.23, $p = 0.8853$), 1 month (3.00 *vs* 0.80, $p = 0.1396$; 2.38 *vs* 0.40, $p = 0.0730$), or 3 months (1.67 *vs* 2.20, $p = 0.7325$; 1.17 *vs* 1.00, $p = 0.8666$) Significantly lower percentage of patients with a perfect-"0" VAS for left-sided middle turbinate lateralization (i.e., totally medialized middle turbinate; 27.3 *vs* 71.4%, $p = 0.030$); no significant difference on the right side (36.4 *vs* 76.9%, $p = 0.095$) No significant difference in mean LKES on the left or right at 8–10 days (1.45 *vs* 1.43, $p = 0.9457$; 1.73 *vs* 1.23, $p = 0.3436$), 20 days (1.70 *vs* 2.08, $p = 0.4384$; 1.56 *vs* 2.08, $p = 0.3144$), 1 month (1.75 *vs* 1.60, $p = 0.8514$; 2.28 *vs* 2.40, $p = 0.8993$), or 3 months (1.83 *vs* 1.50, $p = 0.4848$; 2.33 *vs* 1.17, $p = 0.1204$)

(continued)

Table 22.3 (continued)

Study	Design	Primary inclusion/exclusion criteria	Intervention/comparison (n^a)	Additional study procedures	Results[b]
ADVANCE II [73]	Multi-center, double-blind randomized controlled trial	Adult patients undergoing endoscopic sinus surgery for CRSwNP or CRSsNP after failure of conservative management LM score ≥ 6 No immunodeficiency, invasive fungal sinusitis, acute bacterial sinus infection, type 1 insulin-dependent diabetes or oral steroid-dependent condition No diagnosis of glaucoma, cataracts ≥ grade 3, or posterior subcapsular cataracts	A bioabsorbable, self-expanding, drug-eluting stent placed in the patient's left or right ethmoid sinus cavity (Propel®, 370-μg mometasone furoate in polylactide-co-glycolide [PLGA], $n = 105$) *vs* a non-eluting PLGA stent placed on the other side ($n = 105$) (Intrapatient comparison, with treatment side randomized)	Extent of surgery included ≥ bilateral ethmoidectomy; other turbinate medialization procedures were not permitted Peri-operative care included a 14-day antibiotic course; antibiotic treatment for suspected infections was permitted during the follow-up period Saline nasal sprays and intranasal saline irrigations were allowed after surgery No steroid nasal sprays or oral steroids were allowed in the initial 30-day period after surgery; oral inhaled corticosteroids were allowed for asthma control Endoscopic assessment was performed on recordings by a blinded, 3-member, review panel, and in real time by the study site investigators	*Objective Outcome Measures*: Significantly lower percentage of sinuses having an endoscopic indication for postsurgical intervention (i.e., adhesion lysis or oral steroids) at 30 days, as determined by majority opinion of a blinded panel of sinus surgeons (33.3 *vs* 46.9%, $p = 0.028$); no significant difference as determined by the study site investigators (21.9 *vs* 31.4%, $p = 0.068$) Lower frequency of frank polyposis (i.e., polyp grade ≥ 2) at 30 days, as determined by majority opinion of a blinded panel of sinus surgeons (18.8 *vs* 34.1%, $p = 0.002$); no significant difference when using the scores from the study site investigators (3.8 *vs* 7.7%, $p = 0.344$) No significant difference in the percent of sinuses with a lateralized middle turbinate at 30 days, as per scores from the study site investigators (1.9 *vs* 6.7%, $p = 0.125$) Significantly lower prevalence of dense or severe adhesions at 30 days, as per scores from the study site investigators (4.8 *vs* 12.5%, $p = 0.039$) *Safety Results/Adverse Events*: No clinically significant intraocular pressure or lens opacity changes from baseline

Murr, et al. (2011) [72]	Multi-center, double-blind randomized controlled trial	Adult patients undergoing endoscopic sinus surgery for CRSwNP or CRSsNP after failure of conservative management LM score ≥ 3 per side No immunodeficiency, allergic fungal sinusitis, type 1 insulin-dependent diabetes or oral steroid-dependent condition	A bioabsorbable, self-expanding, drug-eluting stent placed in the patient's left or right ethmoid sinus cavity (Propel®, 370-μg mometasone furoate in polylactide-co-glycolide [PLGA], $n = 38$) vs a non-eluting PLGA stent placed on the other side ($n = 38$) (intrapatient comparison, with treatment side randomized)	Oral steroids were not permitted in the 14-day period before surgery; steroid nasal sprays could be used up until the day before Extent of surgery included at least a bilateral maxillary antrostomy and ethmoidectomy; other turbinate medialization procedures were not permitted Peri-operative care included intravenous dexamethasone administered before the start of surgery, a 14-day antibiotic course (amoxicillin-clavulanate, 875 mg–125 mg, every 12 hours), and saline nasal sprays and/or intranasal saline irrigations as per preference of the physician After 30 days, clinicians were permitted to prescribe steroids if necessary; no steroid nasal sprays or oral steroids were allowed in the initial 30-day period after surgery	*Objective Outcome Measures*: Significantly lower ethmoid sinus inflammation, as measured by mean VAS score, at 21 (23.2 vs 35.3, $p = 0.0032$), 30 (20.2 vs 30.1, $p = 0.0011$), and 45 (15.9 vs 24.0, $p = 0.0022$) days; no significant difference at 7 (29.6 vs 29.4, $p = 0.6038$), 14 (24.7 vs 31.2, $p = 0.0780$), or 60 (12.0 vs 17.5, $p = 0.0855$) days Significantly lower frequencies of polypoid mucosal changes (i.e., polyp grade ≥ 1; 18.4 vs 36.8%, $p = 0.0391$) and dense or severe adhesions (5.3 vs 21.1%, $p = 0.0313$) at 30 days No significant difference in the percent of sinuses with a lateralized middle turbinate at 30 days (5.3 vs 15.8%, $p = 0.2188$) *Safety Results/Adverse Events*: No device-related adverse events

CI confidence interval, *CRSwNP/sNP* CRS with and without nasal polyposis, *eCRSwNP* eosinophilic CRSwNP, *HR* hazard ratio, *LKES* Lund-Kennedy Endoscopic Score, *LM* Lund-Mackay, *NOSE* Nasal Obstruction Symptom Evaluation, *SNOT-22* 22-Item Sino-Nasal Outcome Test, *VAS* visual analog scale

[a]included in the analysis

[b]of intergroup comparisons, unless otherwise stated

postoperative outcomes in blinded, randomized controlled studies [76, 77]. Other randomized controlled trials have evaluated steroid-impregnated packing materials [78–84] and calcium alginate packing [85], with mixed results across studies.

Several early studies [86, 87] showed the safety, efficacy, and feasibility of in-office endoscopic steroid-eluting stent placement in the ethmoid cavity of adult patients with a prior history of sinus surgery. Though there is a case series describing in-office placement of absorbable steroid implants in the ethmoid cavity at 5–7 days after sinus surgery [87], only one nonabsorbable sinus implant is FDA-approved drug-eluting stent specifically developed for in-office insertion (Sinuva®). This sinus implant is a self-expanding stent composed of a mometasone furoate-impregnated polymer, allowing controlled release of 1350 μg of steroid over a 90-day period that was specially designed for in-office endoscopic insertion in formerly operated ethmoid cavities, and is intended to be removed at day 90 or before. Blinded, randomized controlled studies in CRSwNP patients meeting criteria for revision sinus surgery have shown that in-office sinus implant insertion results in greater improvement in ethmoid obstruction, polyp grade, and NOSE (Nasal Obstruction Symptom Evaluation) score, compared to sham insertion with continued benefit noted at 6-month follow-up [88–90]. Moreover, the percentage of patients who remained candidates for revision surgery after 90 days was considerably reduced with sinus implantation versus placebo (39.0 vs 63.3%, $p = 0.0004$) [88].

A new bioabsorbable nasal mesh (LYR-210®) is currently in phase 3 clinical testing. This device is a self-expanding, steroid-eluting, elastomeric mesh, intended for insertion in the middle meatus of CRS patients with no prior history of sinus surgery, and delivers 2500 μg or 7500 μg of mometasone furoate over 24 weeks. Phase 2 study results demonstrated improvement in mean MRI score, patient reported cardinal symptoms, and SNOT-22, as well as lower utilization of rescue therapy, at 24 weeks when compared to sham insertion [91].

Reported rates of successful deployment of sinus implants are high, and routine insertion of an implant at the end of surgery is typically straightforward, though there have been reports of misplaced implants/stents [92]. Studies have shown no significant HPA axis suppression or increases in intraocular pressure or cataract diagnosis with multiple steroid-eluting implants [71, 73, 76, 77, 90, 91]. Device-related adverse events are uncommon but can include infection, facial pain/headache, and stent migration with expulsion or oropharyngeal obstruction [93]. These adverse events should be viewed in context and weighed against possible adverse outcomes from postoperative interventions (e.g., adhesion lysis or oral steroids) or primary or revision sinus surgery. The comfort level with in-office stent placement appears to be provider-dependent, with a recent survey showing that in-office endoscopic steroid-eluting stent placement is performed by only a minority of rhinologists [94].

There are multiple considerations when determining when to use steroid-eluting stents in clinical practice. These stents add a considerable expense to patient care [95] and may be better suited for use in patients at higher risk for surgical or treatment failure. However, subgroup analyses of pooled data from high-quality, industry-sponsored blinded, randomized, placebo-controlled studies were largely unrevealing as to which specific populations would benefit most from steroid-eluting sinus stents [96–98]. A recent Delphi method study of rhinology experts revealed general agreement that steroid-eluting stent placement could be considered in oral steroid-intolerant patients and patients with diabetes (as an alternative to oral steroids) or extended frontal sinus surgery [99]. Ninety-two percent of experts also agreed that in-office stent placement could be considered in CRSwNP patients with recurrent stenosis [99]. While drug-eluting stents may have little utility for routine CRS patients, they are useful tools and beneficial in certain scenarios. However, with the state of the current literature, it is still largely up to individual patients and clinicians to determine individual risks and benefits.

Glucocorticoid Insensitivity

One factor that may influence the efficacy of topical steroid therapy is glucocorticoid resistance. If glucocorticoids are fundamentally ineffective in a subset of patients with CRS, then better delivery methods will be of little use in these patients. There are multiple possible mechanisms of glucocorticoid insensitivity in CRS, including genetic variants in the GR gene [100], disrupted GR function by under- or overexpression of mucins [101, 102], and P-glycoprotein (a multidrug resistance protein) overexpression with accelerated efflux of intracellular steroid [103]. However, the mechanism that has received the most attention concerns alternative splicing of the GR pre-mRNA to generate alpha (GRα) and beta (GRβ) isoforms. GRα is the classical GR isoform that resides in the cellular cytoplasm and mediates the response to glucocorticoids. Conversely, GRβ does not bind to glucocorticoids, is only present in the nucleus, and exerts dominant negative effects on GRα as well as regulates gene expression in a GRα- and steroid-independent manner [28, 29]. Therefore, individual variations in alternative splicing of GR transcripts represent one hypothesis to explain the poor response to nasal corticosteroids of some patients. However, current studies have yielded conflicting results regarding whether and how the relative and/or absolute expression of GRα and GRβ is altered in CRSwNP and CRSsNP tissue relative to control nasal mucosa, following glucocorticoid treatment, and with treatment-resistant CRS [32, 104–113]. Moreover, the comparative contributions of glucocorticoid resistance and suboptimal topical drug delivery (i.e., with simple nasal steroid spray) to the larger problem of refractory CRS are unknown.

Conclusions

Recalcitrant CRS is the product of an aberrant inflammatory response surrounding the sinonasal mucosa, which results in symptoms that significantly diminish a patient's quality of life. Topical corticosteroids, which provide a localized anti-inflammatory effect and avoid many of the undesirable side effects of systemic corticosteroids, are an attractive and useful therapy for many of these patients. By altering the amount and delivery method of corticosteroid, better topical delivery of corticosteroids may assist CRS patients with recalcitrant disease, who failed to respond to initial treatment with intranasal corticosteroid sprays, saline irrigations, and even surgery. The delivery methods described in this chapter, including intranasal corticosteroid irrigations, exhalation delivery systems, and steroid-eluting implants, are all useful tools for the treatment of recalcitrant CRS. However, until more predictive phenotypes or endotypes are described or more robust comparative RCTs are performed, patients and providers will have to rely on general guidelines, anecdotal experience, and trial and error in the treatment of this challenging disease.

References

1. Borish L, Baroody FM, Kim MS, Lieberman JA, Peters A, Stevens WW, et al. Yardstick for the medical management of chronic rhinosinusitis. Ann Allergy Asthma Immunol. 2022;128(2):118–28.
2. Fokkens WJ, Lund VJ, Hopkins C, Hellings PW, Kern R, Reitsma S, et al. European position paper on rhinosinusitis and Nasal Polyps 2020. Rhinology. 2020;58(Suppl S29):1–464.
3. Han JK, Bosso JV, Cho SH, Franzese C, Lam K, Lane AP, et al. Multidisciplinary consensus on a stepwise treatment algorithm for management of chronic rhinosinusitis with nasal polyps. Int Forum Allergy Rhinol. 2021;11(10):1407–16.
4. Orlandi RR, Kingdom TT, Smith TL, Bleier B, DeConde A, Luong AU, et al. International consensus statement on allergy and rhinology: rhinosinusitis 2021. Int Forum Allergy Rhinol. 2021;11(3):213–739.
5. Rosenfeld RM, Piccirillo JF, Chandrasekhar SS, Brook I, Ashok Kumar K, Kramper M, et al. Clinical practice guideline (update): adult sinusitis. Otolaryngol Head Neck Surg. 2015;152(2 Suppl):S1–S39.
6. Rudmik L, Hoy M, Schlosser RJ, Harvey RJ, Welch KC, Lund V, et al. Topical therapies in the management of chronic rhinosinusitis: an evidence-based review with recommendations. Int Forum Allergy Rhinol. 2013;3(4):281–98.
7. Rudmik L, Soler ZM. Medical therapies for adult chronic sinusitis: a systematic review. JAMA. 2015;314(9):926–39.
8. Scadding GK, Durham SR, Mirakian R, Jones NS, Drake-Lee AB, Ryan D, et al. BSACI guidelines for the management of rhinosinusitis and nasal polyposis. Clin Exp Allergy. 2008;38(2):260–75.
9. Chong LY, Head K, Hopkins C, Philpott C, Schilder AG, Burton MJ. Intranasal steroids versus placebo or no intervention for chronic rhinosinusitis. Cochrane Database Syst Rev. 2016;4(4):CD011996.
10. Joe SA, Thambi R, Huang J. A systematic review of the use of intranasal steroids in the treatment of chronic rhinosinusitis. Otolaryngol Head Neck Surg. 2008;139(3):340–7.
11. Rudmik L, Schlosser RJ, Smith TL, Soler ZM. Impact of topical nasal steroid therapy on symptoms of nasal polyposis: a meta-analysis. Laryngoscope. 2012;122(7):1431–7.
12. Young LC, Stow NW, Zhou L, Douglas RG. Efficacy of medical therapy in treatment of chronic rhinosinusitis. Allergy Rhinol (Providence). 2012;3(1):e8–e12.
13. Soler ZM, Wittenberg E, Schlosser RJ, Mace JC, Smith TL. Health state utility values in patients undergoing endoscopic sinus surgery. Laryngoscope. 2011;121(12):2672–8.
14. Rudmik L, Smith TL, Schlosser RJ, Hwang PH, Mace JC, Soler ZM. Productivity costs in patients with refractory chronic rhinosinusitis. Laryngoscope. 2014;124(9):2007–12.
15. Vaidyanathan S, Barnes M, Williamson P, Hopkinson P, Donnan PT, Lipworth B. Treatment of chronic rhinosinusitis with nasal polyposis with oral steroids followed by topical steroids: a randomized trial. Ann Intern Med. 2011;154(5):293–302.

16. Van Zele T, Gevaert P, Holtappels G, Beule A, Wormald PJ, Mayr S, et al. Oral steroids and doxycycline: two different approaches to treat nasal polyps. J Allergy Clin Immunol. 2010;125(5):1069–76.e4
17. Poetker DM, Reh DD. A comprehensive review of the adverse effects of systemic corticosteroids. Otolaryngol Clin N Am. 2010;43(4):753–68.
18. Waljee AK, Rogers MA, Lin P, Singal AG, Stein JD, Marks RM, et al. Short term use of oral corticosteroids and related harms among adults in the United States: population based cohort study. BMJ. 2017;357:j1415.
19. Yao TC, Huang YW, Chang SM, Tsai SY, Wu AC, Tsai HJ. Association between oral corticosteroid bursts and severe adverse events : a nationwide population-based cohort study. Ann Intern Med. 2020;173(5):325–30.
20. Rudman KL, O'Brien EK, Leopold DA. Radiographic distribution of drops and sprays within the sinonasal cavities. Am J Rhinol Allergy. 2011;25(2):94–7.
21. Siu J, Johnston JJ, Pontre B, Inthavong K, Douglas RG. Magnetic resonance imaging evaluation of the distribution of spray and irrigation devices within the sinonasal cavities. Int Forum Allergy Rhinol. 2019;9(9):958–70.
22. Wormald PJ, Cain T, Oates L, Hawke L, Wong I. A comparative study of three methods of nasal irrigation. Laryngoscope. 2004;114(12):2224–7.
23. Djupesland PG, Skretting A. Nasal deposition and clearance in man: comparison of a bidirectional powder device and a traditional liquid spray pump. J Aerosol Med Pulm Drug Deliv. 2012;25(5):280–9.
24. Djupesland PG, Skretting A, Winderen M, Holand T. Breath actuated device improves delivery to target sites beyond the nasal valve. Laryngoscope. 2006;116(3):466–72.
25. Lam K, Tan BK, Lavin JM, Meen E, Conley DB. Comparison of nasal sprays and irrigations in the delivery of topical agents to the olfactory mucosa. Laryngoscope. 2013;123(12):2950–7.
26. Wang X, Zhang N, Bo M, Holtappels G, Zheng M, Lou H, et al. Diversity of TH cytokine profiles in patients with chronic rhinosinusitis: a multicenter study in Europe, Asia, and Oceania. J Allergy Clin Immunol. 2016;138(5):1344–53.
27. Xie X, Xuan L, Zhao Y, Wang X, Zhang L. Diverse endotypes of chronic rhinosinusitis and clinical implications. Clin Rev Allergy Immunol. 2023;65(3):420–32.
28. Cain DW, Cidlowski JA. Immune regulation by glucocorticoids. Nat Rev Immunol. 2017;17(4):233–47.
29. Timmermans S, Souffriau J, Libert C. A general introduction to glucocorticoid biology. Front Immunol. 2019;10:1545.
30. Galon J, Franchimont D, Hiroi N, Frey G, Boettner A, Ehrhart-Bornstein M, et al. Gene profiling reveals unknown enhancing and suppressive actions of glucocorticoids on immune cells. FASEB J. 2002;16(1):61–71.
31. Bai CH, Song SY, Kim YD. Effect of glucocorticoid on the MUC4 gene in nasal polyps. Laryngoscope. 2007;117(12):2169–73.
32. Valera FC, Queiroz R, Scrideli C, Tone LG, Anselmo-Lima WT. Evaluating budesonide efficacy in nasal polyposis and predicting the resistance to treatment. Clin Exp Allergy. 2009;39(1):81–8.
33. Hamilos DL, Thawley SE, Kramper MA, Kamil A, Hamid QA. Effect of intranasal fluticasone on cellular infiltration, endothelial adhesion molecule expression, and proinflammatory cytokine mRNA in nasal polyp disease. J Allergy Clin Immunol. 1999;103(1 Pt 1):79–87.
34. Ahamed S, Samson D, Sundaresan R, Balasubramanya B, Thomas R. Double blinded randomized controlled trial comparing budesonide and saline nasal rinses in the post-operative management of chronic rhinosinusitis. Indian J Otolaryngol Head Neck Surg. 2024;76(1):408–13.
35. Megow A, Bouras G, Ooi EH, Vreugde S, Psaltis A, Wormald PJ. Double blind randomized controlled trial measuring the efficacy of nebulized steroid at half dose in comparison to high volume squeeze bottle steroid irrigation in management of patients with chronic rhinosinusitis. Int Forum Allergy Rhinol. 2024;14(8):1375–7.
36. Jiramongkolchai P, Peterson A, Kallogjeri D, Lee JJ, Kukuljan S, Liebendorfer A, et al. Randomized clinical trial to evaluate mometasone lavage vs spray for patients with chronic

rhinosinusitis without nasal polyps who have not undergone sinus surgery. Int Forum Allergy Rhinol. 2020;10(8):936–43.
37. Harvey RJ, Snidvongs K, Kalish LH, Oakley GM, Sacks R. Corticosteroid nasal irrigations are more effective than simple sprays in a randomized double-blinded placebo-controlled trial for chronic rhinosinusitis after sinus surgery. Int Forum Allergy Rhinol. 2018;8(4):461–70.
38. Tait S, Kallogjeri D, Suko J, Kukuljan S, Schneider J, Piccirillo JF. Effect of budesonide added to large-volume, low-pressure saline sinus irrigation for chronic rhinosinusitis: a randomized clinical trial. JAMA Otolaryngol Head Neck Surg. 2018;144(7):605–12.
39. Rawal RB, Deal AM, Ebert CS, Dhandha VH, Mitchell CA, Hang AX, et al. Post-operative budesonide irrigations for patients with polyposis: a blinded, randomized controlled trial. Rhinology. 2015;53(3):227–34.
40. Rotenberg BW, Zhang I, Arra I, Payton KB. Postoperative care for Samter's triad patients undergoing endoscopic sinus surgery: a double-blinded, randomized controlled trial. Laryngoscope. 2011;121(12):2702–5.
41. Dawson B, Gutteridge I, Cervin A, Robinson D. The effects of nasal lavage with betamethasone cream post-endoscopic sinus surgery: clinical trial. J Laryngol Otol. 2018;132(2):143–9.
42. Kang TW, Chung JH, Cho SH, Lee SH, Kim KR, Jeong JH. The effectiveness of budesonide nasal irrigation after endoscopic sinus surgery in chronic rhinosinusitis with asthma. Clin Exp Otorhinolaryngol. 2017;10(1):91–6.
43. Kosugi EM, Moussalem GF, Simões JC, de Paula e Silva Felici de Souza R, Chen VG, Neto PS, et al. Topical therapy with high-volume budesonide nasal irrigations in difficult-to-treat chronic rhinosinusitis. Braz J Otorhinolaryngol. 2016;82(2):191–7.
44. Sachanandani NS, Piccirillo JF, Kramper MA, Thawley SE, Vlahiotis A. The effect of nasally administered budesonide respules on adrenal cortex function in patients with chronic rhinosinusitis. Arch Otolaryngol Head Neck Surg. 2009;135(3):303–7.
45. Snidvongs K, Pratt E, Chin D, Sacks R, Earls P, Harvey RJ. Corticosteroid nasal irrigations after endoscopic sinus surgery in the management of chronic rhinosinusitis. Int Forum Allergy Rhinol. 2012;2(5):415–21.
46. Pipaliya RM, Duckett KA, Monaghan NP, Miller EM, Young G, Brennan EA, et al. The placebo effect in randomized-controlled trials of medical treatments for chronic rhinosinusitis: a systematic review and meta-analysis. Int Forum Allergy Rhinol. 2024;14(3):695–710.
47. Park DY, Choi JH, Kim DK, Jung YG, Mun SJ, Min HJ, et al. Clinical practice guideline: nasal irrigation for chronic rhinosinusitis in adults. Clin Exp Otorhinolaryngol. 2022;15(1):5–23.
48. Gutierrez JA, Shannon CM, Chapurin N, Schlosser RJ, Soler ZM. Challenges to medication adherence with intranasal corticosteroid irrigations. Int Forum Allergy Rhinol. 2024;14(1):32–40.
49. Eschenbacher WH. Nasal saline irrigation with steroids: reviewing a common practice carefully. Ann Allergy Asthma Immunol. 2023;130(1):2–3.
50. Barham HP, Ramakrishnan VR, Knisely A, Do TQ, Chan LS, Gunaratne DA, et al. Frontal sinus surgery and sinus distribution of nasal irrigation. Int Forum Allergy Rhinol. 2016;6(3):238–42.
51. Beule A, Athanasiadis T, Athanasiadis E, Field J, Wormald PJ. Efficacy of different techniques of sinonasal irrigation after modified Lothrop procedure. Am J Rhinol Allergy. 2009;23(1):85–90.
52. Mozzanica F, Preti A, Bandi F, Fazio E, Cardella A, Gallo S, et al. Effect of surgery, delivery device and head position on sinus irrigant penetration in a cadaver model. J Laryngol Otol. 2021;135(3):234–40.
53. Singhal D, Weitzel EK, Lin E, Feldt B, Kriete B, McMains KC, et al. Effect of head position and surgical dissection on sinus irrigant penetration in cadavers. Laryngoscope. 2010;120(12):2528–31.
54. Sumaily I, Jomaah M, Alarifi I, Alromaih S, Aloulah M, Ajlan A, et al. Extent of nasal irrigation in non-operated sinuses: a cadaveric trial. Ear Nose Throat J. 2022;1455613221081567

55. Barham HP, Hall CA, Hernandez SC, Zylicz HE, Stevenson MM, Zito BA, et al. Impact of Draf III, Draf IIb, and Draf IIa frontal sinus surgery on nasal irrigation distribution. Int Forum Allergy Rhinol. 2020;10(1):49–52.
56. Grayson JW, Cavada M, Wong E, Lien B, Duvnjak M, Campbell R, et al. Effects of sphenoid surgery on nasal irrigation delivery. Int Forum Allergy Rhinol. 2019;9(9):971–6.
57. Wong E, Sansoni ER, Do TQ, Matchett I, Kalish LH, Sacks R, et al. Cadaveric assessment of the efficacy of sinus irrigation after staged clearance of the medial maxillary wall. Am J Rhinol Allergy. 2020;34(2):290–6.
58. Hansen FS, Djupesland PG, Fokkens WJ. Preliminary efficacy of fluticasone delivered by a novel device in recalcitrant chronic rhinosinusitis. Rhinology. 2010;48(3):292–9.
59. Vlckova I, Navrátil P, Kana R, Pavlicek P, Chrbolka P, Djupesland PG. Effective treatment of mild-to-moderate nasal polyposis with fluticasone delivered by a novel device. Rhinology. 2009;47(4):419–26.
60. Leopold DA, Elkayam D, Messina JC, Kosik-Gonzalez C, Djupesland PG, Mahmoud RA. NAVIGATE II: randomized, double-blind trial of the exhalation delivery system with fluticasone for nasal polyposis. J Allergy Clin Immunol. 2019;143(1):126–34.e5
61. Palmer JN, Jacobson KW, Messina JC, Kosik-Gonzalez C, Djupesland PG, Mahmoud RA. EXHANCE-12: 1-year study of the exhalation delivery system with fluticasone (EDS-FLU) in chronic rhinosinusitis. Int Forum Allergy Rhinol. 2018;8(8):869–76.
62. Sher MR, Steven GC, Romett JL, Pien G, LeBenger K, Messina JC, et al. EXHANCE-3: a cohort study of the exhalation delivery system with fluticasone for chronic sinusitis with or without nasal polyps. Rhinology. 2020;58(1):25–35.
63. Palmer JN, Adappa ND, Chandra RK, Davis GE, Mahdavinia M, Messina J, et al. Efficacy of EDS-FLU for chronic rhinosinusitis: two randomized controlled trials (ReOpen1 and ReOpen2). J Allergy Clin Immunol Pract. 2024;12(4):1049–61.
64. Sindwani R, Han JK, Soteres DF, Messina JC, Carothers JL, Mahmoud RA, et al. NAVIGATE I: randomized, placebo-controlled, double-blind trial of the exhalation delivery system with fluticasone for chronic rhinosinusitis with nasal polyps. Am J Rhinol Allergy. 2019;33(1):69–82.
65. Messina JC, Offman E, Carothers JL, Mahmoud RA. A randomized comparison of the pharmacokinetics and bioavailability of fluticasone propionate delivered via Xhance exhalation delivery system versus Flonase nasal spray and Flovent HFA inhalational aerosol. Clin Ther. 2019;41(11):2343–56.
66. Senior BA, Schlosser RJ, Bosso J, Soler ZM. Efficacy of the exhalation delivery system with fluticasone in patients who remain symptomatic on standard nasal steroid sprays. Int Forum Allergy Rhinol. 2021;11(5):837–45.
67. Yao WC, Ramakrishnan VR, Luong AU, Citardi MJ. VISUALIZE: a 24-week, open-label study using nasal endoscopy video to evaluate the efficacy and safety of EDS-FLU 186 μg twice daily in adults with bilateral nasal polyps. Rhinology Online. 2020;3:58–66.
68. Ow RA, Soler ZM, Sindwani R, Leopold DA, Lee JT, Mahmoud RA, et al. Efficacy of the exhalation delivery system with fluticasone in patients with chronic rhinosinusitis with nasal polyps whose symptoms recur after sinus surgery. Int Forum Allergy Rhinol. 2023;13(1):31–41.
69. Wise SK, Adappa ND, Chandra RK, Davis GE, Mahdavinia M, Mahmoud R, et al. EDS-FLU efficacy in patients with chronic rhinosinusitis with or without prior sinus surgery in ReOpen1 and ReOpen2 randomized controlled trials. Int Forum Allergy Rhinol. 2024;
70. Li PM, Downie D, Hwang PH. Controlled steroid delivery via bioabsorbable stent: safety and performance in a rabbit model. Am J Rhinol Allergy. 2009;23(6):591–6.
71. Forwith KD, Chandra RK, Yun PT, Miller SK, Jampel HD. ADVANCE: a multisite trial of bioabsorbable steroid-eluting sinus implants. Laryngoscope. 2011;121(11):2473–80.
72. Murr AH, Smith TL, Hwang PH, Bhattacharyya N, Lanier BJ, Stambaugh JW, et al. Safety and efficacy of a novel bioabsorbable, steroid-eluting sinus stent. Int Forum Allergy Rhinol. 2011;1(1):23–32.

73. Marple BF, Smith TL, Han JK, Gould AR, Jampel HD, Stambaugh JW, et al. Advance II: a prospective, randomized study assessing safety and efficacy of bioabsorbable steroid-releasing sinus implants. Otolaryngol Head Neck Surg. 2012;146(6):1004–11.
74. Luong A, Ow RA, Singh A, Weiss RL, Han JK, Gerencer R, et al. Safety and effectiveness of a bioabsorbable steroid-releasing implant for the paranasal sinus ostia: a randomized clinical trial. JAMA Otolaryngol Head Neck Surg. 2018;144(1):28–35.
75. Smith TL, Singh A, Luong A, Ow RA, Shotts SD, Sautter NB, et al. Randomized controlled trial of a bioabsorbable steroid-releasing implant in the frontal sinus opening. Laryngoscope. 2016;126(12):2659–64.
76. Wang C, Yu L, Chu X, Wang K, Li J, Lai Y, et al. Short-term postoperative efficacy of steroid-eluting stents for eosinophilic chronic rhinosinusitis with nasal polyps: a randomized clinical trial. Int Forum Allergy Rhinol. 2023;13(5):899–909.
77. Huang Z, Zhou B, Wang D, Zang H, Zhang H, Wang H, et al. Comparison of bioabsorbable steroid-eluting sinus stents versus nasopore after endoscopic sinus surgery: a multicenter, randomized, controlled, single-blinded clinical trial. Ear Nose Throat J. 2022;101(4):260–7.
78. Sow YL, Tang IP, Kho JP, Prepageran N. Pilot study comparing steroid-impregnated and non-steroid-impregnated absorbable nasal dressing following endoscopic sinus surgery. Med J Malaysia. 2018;73(4):244–8.
79. Adriaensen GF, Lim KH, Fokkens WJ. Safety and efficacy of a bioabsorbable fluticasone propionate-eluting sinus dressing in postoperative management of endoscopic sinus surgery: a randomized clinical trial. Int Forum Allergy Rhinol. 2017;7(8):813–20.
80. Côté DW, Wright ED. Triamcinolone-impregnated nasal dressing following endoscopic sinus surgery: a randomized, double-blind, placebo-controlled study. Laryngoscope. 2010;120(6):1269–73.
81. Grzeskowiak B, Wierzchowska M, Walorek R, Seredyka-Burduk M, Wawrzyniak K, Burduk PK. Steroid vs. antibiotic impregnated absorbable nasal packing for wound healing after endoscopic sinus surgery: a randomized, double blind, placebo-controlled study. Braz J Otorhinolaryngol. 2019;85(4):473–80.
82. Promentilla SM, Onofre RD, Campomanes BS. Effects of dexamethasone versus saline-impregnated nasal packing on the postoperative outcome of patients with chronic rhinosinusitis and nasal polyps after endoscopic sinus surgery: a randomized controlled trial. Philipp J Otolaryngol Head Neck Surg. 2016;31(1):10–3.
83. Zhao KQ, Yu YQ, Yu HM. Effects of mometasone furoate-impregnated biodegradable nasal dressing on endoscopic appearance in healing process following endoscopic sinus surgery: a randomized, double-blind, placebo-controlled study. Int Forum Allergy Rhinol. 2018;8(11):1233–41.
84. Rudmik L, Mace J, Mechor B. Effect of a dexamethasone Sinu-Foam™ middle meatal spacer on endoscopic sinus surgery outcomes: a randomized, double-blind, placebo-controlled trial. Int Forum Allergy Rhinol. 2012;2(3):248–51.
85. Hwang CS, Al Sharhan SS, Kim BR, Kim SI, Kim JW, Cho HJ, et al. Randomized controlled trial of steroid-soaked absorbable calcium alginate nasal packing following endoscopic sinus surgery. Laryngoscope. 2018;128(2):311–6.
86. Lavigne F, Miller SK, Gould AR, Lanier BJ, Romett JL. Steroid-eluting sinus implant for in-office treatment of recurrent nasal polyposis: a prospective, multicenter study. Int Forum Allergy Rhinol. 2014;4(5):381–9.
87. Matheny KE, Carter KB, Tseng EY, Fong KJ. Safety, feasibility, and efficacy of placement of steroid-eluting bioabsorbable sinus implants in the office setting: a prospective case series. Int Forum Allergy Rhinol. 2014;4(10):808–15.
88. Kern RC, Stolovitzky JP, Silvers SL, Singh A, Lee JT, Yen DM, et al. A phase 3 trial of mometasone furoate sinus implants for chronic sinusitis with recurrent nasal polyps. Int Forum Allergy Rhinol. 2018;8(4):471–81.
89. Forwith KD, Han JK, Stolovitzky JP, Yen DM, Chandra RK, Karanfilov B, et al. RESOLVE: bioabsorbable steroid-eluting sinus implants for in-office treatment of recurrent sinonasal

polyposis after sinus surgery: 6-month outcomes from a randomized, controlled, blinded study. Int Forum Allergy Rhinol. 2016;6(6):573–81.
90. Han JK, Forwith KD, Smith TL, Kern RC, Brown WJ, Miller SK, et al. RESOLVE: a randomized, controlled, blinded study of bioabsorbable steroid-eluting sinus implants for in-office treatment of recurrent sinonasal polyposis. Int Forum Allergy Rhinol. 2014;4(11):861–70.
91. Cervin A, Rimmer J, Wrobel A, Abelak Y, Brayton L, Kuang Y. Long-acting implantable corticosteroid matrix for chronic rhinosinusitis: results of LANTERN Phase 2 randomized controlled study. Int Forum Allergy Rhinol. 2022;12(2):147–59.
92. Tang DM, Roxbury CR, Sindwani R, Kshettry VR, Recinos P, Woodard TD. Multiple bioabsorbable corticosteroid-eluting stent placement with associated skull base injury. Laryngoscope. 2019;129(7):1494–6.
93. Shah VN, Pasick LJ, Benito DA, Ghiam MK, D'Aguillo C. Complications associated with PROPEL Mometasone Furoate bioabsorbable drug-eluting sinus stents from 2012 to 2020. Am J Rhinol Allergy. 2022;36(2):185–90.
94. Lee JT, DelGaudio J, Orlandi RR. Practice patterns in office-based rhinology: survey of the American Rhinologic Society. Am J Rhinol Allergy. 2019;33(1):26–35.
95. Rudmik L, Smith TL. Economic evaluation of a steroid-eluting sinus implant following endoscopic sinus surgery for chronic rhinosinusitis. Otolaryngol Head Neck Surg. 2014;151(2):359–66.
96. Han JK, Marple BF, Smith TL, Murr AH, Lanier BJ, Stambaugh JW, et al. Effect of steroid-releasing sinus implants on postoperative medical and surgical interventions: an efficacy meta-analysis. Int Forum Allergy Rhinol. 2012;2(4):271–9.
97. Singh A, Luong AU, Fong KJ, Ow RA, Han JK, Gerencer R, et al. Bioabsorbable steroid-releasing implants in the frontal sinus ostia: a pooled analysis. Int Forum Allergy Rhinol. 2019;9(2):131–9.
98. Stolovitzky JP, Kern RC, Han JK, Forwith KD, Ow RA, Wright SK, et al. In-office placement of mometasone furoate sinus implants for recurrent nasal polyps: a pooled analysis. Am J Rhinol Allergy. 2019;33(5):545–58.
99. Lee VS, Patel P, O'Brien D, Scangas GA, Campbell RG, Chandra R, et al. Indications for absorbable steroid-eluting sinus implants: viewpoint via the Delphi method. Int Forum Allergy Rhinol. 2022;12(10):1225–31.
100. Wu C, Fang F, Zhan X, Wei Y. The association between glucocorticoid receptor (NR3C1) gene polymorphism and difficult-to-treat rhinosinusitis. Eur Arch Otorrinolaringol. 2022;279(8):3981–7.
101. Milara J, Morell A, Ballester B, Armengot M, Morcillo E, Cortijo J. MUC4 impairs the anti-inflammatory effects of corticosteroids in patients with chronic rhinosinusitis with nasal polyps. J Allergy Clin Immunol. 2017;139(3):855–862.e13.
102. Milara J, Peiró T, Armengot M, Frias S, Morell A, Serrano A, et al. Mucin 1 downregulation associates with corticosteroid resistance in chronic rhinosinusitis with nasal polyps. J Allergy Clin Immunol. 2015;135(2):470–6.
103. Kocharyan A, Feldman R, Singleton A, Han X, Bleier BS. P-glycoprotein inhibition promotes prednisone retention in human sinonasal polyp explants. Int Forum Allergy Rhinol. 2014;4(9):734–8.
104. An YH, Hong SL, Han DH, Lee CH, Min YG, Rhee CS. Expression of the cysteinyl leukotriene 1 receptor and glucocorticoid receptor-β in nasal polyps. Eur Arch Otorrinolaringol. 2013;270(4):1373–8.
105. Choi BR, Kwon JH, Gong SJ, Kwon MS, Cho JH, Kim JH, et al. Expression of glucocorticoid receptor mRNAs in glucocorticoid-resistant nasal polyps. Exp Mol Med. 2006;38(5):466–73.
106. Hamilos DL, Leung DY, Muro S, Kahn AM, Hamilos SS, Thawley SE, et al. GRbeta expression in nasal polyp inflammatory cells and its relationship to the anti-inflammatory effects of intranasal fluticasone. J Allergy Clin Immunol. 2001;108(1):59–68.
107. Li P, Li Y, Li YQ, Yang QT, Zhang GH. Glucocorticoid receptor expression and glucocorticoid therapeutic effect in nasal polyps. Clin Invest Med. 2010;33(3):E181–8.

108. Pujols L, Alobid I, Benítez P, Martínez-Antón A, Roca-Ferrer J, Fokkens WJ, et al. Regulation of glucocorticoid receptor in nasal polyps by systemic and intranasal glucocorticoids. Allergy. 2008;63(10):1377–86.
109. Pujols L, Mullol J, Benítez P, Torrego A, Xaubet A, de Haro J, et al. Expression of the glucocorticoid receptor alpha and beta isoforms in human nasal mucosa and polyp epithelial cells. Respir Med. 2003;97(1):90–6.
110. Valera FC, Scrideli C, Queinoz, Tone LG, Anselmo-Lima. NF-kappaB expression predicts clinical outcome for nasal polyposis. Rhinology. 2010;48(4):408–41.
111. Wang SB, Chen SM, Zhu KS, Zhou B, Chen L, Zou XY. Increased lipopolysaccharide content is positively correlated with glucocorticoid receptor-beta expression in chronic rhinosinusitis with nasal polyps. Immun Inflamm Dis. 2020;8(4):605–14.
112. Wang M, Shi P, Chen B, Shi G, Li H, Wang H. Superantigen-induced glucocorticoid insensitivity in the recurrence of chronic rhinosinusitis with nasal polyps. Otolaryngol Head Neck Surg. 2011;145(5):717–22.
113. Watanabe S, Suzaki H. Changes of glucocorticoid receptor expression in the nasal polyps of patients with chronic sinusitis following treatment with glucocorticoid. In Vivo. 2008;22(1):37–42.
114. Rawl JW, McQuitty RA, Khan MH, Reichert LK, Kuo YF, Chaaban MR. Comparison of steroid-releasing stents vs nonabsorbable packing as middle meatal spacers. Int Forum Allergy Rhinol. 2020;10(3):328–33.

Aspirin Desensitization for Recalcitrant Chronic Rhinosinusitis with Nasal Polyposis

23

Anthony F. LaCava and John V. Bosso

Key Points
- Aspirin-exacerbated respiratory disease (AERD) consists of the triad of asthma, chronic rhinosinusitis with nasal polyposis, and respiratory reactions to COX-1 inhibitors/allergy to nonsteroidal anti-inflammatory drugs.
- Aspirin desensitization in patients with AERD is an effective means to control inflammatory symptoms.
- Aspirin therapy after desensitization improves sinus and respiratory symptoms, reduces polyp formation, and reduces the need for oral and inhaled corticosteroids and revision sinus surgery.
- Aspirin therapy is affordable and cost-effective as first-line therapy after complete endoscopic sinus surgery.

Background

Pseudonyms, Prevalence, and Clinical Manifestations

Aspirin-exacerbated respiratory disease (AERD), also known as Samter's triad, aspirin-sensitive rhinosinusitis asthma, aspirin triad, aspirin idiosyncrasy, and nonsteroidal anti-inflammatory drug (NSAID)-exacerbated respiratory disease, is an

A. F. LaCava
Section of Allergy & Immunology, Division of Pulmonary, Allergy, & Critical Care Medicine, Perelman School of Medicine, University of Pennsylvania, Philadelphia, PA, USA

J. V. Bosso (✉)
Division of Rhinology, Department of Otolaryngology, Perelman School of Medicine, University of Pennsylvania, Philadelphia, PA, USA
e-mail: john.bosso@pennmedicine.upenn.edu

J. T. Lee et al. (eds.), *Advances in Surgical and Medical Interventions for Recalcitrant Chronic Rhinosinusitis*,
https://doi.org/10.1007/978-3-031-89191-5_23

Table 23.1 Medications that inhibit COX-1 and COX-2

Highly selective COX-1 inhibitors		
Acetylsalicylic acid	Flurbiprofen	Dipyrone
Antipyrine-benzocaine	Ibuprofen	Mefenamic acid
Benoxaprofen	Indomethacin	Naproxen
Diclofenac	Ketoprofen	Oxaprozin
Etodolac	Ketorolac	Piroxicam
Fenoprofen	Meclofenamate	Tolmetin
Weakly selective COX-1 inhibitors		
Acetaminophen	Diflunisal	
Choline magnesium trisalicylate	Salsalate	
Highly selective COX-2 inhibitors		
Celecoxib	Lumiracoxib	
Etoricoxib	Parecoxib	
Preferentially selective COX-2 inhibitors		
Meloxicam		
Nabumetone		
Nimesulide		

inflammatory syndrome characterized by the combination of asthma, chronic rhinosinusitis with nasal polyposis (CRSwNP), and acute respiratory reactions following exposure to cyclooxygenase (COX)-1 inhibitors. Table 23.1 lists the medications that are known to inhibit COX-1 and COX-2 enzymes. In AERD patients, challenges with highly selective COX-2 inhibitors have demonstrated that these medications are well tolerated [1]. There is variable cross-reactivity among the weakly selective COX-1 inhibitors, and these reactions tend to be less severe. Settipane demonstrated 34% cross-reactivity in AERD patients with acetaminophen doses at or above 1000 mg [2]. Lower doses did not seem to trigger respiratory reactions.

AERD is often first noted following an upper respiratory infection in early adulthood, with progression to chronic rhinosinusitis and recurrent nasal polyposis. As the sinus disease develops, lower respiratory tract symptoms also begin, and asthma is diagnosed. In some cases, respiratory symptoms are more notable, and asthma may be diagnosed before nasal polyposis. Respiratory sensitivity to COX-1-inhibiting NSAIDs often manifests after the establishment of upper and lower respiratory disease. The syndrome can take 2–4 years to clinically manifest its full triad, thereby leading to diagnostic confusion and delays [3]. Rarely, a patient with AERD does not demonstrate clinical asthma, the so-called upper airway variant. When patients with AERD ingest aspirin or an NSAID, they develop acute upper and/or lower respiratory symptoms. Other clinical associations include anosmia or hyposmia, respiratory reactions to alcoholic beverages especially beer and wine, atopic disorders, and peripheral blood eosinophilia. AERD affects between 7% and 15% of patients with asthma and up to 16% of patients with CRSwNP [4, 5]. Atopy is present in a higher-than-expected number of AERD patients; however, the clinical significance of this finding is still unclear [6]. Exposure to passive cigarette smoke in early life and a personal history of smoking have been associated with more than a threefold increase in the odds of developing AERD [7]. Atopy, cigarette smoke, and viral or bacterial insults to the sinonasal epithelium could be initial catalysts in igniting the dysregulated inflammation seen in AERD. Unfortunately, despite an avalanche of recent publications, AERD is often underdiagnosed due to a lack of physician recognition [8].

Pathophysiology

Arachidonic acid metabolism is chronically dysregulated in AERD (Fig. 23.1). There is overproduction of cysteinyl leukotrienes (LTC_4, LTD_4, LTE_4) and PGD_2, which leads to the development of bronchospasm, increased mucus production, increased vascular permeability, and recruitment of inflammatory cells [9–11]. Levels of PGE_2, which has anti-inflammatory effects and suppresses leukotriene production, are reduced in AERD [11]. Abnormal aggregates of platelets and leukocytes (i.e., neutrophils, eosinophils, and monocytes) can share metabolic processes (i.e., through transcellular transfer of metabolic intermediates) to produce high amounts of inflammatory leukotrienes [12]. Eosinophils and mast cells have been

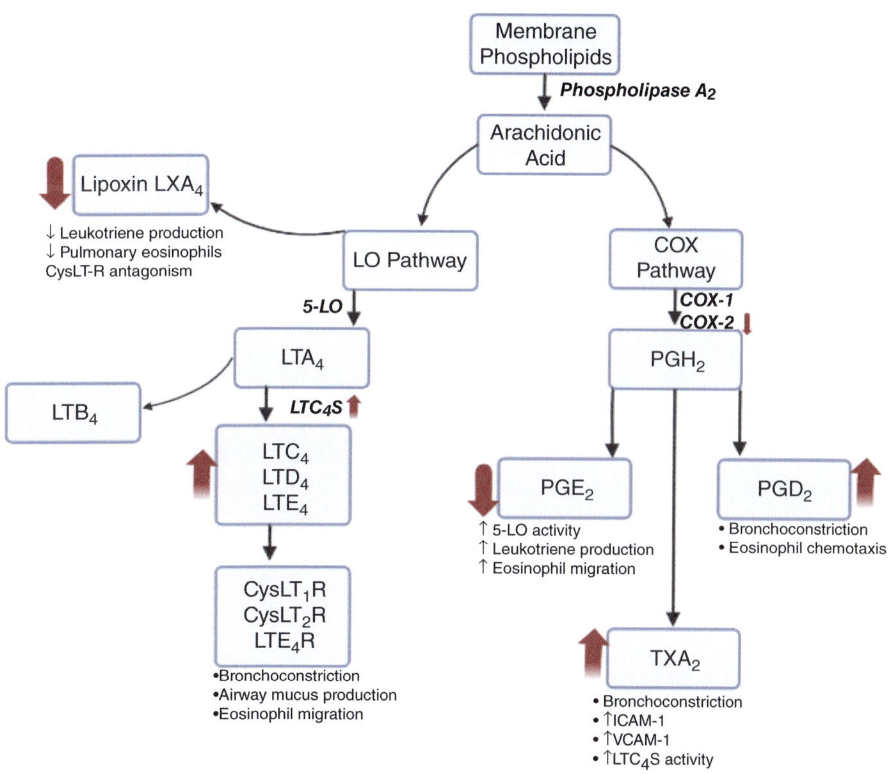

Fig. 23.1 Pathways of arachidonic acid metabolism involved in the pathogenesis of AERD Italicized words represent enzymes involved in this pathway. Signaling effects are listed in bullet points. Red arrows represent mediators that are either increased or decreased in AERD patients

shown to be primary sources of excess leukotrienes in patients with AERD [13–15]. Basophils have also been demonstrated to contribute to AERD pathogenesis, although their involvement in AERD pathophysiology remains unclear [16]. Recently, it has been demonstrated that there may be inflammatory heterogeneity within AERD, which can be differentiated into three inflammatory sub-endotypes: (1) low inflammatory burden, (2) very high type 2 cytokines (IL-4, IL-5, IL-13), and (3) low type 2 cytokines with high levels of type 1 (IFN-γ) and type 3 cytokines (IL-17A). The concept of sub-endotypes within AERD may explain some of the differential responses to treatments.

Radiographic and Histologic Findings

CT imaging of the sinuses reveals pan-sinus opacification in most AERD patients secondary to diffuse mucosal inflammation [6]. Bony thickening of the intersinus septum and sphenoid bone is also seen in increased frequency [17]. The evolution of sinus polypoid opacification typically starts in the ethmoid and frontal sinuses [18]. Normal preoperative imaging of the sinuses rules out the diagnosis of AERD. Histologically, AERD is characterized by increased inflammation within the upper and lower respiratory tracts. Bronchial and nasal/sinus tissue examination reveals an increased number of eosinophils and degranulated mast cells [13, 19].

Diagnosis

A clinical diagnosis of AERD can be made based on a history of asthma and nasal polyposis, in addition to adverse reactions caused by aspirin, NSAIDs, or other COX-1 inhibitors. Many patients do not have a clear history of adverse reactions to COX-1 inhibitors or other NSAIDs. In patients without a clear history, aspirin challenge can confirm or exclude hypersensitivity and is considered the gold standard for diagnosing AERD [20]. Urinary leukotriene E4 measurements are poorly predictive of AERD [21]. Diagnostic aspirin challenges should be offered to patients with suspected AERD prior to endoscopic sinus surgery to increase diagnostic accuracy and to minimize the risk of false-negative aspirin challenges, which are sometimes seen in the early postoperative period [22].

Aspirin Challenge

Indications for Aspirin Challenge

An aspirin challenge should be considered in all chronic rhinosinusitis with nasal polyposis patients with an unclear clinical presentation. A list of clinical scenarios where an aspirin challenge should be considered is shown in Table 23.2.

Table 23.2 Indications for aspirin challenge

Clinical indications for aspirin challenge
CRSwNP, asthma without prior exposure to aspirin or COX-1 inhibitor during the time of the inflammatory disease
CRSwNP, asthma receiving a leukotriene receptor antagonist (i.e., montelukast, zafirlukast) or 5-lipooxygenase inhibitor (i.e., zileuton)
CRSwNP, asthma on daily low-dose aspirin
CRSwNP, asthma and is a poor perceiver of nasal or respiratory symptoms
CRSwNP, asthma with suggestive radiographic (pansinusitis, intersphenoid septal thickening) or histopathologic findings (intense eosinophilic infiltration on structured histopathologic examination)
CRSwNP, asthma requiring frequent bursts of systemic corticosteroids to control respiratory or sinus symptoms
CRSwNP, asthma with one reaction associated with aspirin or COX-1 inhibitor which was atypical in nature and not serious
Uncontrolled chronic rhinosinusitis with nasal polyposis despite the use of standard medical therapy
Recurrent nasal polyposis requiring repeat endoscopic sinus surgery
Any patient with pansinusitis

Abbreviations: *CRSwNP* chronic rhinosinusitis with nasal polyposis, *COX-1* cyclooxygenase-1

A common clinical scenario that would warrant an aspirin challenge includes patients with chronic rhinosinusitis with nasal polyposis (CRSwNP) and asthma without a previous exposure to aspirin or COX-1 inhibitor during the time of the inflammatory disease. Leukotriene receptor antagonists can modify upper airway symptoms in AERD and can decrease nasal symptoms with aspirin exposure, which can potentially mask an underlying hypersensitivity. Therefore, an aspirin challenge can be considered in patients with CRSwNP and asthma who have tolerated aspirin or COX-1 inhibitors while receiving concomitant leukotriene or 5-lipoxygenase inhibitor treatment [23]. There is also a subset of patients who are desensitized to aspirin through low-dose daily use; these patients would also benefit from an aspirin challenge after holding their daily aspirin for 10 days [24]. An aspirin challenge may also be considered in patients who are poor perceivers of symptoms, patients with suggestive radiographic or histopathologic findings, and patients with refractory sinus disease. It is possible to have AERD without asthma; therefore, aspirin challenge can be considered in carefully selected patients with a history of chronic pansinusitis alone.

A study by Dursun et al. evaluated 243 consecutive referrals for aspirin challenges and desensitization. They found that patients with at least two prior aspirin- and NSAID-associated respiratory reactions had an 89% chance of having a positive oral aspirin challenge [25]. Therefore, aspirin challenge is typically unnecessary in patients with CRSwNP and asthma who report a history of two previous hypersensitivity reactions to aspirin or COX-1 inhibitors. In this same study, patients who had one serious respiratory reaction associated with aspirin/NSAID ingestion had a 100% likelihood of a positive challenge, thereby eliminating the need to challenge patients with this history.

Absolute and Relative Contraindications to Aspirin Challenge

Absolute contraindications to aspirin challenge include pregnancy, active gastrointestinal bleeding due to peptic ulcer disease, eosinophilic esophagitis, and bleeding disorders. Ideally, asthma should be controlled (i.e., ACT >19,) with an FEV1 value of at least 1.5 L and >70% of predicted, although exceptions can be made in patients with concomitant restrictive disease or fixed obstructive disease [26]. Concomitant beta blockade is a relative contraindication, with a greater caution associated with non-cardioselective agents. At the Penn AERD Center, in order to prevent difficult-to-treat refractory asthma or anaphylaxis, we typically do not challenge patients actively ingesting these non-cardioselective beta-blocker agents. A temporary hold equal to five drug half-lives is suggested, if clinically feasible.

Aspirin Challenge Procedure

A protocol for oral aspirin challenges for the diagnosis of AERD is detailed in Table 23.3. In order to optimize safety, asthma should be stable prior to starting an aspirin challenge procedure. Patients should be instructed to stop antihistamines for 48 hours, leukotriene antagonists for 7 days, and oral corticosteroids for 7 days if possible. In cases where steroid cessation would lead to adrenal suppression or destabilization of asthma, patients may remain on the lowest possible dose of oral corticosteroids leading up to the challenge. Patients may continue to take their prescribed inhaled corticosteroids (ICS) with or without long-acting beta-agonists. Topical intranasal steroids may also be continued.

Spirometry, nasal inspiratory peak flow values, and upper and lower respiratory symptoms should be recorded at baseline and at 60-min intervals. Symptom scores, using the composite score outlined by Cook et al. should also be recorded at baseline and at 60-min intervals [Table 23.4] [27].

For the aspirin challenge, 40.5 mg of aspirin (1/2 of an 81 mg aspirin tablet) is initially administered. After a 60-min observation period, if there is no reaction, the dose is doubled to 81 mg, and after an additional 90-min observation period, a dose of 325 mg is administered again, provided there is no clinical reaction. A three-hour observation period after the 325 mg oral dose is recommended before discharging the patient in the case of a negative challenge. The diagnosis of AERD is confirmed by the presence of a positive aspirin challenge response, defined as a hypersensitivity reaction manifesting with at least one of the following symptoms: (a) ≥15% decline in FEV1; (b) ≥20% decline in peak nasal inspiratory flow; and (c) ≥5-point

Table 23.3 Recommended protocol for oral aspirin challenges in patients with suspected AERD

Aspirin challenge protocol		
Challenge step	Time	Aspirin dosage
1	8:00 a.m.	40.5 mg
2	9:00 a.m.	81 mg
3	10:30 a.m.	325 mg

Table 23.4 Composite symptom score during aspirin challenge [27]

Symptoms[a]
Nasal congestion
Runny nose
Sneezing
Itchy nose
Itchy, watery eyes
Itchy ears
Itchy mouth, tongue
Tight throat
Wheezing
Chest tightness

[a]Instructions:
1. Patients self-record the above symptoms on a scale from 0 to 10 (0 = no symptoms, 1–3 = mild or barely noticeable, 4–7 = moderate or somewhat troublesome, 8–10 = much worse than you generally experience, making you very uncomfortable)
2. The composite score is calculated based on the sum of all individual scores. A change of 5 points in the composite score from baseline is considered positive.

Table 23.5 Treatment of aspirin-induced reactions

Organ involvement	Treatment options
Ocular	Intraocular or oral H1-receptor antagonists
Nasal	Intranasal, oral, or intravenous H1-receptor antagonists Intranasal decongestants Intranasal corticosteroids
Laryngeal	Racemic or intramuscular epinephrine
Respiratory	Inhaled B_2-agonists Inhaled anticholinergics Intramuscular epinephrine
Gastrointestinal	Intravenous H1- and H2-receptor antagonists Antiemetics (e.g., ondansetron) Intramuscular epinephrine
Skin	Oral or intravenous H1-receptor antagonists
Systemic (multisystem or hypotension)	Intramuscular epinephrine Intravenous saline or lactated ringer's

change in composite symptom score [27]. Clinical judgment may be used when determining a positive aspirin challenge response. All positive challenges should be medically treated until the patient is stabilized. Systemic symptoms such as gastrointestinal distress or urticaria/angioedema and rarely hypotension may occur in addition to respiratory symptoms and should be treated until resolution, as well. See Table 23.5 for the recommended treatment of aspirin-induced reactions, which will be discussed in more detail below.

Aspirin Desensitization

Preparation

As stated previously, aspirin is contraindicated in pregnancy, gastric ulcers or bleeding disorders, and eosinophilic esophagitis. In order to optimize safety, asthma should be stable prior to starting an aspirin challenge procedure with a post-bronchodilator FEV1 of at least 1.5 L and > 70% of predicted. Spirometry is recommended 1–2 weeks prior to the planned procedure. Exceptions to this may be made using clinical judgment in cases of fixed obstructive airways or restrictive airways; however, the baseline FEV1 should ideally be less than 12% lower than the post-bronchodilator value to assure airway stability prior to the procedure. Although optional, the authors prefer to stop antihistamines for 48 h prior to desensitization in order to prevent masking mild and earlier nasal reactions in favor of forcing reactions to occur at higher doses. Patients should refrain from using short-acting bronchodilators for at least 12 h before the desensitization (this might mask a milder earlier bronchial reaction and allow a stronger reaction to occur later), but they may continue to take their prescribed inhaled corticosteroids (ICS) with or without long-acting beta-agonists and leukotriene modifiers. Leukotriene modifiers will blunt the level of FEV1 decline, and their use during the procedure often prevents more serious respiratory reactions from occurring during desensitization and is therefore recommended.

Logistics

Aspirin desensitization generally can be performed in an outpatient setting which is adequately equipped to manage severe asthma and anaphylaxis. Prior to aspirin desensitization, written informed consent should be obtained from the patient. The patient should be seated in a comfortable chair. Providers should consider obtaining intravenous access, as the procedure involves administering a suspected allergen to the patient. A 1:2 nursing-to-patient ratio is also suggested. A baseline urine or serum HCG test should be negative for females of childbearing potential. Emergency medications should be readily available, including intramuscular epinephrine, intravenous and oral diphenhydramine, intravenous methylprednisolone, intravenous famotidine, oral dissolving ondansetron tablets, nebulized albuterol and ipratropium, normal saline or Lactated Ringer's solution, and intravenous glucagon (for patients who cannot stop beta-blocker treatment). Additional medications that should be available for symptomatic relief include intranasal oxymetazoline and azelastine, ocular antihistamines, and oral second-generation antihistamines.

Monitoring

Spirometry, nasal inspiratory peak flow values, and respiratory symptoms should be recorded at baseline, prior to each successive dose, and with any changes in signs or symptoms suggestive of an allergic reaction. Symptom scores, using the composite score outlined by Cook et al., should also be recorded at baseline and prior to each successive dose [Table 23.4] [27].

Protocols

Select desensitization protocols are detailed in Table 23.6. The first protocol outlined in Table 23.6a outlines a modified two-day intranasal ketorolac and oral aspirin desensitization protocol. The ketorolac nasal spray can be prepared by mixing ketorolac tromethamine (60 mg/2 mL) with preservative-free normal saline (2.75 mL) in an empty nasal spray bottle. Each spray actuates 1.26 mg of solution. Providers should prime with five sprays before use and administer using appropriate nasal spray technique. Varying doses of aspirin (60, 150 mg) will require advanced preparation through a compounding pharmacy. The second and third protocols shown in Table 23.6b and c can be performed with over-the-counter aspirin tablets which may be cut using a pill-cutter or doubled to achieve the desired doses. The fourth protocol shown in Table 23.6d uses dissolved original Alka-Seltzer.

The obvious advantage of a 1-day desensitization protocol is that it can be completed in a single office visit, but these protocols are often prolonged due to aspirin-induced reactions. After a clinical reaction has occurred, the patient should be treated and observed for 3 h to ensure complete resolution of symptoms prior to repeating the provocative dose (discussed in more detail below). If there are multiple reactions, a 1-day desensitization protocol can unfortunately become very lengthy. Two-day desensitization protocols can be advantageous from this perspective, as these protocols can better accommodate clinical reactions since it is extended over a longer period of time

Aspirin-Induced Reactions

Most patients with AERD should develop clinical symptoms during an aspirin desensitization. Reactions are observed between 45 mg and 100 mg of aspirin, but this differs between individuals and can occur at any dosage [31]. Proper stabilization of asthma prior to the procedure combined with performing the procedure in the first 6–8 weeks postoperatively can occasionally result in a “silent desensitization” (discussed further below). Therefore, establishing the diagnosis before

Table 23.6 Select aspirin desensitization protocols[a,b]

(a) Modified two-day intranasal ketorolac and oral aspirin desensitization protocol [28]		
Day	**Time**	**Intranasal ketorolac and oral aspirin**
Day 1		
	8:00 a.m.	1 spray (1 in 1 nostril)
	8:30 a.m.	2 sprays (1 in each nostril)
	9:00 a.m.	4 sprays (2 in each nostril)
	9:30 a.m.	6 sprays (3 in each nostril)
	10:30 a.m.	60 mg of aspirin
	12:00 p.m.	60 mg of aspirin
	3:00 p.m.	Instructions and discharge
Day 2		
	8:00 a.m.	150 mg of aspirin
	11:00 a.m.	325 mg of aspirin
	2:00 p.m.	Instructions and discharge
(b) Two-day oral aspirin desensitization protocol [29]		
Day	**Time**	**Oral aspirin**
Day 1		
	8:00 a.m.	40.5 mg of aspirin (1/2 of 81 mg tab)
	11:00 a.m.	81 mg of aspirin
	2:00 p.m.	162 mg of aspirin
	5:00 p.m.	Instructions and discharge
Day 2		
	8:00 a.m.	325 mg of aspirin
	11:00 a.m.	Instructions and discharge

(c) One-day, 90-min oral aspirin desensitization protocol [26]	
Time	**Oral aspirin**
8:00 a.m.	40.5 mg of aspirin (1/2 of 81 mg tab)
9:30 a.m.	81 mg of aspirin
11:00 a.m.	162.5 mg of aspirin
12:30 p.m.	325 mg of aspirin
(d) One-day, 60-min oral aspirin protocol [30]	
Time	**Oral aspirin** (dissolved original Alka-Seltzer®)[c]
8:00 a.m.	40 mg of aspirin (4 mL of 10 mg/mL solution)
9:30 a.m.	80 mg of aspirin (8 mL of 10 mg/mL solution)
11:00 a.m.	160 mg of aspirin (16 mL of 10 mg/mL solution)
12:30 p.m.	325 mg of aspirin (1 full Alka-Seltzer tablet)

[a]Clinical and objective evaluation performed every 30 min and as-needed
[b]Listed times assume no reactions; provoking dose is repeated; symptoms are treated as indicated
[c]Dissolve 1 Alka-seltzer tablet in 32.5 mL water for a 10 mg/mL solution

surgery is critical. Immediate reactions typically include upper respiratory tract symptoms (i.e., nasal congestion, rhinorrhea, postnasal drip, sneezing, nasal or ocular pruritus, conjunctival redness, lacrimation) or lower respiratory tract symptoms (i.e., cough, wheezing, chest tightness, shortness of breath). Patients may also develop cutaneous symptoms (i.e., flushing, urticaria, angioedema, maculopapular rashes), and/or gastrointestinal symptoms (cramping abdominal pain, nausea, vomiting). Hypotension is a rare complication that clinicians also need to be prepared to treat. Acute pancreatitis has also been reported as a very rare complication during desensitization [64].

Treatment of Aspirin-Induced Reactions

Treatment of aspirin-induced reactions is dependent upon the symptoms reported by the patient and the objective findings on physical examination [Table 23.5].

Ocular reactions can be treated with intraocular or oral antihistamines. Nasal reactions can be treated with intranasal, intravenous, or oral antihistamines, intranasal decongestants, or intranasal corticosteroids. Laryngeal symptoms can be treated with racemic or intramuscular epinephrine. Respiratory symptoms can be treated with inhaled short-acting B_2-agonists, short-acting antimuscarinics, or intramuscular epinephrine. Oral leukotriene antagonists may be given if the patient is not currently taking one. A 5-lipoxygenase inhibitor may be given to patients currently taking leukotriene receptor antagonists. Although the onset of action is 1–2 h, it is often beneficial in patients experiencing prolonged bronchospasm during the protocol. Gastrointestinal symptoms can be treated with oral H1- and H2-receptor antagonists, antiemetics, or intramuscular epinephrine. Urticaria, angioedema, or flushing may be treated with oral or intravenous H1-receptor antagonists. Systemic (i.e., multisystem) reactions require intramuscular epinephrine 1:1000. Hypotension is rare, but treatment requires intramuscular epinephrine, intravenous saline or Lactated Ringer's, and, if refractory, transfer to an intensive care unit for vasopressor therapy.

Evidence Supporting the Role of Aspirin Desensitization and Continued Aspirin Therapy

Case Reports, Case Series, and Retrospective Analyses

The first aspirin desensitization was described in 1922 in a 37-year-old woman with Samter's triad, allowing the patient to tolerate aspirin subsequently without adverse reactions [32]. This was again described in the 1970s by Zeiss and Lockey [33] in a patient with aspirin-induced asthma and nasal polyps who had reacted during an initial challenge but tolerated subsequent doses of aspirin the following day. In 1980, Stevenson et al. [34] published a report on two patients with AERD who underwent aspirin desensitization and were maintained on daily aspirin. Both patients showed improvement in their asthma and rhinitis symptoms, suggesting that aspirin therapy after desensitization (ATAD) could provide clinical benefits for these patients. Cross-desensitization to other COX-1-inhibiting NSAIDs was demonstrated by the same investigators, allowing patients to ingest other NSAIDs with impunity [35].

Observational studies then examined large cohorts of patients with AERD who underwent aspirin desensitization and were maintained on daily aspirin for weeks, months, or years [Table 23.7]. ATAD for patients with AERD was associated with

Table 23.7 —Summary of nonrandomized studies evaluating the clinical efficacy of ATAD in patients with AERD

Study	Study description, level of evidence[a]	Duration of study	No. of patients who completed the study	Sinus surgery required prior to desensitization?	Maintenance oral aspirin dosage	Results
Lumry et al. [38], 1983	Prospective (4)	2–12 months	17	No	325–2600 mg	47% had persistent sinonasal symptom improvement and tolerated daily aspirin
Sweet et al. [39], 1990	Retrospective (4)	32–102 months	65 (on ATAD) and 42 (avoiding aspirin)	No	325–2600 mg	54% tolerated aspirin. ATAD resulted in fewer ER visits, reduced OCS, improved nasal symptoms, and fewer sinus surgeries (compared to patients avoiding aspirin)
Stevenson et al. [40], 1996	Longitudinal (4)	1–6 year	65	No	325–1950 mg	83% tolerated aspirin. ATAD resulted in fewer sinus surgeries, reduced oral and intranasal steroid use, and an improved sense of smell (compared to before ATAD)
Berges-Gimeno et al. [41], 2003	Longitudinal (4)	4 week	38	No	1300 mg	ATAD improved nasal and asthma symptoms and reduced oral steroid use (compared to before ATAD)
Berges-Gimeno et al. [42], 2003	Longitudinal (4)	1–5 year	126	No	1300 mg	67% tolerated aspirin. ATAD improved upper and lower respiratory tract symptoms, reduced steroid use, reduced sinus surgeries, and decreased ED visits for asthma (compared to before ATAD)
Lee et al. [43], 2007	Longitudinal (4)	1 year	105	No	650–1300 mg	ATAD was associated with improved nasal and asthma symptoms, reduced need for sinus surgery, & reduced hospitalizations for asthma. Some patients on the lower aspirin dose required an increase to 1300 mg daily to have improvement
Rozsasi et al. [44], 2008	Prospective (4)	1 year	14	No	100 mg & 300 mg	*100 mg*: 100% had recurrence of nasal polyps and no change in sense of smell or lung function *300 mg*: 0% had recurrence of nasal polyps. All had improvement in sense of smell and lung function

Havel et al. [45], 2013	Retrospective (4)	18–84 months	51 (on ATAD) and 53 (avoiding aspirin)	Yes	500 mg	ATAD was associated with less polyp regrowth, improved sinus and asthma symptoms (compared to avoidance)
Comert et al. [46], 2013	Prospective (4)	3 year	18	No	300 mg	ATAD improved sinonasal symptoms, reduced oral corticosteroids, and decreased sinus surgeries (compared to before ATAD)
Cho et al. [47], 2014	Retrospective (4)	6 month	21	Yes	650–975 mg	95% tolerated aspirin. ATAD further improved sinonasal symptoms after sinus surgery
Jerschow et al. [48], 2017	Prospective (4)	4 week	39	Yes	1300 mg	ATAD improved symptoms and lung function in 31% 49% either failed to complete desensitization and had worsening symptoms or lung function on ATAD
Adappa et al. [49], 2018	Retrospective (4)	30 months	32	Yes	325–1300 mg	85% tolerated aspirin. ATAD further improved sinonasal symptoms after sinus surgery
Walters et al. [50], 2018	Retrospective (4)	10 year	57	No	325–650 mg	85% of patients on ATAD found it helpful in improving airway disease and QOL
Shah et al. [51], 2019	Prospective (4)	6 months	40	Yes	1300 mg (first mo.) then 650 mg	19 patients who benefited and 21 patients who failed ATAD with a distant history of ESS were identified. 24 of these patients had repeat ESS and underwent ATAD 3–4 week later, which was tolerated

[a]Level of evidence: 1 (systematic review of randomized trials); 2 (randomized clinical trial or observational study with dramatic effect); 3 (nonrandomized controlled cohort study); 4 (case series, case-control studies)

symptomatic improvement of upper and lower respiratory tract symptoms and reduced the need for oral corticosteroids. Clinical improvement was seen with maintenance therapy as early as 4 weeks after desensitization [41] and was maintained even 10 years later [50]. Additional clinical benefits observed in AERD patients receiving ATAD include a reduced need for additional sinus surgery [39, 40, 42, 43, 46], a slower rate of polyp regrowth [45], reduced oral and inhaled corticosteroids [36], improved tolerance to alcohol [37], and reduced ER visits for asthma [39, 42, 43].

Randomized-Controlled Trials and Meta-analyses

There have been several published double-blind placebo-controlled trials involving aspirin desensitization and maintenance aspirin therapy in AERD patients [Table 23.8]. In these studies, most patients experienced symptomatic improvement of upper and lower respiratory tract symptoms as well as improved disease control while on aspirin maintenance therapy compared with placebo.

There have been two meta-analyses which have evaluated outcomes in AERD patients who underwent aspirin desensitization and maintenance aspirin therapy. Both reviews found that patients experienced symptomatic improvement with aspirin maintenance therapy [56, 57].The meta-analysis by Ryan et al. [57] included patients with AERD who underwent sinus surgery with subsequent aspirin desensitization. It was found that aspirin desensitization allowed for long-term stability of symptom improvement following sinus surgery and reduced the need for revision surgery. These studies highlight the usefulness of aspirin desensitization and maintenance of daily aspirin therapy in patients with AERD.

Table 23.8 Summary of blinded placebo-controlled studies and meta-analyses evaluating the clinical efficacy of ATAD in patients with AERD

Study	Study description, level of evidence[a]	Duration of study	No. of patients who completed the study	Sinus surgery required prior to desensitization?	Maintenance oral aspirin dosage	Results
Stevenson et al. [29], 1984	Double-blind placebo-controlled crossover (3)	7 months	25	No	325 mg, 1300 mg, 2600 mg	*325 mg*: 57% (4 of 7) had improved sinonasal and/or asthma symptoms and tolerated daily aspirin *1300 mg*: 60% (3 of 5) had improved sinonasal and/or asthma symptoms and tolerated daily aspirin *2600 mg*: 69% (9 of 13) had improved sinonasal and/or asthma symptoms and tolerated daily aspirin
Fruth et al. [52], 2013	Double-blind placebo-controlled (2)	36 months	31	Yes	100 mg	ATAD improved QOL compared with controls, but no significant difference in rate of polyp regrowth or size
Swierczynska-Krepa et al. [53], 2014	Double-blind placebo-controlled (2)	6 months	15	No	624 mg	ATAD improved sinonasal symptoms, asthma control, and reduced inhaled steroid dose (compared with placebo)
Esmaeilzadeh et al. [54], 2015	Double-blind placebo-controlled (2)	6 months	32	No	650–1300 mg	ATAD had improved sinonasal symptoms & lung function (compared with placebo)
Mortazavi et al. [55], 2017	Double-blind placebo-controlled (2)	6 months	38	No	1300 mg (first 4 week) then 650 daily	ATAD reduced symptoms, improved FEV1, and improved QOL (compared with placebo)
Chu et al. [56], 2019	Meta-analysis (1)	N/A	N/A	N/A	N/A	Aspirin desensitization reduced symptoms of rhinosinusitis and improved QOL. Adverse event rates higher than in placebo group
Ryan et al. [57], 2020	Meta-analysis (1)	N/A	N/A	Yes	N/A	Surgery followed by aspirin desensitization in AERD improved symptoms. Aspirin desensitization allows for long-term stability in symptomatic improvement and reduces need for revision surgery

[a]Level of evidence: 1 (systematic review of randomized trials); 2 (randomized clinical trial or observational study with dramatic effect); 3 (nonrandomized controlled cohort study); 4 (case series, case-control studies)

Maintenance Aspirin Therapy after Desensitization

Dosage and Duration of Maintenance Aspirin Therapy after Desensitization

Currently there are no known clinical factors which can determine the optimal maintenance dosage of aspirin in patients with AERD. A dose as low as 81 mg may maintain the desensitized state in a cardiac patient, but this dosage is suboptimal in hindering the inflammatory disease within the respiratory tract. Furthermore, a dose of 325 mg is required to maintain cross-desensitization to other COX-1-inhibiting NSAIDs [58]. A study by Rozsasi et al. randomized AERD patients to receive either 100 mg or 300 mg of aspirin daily. They found nasal polyp regrowth after 1 year in all seven patients who were randomized to receive aspirin 100 mg daily, whereas patients randomized to aspirin 300 mg daily did not experience polyp regrowth [44]. This suggests that patients should be maintained at a dosage of at least 300 mg of daily aspirin, which has been recommended by several groups. Most authors recommend that patients receive aspirin 650 mg twice daily for the first 6 months after desensitization. This dose can be decreased to 325 mg twice daily if the patient is clinically improved, and the dose can be further decreased to 325 mg daily if there is continued clinical improvement. The dose of aspirin can always be increased back to 650 mg twice daily if there is worsening of disease control. Recently, we have adopted a new strategy based upon the average dosage required for patients of various age groups. In our retrospective analysis, we published maintenance aspirin dose averages based on age and found that patients 60 years or older required lower maintenance doses [59]. Patients aged 18–39 years required a mean dose of 928.6 mg, those aged 40–59 required a mean dose of 907 mg, and those aged 60 years or older required a mean dose of just 669.3 mg. Based on these results, our new approach starts with a dosage of 975 mg per day in divided doses for patients under 60 years and 650 mg per day for patients aged 60 and older.

Maintenance aspirin therapy should be continued indefinitely in patients who improve clinically and tolerate the medication. A six-month trial of maintenance aspirin therapy is sufficient to determine if there is a clinical benefit. If there is no clinical improvement after this time period, aspirin therapy can be discontinued. These patients will eventually become re-sensitized, and thus the provider should counsel them to strictly avoid all COX-1 inhibitors. There may be some patients who do not experience improvement in their upper and lower respiratory tract symptoms but may choose to maintain aspirin therapy for cardiac protection or the freedom to use other NSAIDs. Patients who experience intolerable side effects with aspirin despite medical management should discontinue aspirin therapy. Patients who disrupt aspirin treatment for more than 48 hours require repeat desensitization.

Silent Desensitization

The diagnosis of AERD should be established prior to surgical intervention by a firm history or a confirmatory challenge. Surgery has been shown to reduce the severity of ASA-/NSAID-induced respiratory reactions [22]. Occasionally, it is not feasible to do this, and the challenge may be performed after the surgery or as part of the desensitization protocol. In this setting, physicians may encounter the clinical dilemma of a "silent desensitization," referring to a situation in which the patient does not react during aspirin challenge or aspirin desensitization, despite a strong suspicion of AERD. This may be due to several factors, including medications that suppress reactions such as leukotriene modifiers and antihistamines, dampening of responses during the immediate postoperative period, and the type of protocol used and/or the timing between doses. There are two strategies that can be employed in this scenario [60]. The first strategy includes assuming that the patient has AERD and has undergone a silent desensitization. In this strategy, a trial of aspirin therapy can be attempted, and if there is a clinical response, aspirin therapy can be continued. The drawback to this strategy is the remaining question of whether aspirin truly helped, leading to uncertainty regarding need for long-term aspirin use. An alternative strategy would include instructing the patient to stop aspirin for 2 weeks and return for a full-dose (325 mg) aspirin challenge while off antihistamines, leukotriene-receptor antagonists, oral corticosteroids (or lowest possible dose), and mast cell stabilizers for at least 7 days. The benefit of this strategy is that there is no remaining uncertainty—if the patient reacts during the full-dose challenge, AERD is diagnosed, the reaction is treated, and desensitization can be initiated on the same day. Aspirin therapy would be indicated indefinitely, and if the patient does not react, AERD is exceedingly unlikely, and aspirin therapy would not be indicated for its treatment.

Safety Profile of Aspirin Therapy

There are several potential side effects associated with aspirin therapy. The most common adverse reaction is gastritis, which occurs in approximately 10% of patients. Patients should be counseled to always take aspirin with meals. Patients who develop gastritis require dose adjustment or potential aspirin discontinuation. Other gastrointestinal side effects include peptic ulcer disease and gastrointestinal bleeding which are less common and are contraindications to aspirin therapy. Non-gastrointestinal side effects include epistaxis, bruising, and tinnitus. Urticaria is another possible adverse event, typically seen in patients with concomitant chronic spontaneous urticaria (CSU). AERD patients who experience exacerbation of CSU with aspirin therapy may benefit from concomitant omalizumab [61]. Some patients develop an erythematous, pruritic, macular rash with aspirin that is associated with high levels of PGD_2. These patients almost always fail to maintain aspirin desensitization [62]. Acute pancreatitis has been described in AERD patients who recently underwent aspirin desensitization [63], and it has also been described with intranasal ketorolac during a modified aspirin desensitization protocol [64]. Clinicians should be aware of this rare potential complication and be prepared to diagnose and treat it appropriately.

Summary and Recommendations

Strong evidence supports the efficacy and safety of aspirin desensitization and maintenance aspirin therapy for the treatment of AERD. Aspirin therapy after desensitization improves sinus and respiratory symptoms, reduces polyp formation, and reduces the need for oral and inhaled corticosteroids and revision sinus surgery. Biologic therapies show promise for the treatment of AERD, but these agents are extremely expensive with annual costs between $30,000 and $40,000 USD [65]. Additionally, there are no double-blind or placebo-controlled studies that have examined the efficacy of biologics for the treatment of AERD. Aspirin therapy is affordable and cost-effective as first-line therapy after complete endoscopic sinus surgery [66]. It is supported by many double-blind placebo-controlled trials. Aspirin therapy after aspirin desensitization should remain the mainstay of medical therapy for most patients with AERD. The availability of biologic therapies will provide clinicians with additional options for the treatment of AERD, particularly in patients who have failed or have not tolerated aspirin therapy.

References

1. Woessner KM, Simon RA, Stevenson DD. The safety of celecoxib in patients with aspirin-sensitive asthma. Arthritis Rheum. 2002;46(8):2201–6.
2. Settipane R, Stevenson D. Cross sensitivity with acetaminophen in aspirin-sensitive subjects with asthma. J Allergy Clin Immunol. 1989;84(1):26–33.
3. Berges-Gimeno MP. The natural history and clinical characteristics of AERD. Ann Allergy Clin Immunol. 2002;89:474–8.
4. Rajan JP, Wineinger NE, Stevenson DD, White AA. Prevalence of aspirin-exacerbated respiratory disease among asthmatic patients: a meta-analysis of the literature. J Allergy Clin Immunol. 2015;135(3):676–681.e1.
5. Stevens WW, Peters AT, Hirsch AG, Nordberg CM, Schwartz BS, Mercer DG, et al. Clinical characteristics of patients with chronic rhinosinusitis with nasal polyps, asthma, and aspirin-exacerbated respiratory disease. J Allergy Clin Immunol: In Pract. 2017;5(4):1061–1070.e3.
6. Berges-Gimeno MP, Simon RA, Stevenson DD. The natural history and clinical characteristics of aspirin-exacerbated respiratory disease. Ann Allergy Asthma Immunol. 2002;89(5):474–8.
7. Chang JE, Ding D, Martin-Lazaro J, White A, Stevenson DD. Smoking, environmental tobacco smoke, and aspirin-exacerbated respiratory disease. Ann Allergy Asthma Immunol. 2012;108(1):14–9.
8. Cahill KN, Johns CB, Cui J, Wickner P, Bates DW, Laidlaw TM, et al. Automated identification of an aspirin-exacerbated respiratory disease cohort. J Allergy Clin Immunol. 2017;139(3):819–825.e6.
9. Laidlaw TM, Boyce JA. Platelets in patients with aspirin-exacerbated respiratory disease. J Allergy Clin Immunol. 2015;135(6):1407–14.
10. Lyly A, Laidlaw TM, Lundberg M. Pathomechanisms of AERD—recent advances. Front Allergy. 2021;10:2.

11. Laidlaw TM, Boyce JA. Aspirin-exacerbated respiratory disease—new prime suspects. Longo DL, editor. N Engl J Med. 2016;374(5):484–8.
12. Laidlaw TM, Kidder MS, Bhattacharyya N, Xing W, Shen S, Milne GL, et al. Cysteinyl leukotriene overproduction in aspirin-exacerbated respiratory disease is driven by platelet-adherent leukocytes. Blood. 2012;119(16):3790–8.
13. Cowburn AS, Sladek K, Soja J, Adamek L, Nizankowska E, Szczeklik A, et al. Overexpression of leukotriene C4 synthase in bronchial biopsies from patients with aspirin-intolerant asthma. J Clin Invest. 1998;101(4):834–46.
14. Choi G-S, Kim J-H, Shin Y-S, Ye Y-M, Kim S-H, Park H-S. Eosinophil activation and novel mediators in the aspirin-induced nasal response in AERD. Clin Exp Allergy. 2013;43(7):730–40.
15. Kuruvilla ME, Vanijcharoenkarn K, Levy JM. The role of mast cells in aspirin-exacerbated respiratory disease (AERD) pathogenesis: implications for future therapeutics. J Asthma Allergy. 2020;13:463–70.
16. Stevens WW, Staudacher AG, Hulse KE, Poposki JA, Kato A, Carter RG, et al. Studies of the role of basophils in aspirin-exacerbated respiratory disease pathogenesis. J Allergy Clin Immunol. 2021;148(2):439–449.e5.
17. Malfitano MJ, Santarelli GD, Gelpi M, Brown WC, Stepp WH, Hernandez S, et al. A comparison of sphenoid sinus osteoneogenesis in aspirin-exacerbated respiratory disease. Am J Rhinol Allergy. 2020;35(2):172–8.
18. Kim MB, Lim GC, Park JA, Kim YS, Kim JH, Kang JW. Computed tomography findings in patients with Samter's Triad: an observational study. Open Med. 2019;14(1):241–6.
19. Yamashita T, Tsuji H, Maeda N, Tomoda K, Kumazawa T. Etiology of nasal polyps associated with aspirin-sensitive asthma. Rhinol Suppl. 1989;8:15–24.
20. Park HS, Kowalski M, Laidlaw T. Hypersensitivity to aspirin and other nonsteroidal anti-inflammatory drugs. In: Burks AW, Holgate ST, O'Hehir RE, Broide DH, Bacharier LB, Khurana Hershey GK, Peebles RS, editors. Middleton's allergy: principles and practice. 9th ed. Edinburgh: Elsevier; 2020. p. 1283–92.
21. Bochenek G, Stachura T, Szafraniec K, Plutecka H, Sanak M, Nizankowska-Mogilnicka E, et al. Diagnostic accuracy of urinary LTE4 measurement to predict aspirin-exacerbated respiratory disease in patients with asthma. J Allergy Clin Immunol: In Pract. 2018;6(2):528–35.
22. Jerschow E, Edin ML, Chi Y, Hurst B, Abuzeid WM, Akbar NA, et al. Sinus surgery is associated with a decrease in aspirin-induced reaction severity in patients with aspirin exacerbated respiratory disease. J Allergy Clin Immunol: In Pract. 2019;7(5):1580–8.
23. Lee DKC, Haggart K, Robb FM, Lipworth BJ. Montelukast protects against nasal lysine-aspirin challenge in patients with aspirin-induced asthma. Eur Respir J. 2004;24(2):226–30.
24. Lee-Sarwar K, Johns C, Laidlaw TM, Cahill KN. Tolerance of daily low-dose aspirin does not preclude aspirin-exacerbated respiratory disease. J Allergy Clin Immunol: In Pract. 2015;3(3):449–51.
25. Dursun AB, Woessner KA, Simon RA, Karasoy D, Stevenson DD. Predicting outcomes of oral aspirin challenges in patients with asthma, nasal polyps, and chronic sinusitis. Ann Allergy Asthma Immunol. 2008;100(5):420–5.
26. DeGregorio GA, Singer J, Cahill KN, Laidlaw T. A 1-day, 90-minute aspirin challenge and desensitization protocol in aspirin-exacerbated respiratory disease. J Allergy Clin Immunol Pract. 2019;7(4):1174–80.
27. Cook KA, Modena BD, Wineinger NE, Woessner KM, Simon RA, White AA. Use of a composite symptom score during challenge in patients with suspected aspirin-exacerbated respiratory disease. Ann Allergy Asthma Immunol. 2017;118(5):597–602.
28. Lee RU, White AA, Ding D, Dursun AB, Woessner KM, Simon RA, et al. Use of intranasal ketorolac and modified oral aspirin challenge for desensitization of aspirin-exacerbated respiratory disease. Ann Allergy Asthma Immunol. 2010;105(2):130–5.
29. Stevenson DD, Pleskow WW, Simon RA, Mathison DA, Lumry WR, Schatz M, et al. Aspirin-sensitive rhinosinusitis asthma: a double-blind crossover study of treatment with aspirin. J Allergy Clin Immunol. 1984;73(4):500–7.

30. Jerschow E, Ren Z, Hudes G, Sanak M, Morales E, Schuster V, et al. Utility of low-dose oral aspirin challenges for diagnosis of aspirin-exacerbated respiratory disease. Ann Allergy Asthma Immunol. 2016;116(4):321–328.e1.
31. Hope AP, Woessner KA, Simon RA, Stevenson DD. Rational approach to aspirin dosing during oral challenges and desensitization of patients with aspirin-exacerbated respiratory disease. J Allergy Clin Immunol. 2009;123(2):406–10.
32. Widal F, Abrami P, Lermoyez J. First complete description of the aspirin idiosyncrasy-asthma-nasal polyposis syndrome (plus urticaria)--1922 (with a note on aspirin desensitization). J Asthma. 1987;24(5):297–300.
33. Zeiss CR, Lockey RF. Refractory period to aspirin in a patient with aspirin-induced asthma. J Allergy Clin Immunol. 1976;57(5):440–8.
34. Stevenson DD, Simon RA, Mathison DA. Aspirin-sensitive asthma: tolerance to aspirin after positive oral aspirin challenges. J Allergy Clin Immunol. 1980;66(1):82–8.
35. Bosso JV, Creighton D, Stevenson DD. Flurbiprofen (Ansaid) cross-sensitivity in an aspirin-sensitive asthmatic patient. Chest. 1992;101(3):856–8.
36. Bosso JV, Locke TB, Kuan EC, Tripathi SH, Ig-Izevbekhai KI, Kalaf LT, et al. Complete endoscopic sinus surgery followed by aspirin desensitization is associated with decreased overall corticosteroid use. Int Forum Allergy Rhinol. 2020;10(9):1043–8.
37. Glicksman JT, Parasher AK, Doghramji L, Brauer D, Waldram J, Walters K, et al. Alcohol-induced respiratory symptoms improve after aspirin desensitization in patients with aspirin-exacerbated respiratory disease. Int Forum Allergy Rhinol. 2018;8(10):1093–7.
38. Lumry WR, Curd JG, Zeiger RS, Pleskow WW, Stevenson DD. Aspirin sensitive rhinosinusitis: the clinical syndrome and effects of aspirin administration. J Allergy Clin Immunol. 1983;71(6):580–7.
39. Sweet JM, Stevenson DD, Simon RA, Mathison DA. Long-term effects of aspirin desensitization—treatment for aspirin-sensitive rhinosinusitis-asthma. J Allergy Clin Immunol. 1990;85(1):59–65.
40. Stevenson DD, Hankammer MA, Mathison DA, Christiansen SC, Simon RA. Aspirin desensitization treatment of aspirin-sensitive patients with rhinosinusitis-asthma: long-term outcomes. J Allergy Clin Immunol. 1996;98(4):751–8.
41. Berges-Gimeno MP, Simon RA, Stevenson DD. Early effects of aspirin desensitization treatment in asthmatic patients with aspirin-exacerbated respiratory disease. Ann Allergy Asthma Immunol. 2003;90(3):338–41.
42. Berges-Gimeno MP, Simon RA, Stevenson DD. Long-term treatment with aspirin desensitization in asthmatic patients with aspirin-exacerbated respiratory disease. J Allergy Clin Immunol. 2003;111(1):180–6.
43. Lee JY, Simon RA, Stevenson DD. Selection of aspirin dosages for aspirin desensitization treatment in patients with aspirin-exacerbated respiratory disease. J Allergy Clin Immunol. 2007;119(1):157–64.
44. Rozsasi A, Polzehl D, Deutschle T, Smith E, Wiesmiller K, Riechelmann H, et al. Long-term treatment with aspirin desensitization: a prospective clinical trial comparing 100 and 300 mg aspirin daily. Allergy. 2008;63(9):1228–34.
45. Havel M, Ertl L, Braunschweig F, Markmann S, Leunig A, Gamarra F, et al. Sinonasal outcome under aspirin desensitization following functional endoscopic sinus surgery in patients with aspirin triad. Eur Arch Otorrinolaringol. 2012;270(2):571–8.
46. Comert S, Celebioglu E, Yucel T, Erdogan T, Karakaya G, Onerci M, et al. Aspirin 300 mg/day is effective for treating aspirin-exacerbated respiratory disease. Allergy. 2013;68(11):1443–51.
47. Cho K-S, Soudry E, Psaltis AJ, Nadeau KC, McGhee SA, Nayak JV, et al. Long-term sinonasal outcomes of aspirin desensitization in aspirin exacerbated respiratory disease. Otolaryngol Head Neck Surg. 2014;151(4):575–81.
48. Jerschow E, Edin ML, Pelletier T, Abuzeid WM, Akbar NA, Gibber M, et al. Plasma 15-Hydroxyeicosatetraenoic acid predicts treatment outcomes in aspirin-exacerbated respiratory disease. J Allergy Clin Immunol: In Pract. 2017;5(4):998–1007.e2.

49. Adappa ND, Ranasinghe VJ, Trope M, Brooks SG, Glicksman JT, Parasher AK, et al. Outcomes after complete endoscopic sinus surgery and aspirin desensitization in aspirin-exacerbated respiratory disease. Int Forum Allergy Rhinol. 2017;8(1):49–53.
50. Walters KM, Waldram JD, Woessner KM, White AA. Long-term clinical outcomes of aspirin desensitization with continuous daily aspirin therapy in aspirin-exacerbated respiratory disease. Am J Rhinol Allergy. 2018;32(4):280–6.
51. Shah SJ, Abuzeid WM, Ponduri A, Pelletier T, Ren Z, Keskin T, et al. Endoscopic sinus surgery improves aspirin treatment response in aspirin-exacerbated respiratory disease patients. Int Forum Allergy Rhinol. 2019;9(12):1401–8.
52. Fruth K, Pogorzelski B, Schmidtmann I, Springer J, Fennan N, Fraessdorf N, et al. Low-dose aspirin desensitization in individuals with aspirin-exacerbated respiratory disease. Allergy. 2013;68(5):659–65.
53. Świerczyńska-Krępa M, Sanak M, Bochenek G, Stręk P, Ćmiel A, Gielicz A, et al. Aspirin desensitization in patients with aspirin-induced and aspirin-tolerant asthma: a double-blind study. J Allergy Clin Immunol. 2014;134(4):883–90.
54. Esmaeilzadeh H, Nabavi M, Aryan Z, Arshi S, Bemanian MH, Fallahpour M, et al. Aspirin desensitization for patients with aspirin-exacerbated respiratory disease: A randomized double-blind placebo-controlled trial. Clin Immunol. 2015;160(2):349–57.
55. Mortazavi N, Esmaeilzadeh H, Abbasinazari M, Babaie D, Alyasin S, et al. Clinical and immunological efficacy of aspirin desensitization in nasal polyp patients with aspirin-exacerbated respiratory disease. Iran J Pharmaceut Res. 2017;16(4):1639–47.
56. Chu DK, Lee DJ, Lee KM, Schünemann HJ, Szczeklik W, Lee JM. Benefits and harms of aspirin desensitization for aspirin-exacerbated respiratory disease: a systematic review and meta-analysis. Int Forum Allergy Rhinol. 2019;9(12):1409–19.
57. Ryan L, Segarra D, Tabor M, Parasher A. Systematic review of outcomes for endoscopic sinus surgery and subsequent aspirin desensitization in aspirin-exacerbated respiratory disease. World J Otorhinolaryngol—Head Neck Surg. 2020;6(4):220–9.
58. Pleskow W, Stevenson D, Mathison D, Simon R, Schatz M, Zeiger R. Aspirin desensitization in aspirin-sensitive asthmatic patients: clinical manifestations and characterization of the refractory period. J Allergy Clin Immunol. 1982;69(1):11–9.
59. Locke TB, Sweis AM, Gleeson PK, Lin TC, Civantos AM, Parhar HS, et al. Age as a factor in treatment of aspirin-exacerbated respiratory disease: relationship to required aspirin maintenance dose after desensitization. Int Forum Allergy Rhinol. 2020;10(10):1180–1.
60. White AA, Bosso JV, Stevenson DD. The clinical dilemma of "silent desensitization" in aspirin-exacerbated respiratory disease. Allergy Asthma Proc. 2013;34(4):378–82.
61. Porcaro F, Di Marco A, Cutrera R. Omalizumab in patient with aspirin exacerbated respiratory disease and chronic idiopathic urticaria. Pediatr Pulmonol. 2016;52(5):E26–8.
62. Cahill KN, Bensko JC, Boyce JA, Laidlaw TM. Prostaglandin D2: a dominant mediator of aspirin-exacerbated respiratory disease. J Allergy Clin Immunol. 2015;135(1):245–52.
63. Hoyte FCL, Weber RW, Katial RK. Pancreatitis as a novel complication of aspirin therapy in patients with aspirin-exacerbated respiratory disease. J Allergy Clin Immunol. 2012;129(6):1684–6.
64. Luskin KT, Bosso JV, Simon RA. Intranasal ketorolac-induced pancreatitis as a complication of modified oral aspirin desensitization in a patient with aspirin-exacerbated respiratory disease. J Allergy Clin Immunol: In Pract. 2020;8(3):1147–8.
65. Anderson WC, Szefler SJ. Cost-effectiveness and comparative effectiveness of biologic therapy for asthma. Ann Allergy Asthma Immunol. 2019;122(4):367–72.
66. Yong M, Wu YQ, Howlett J, Ballreich J, Walgama E, Thamboo A. Cost-effectiveness analysis comparing dupilumab and aspirin desensitization therapy for chronic rhinosinusitis with nasal polyposis in aspirin-exacerbated respiratory disease. Int Forum Allergy Rhinol. 2021;11(12):1626–36.

Leukotriene Modifiers for Recalcitrant Chronic Rhinosinusitis

24

Akaansha Ganju, Vivian Wang, and Joseph Yusin

Key Points

- Although approved only for asthma and allergic rhinitis for over 20 years, leukotriene antagonists have been utilized to treat multiple diseases, including chronic sinusitis with nasal polyps.
- Inflammatory polyps produce proinflammatory prostaglandins, and leukotrienes can contribute to nasal edema and mucus production as well as signaling eosinophil chemotaxis.
- Although montelukast is a well-known therapeutic in AERD, there is insufficient evidence to support its use for improving nasal symptoms and polyps. Further investigations are necessary.

Background

Upon activation, mast cells release an abundance of mediators that are involved in allergic pathways. These mediators include preformed mediators and newly formed lipid mediators, in addition to cytokines and chemokines. In this chapter, we will focus primarily on lipid mediators, the target of leukotriene modifiers.

Lipid mediators are derived from the activation of the arachidonic acid pathway and play a major role in the late phase of the allergic reaction. Membrane phospholipids provide mast cells with arachidonic acid to synthesize eicosanoids. Eicosanoids are inflammatory mediators that include prostaglandins (PG) and leukotrienes (LT), which eventually become cysteinyl leukotrienes (cysLTs) [1].

A. Ganju (✉) · V. Wang · J. Yusin
Department of Allergy and Immunology, Veterans Affairs Greater Los Angeles Healthcare System, Los Angeles, CA, USA
e-mail: Vivian.Wang@va.gov; Joseph.Yusin2@va.gov

J. T. Lee et al. (eds.), *Advances in Surgical and Medical Interventions for Recalcitrant Chronic Rhinosinusitis*,
https://doi.org/10.1007/978-3-031-89191-5_24

Compared to preformed mediators which are released immediately upon cell activation, eicosanoids are generated at the time of cell activation and can take minutes to hours to appear. These mediators contribute to the late symptoms and signs of allergic reactions. Phospholipase (PL) A2 enzymes release arachidonic acid from membrane phospholipids. Arachidonic acid can be metabolized via two pathways: the cyclooxygenase (COX) pathway and the lipoxygenase (LO) pathway. Arachidonic acid is converted into 5-hydroperoxyeicosatetraenoic acid (5-HPETE) and then into LTA4 by 5-lipoxygenase (5-LO). LTA4 is subsequently converted into LTB4 by LTA4 hydrolase and into LTC4, LTD4, and LTE4 by LTC4 synthase [2].

There are two types of leukotriene receptors: cysteinyl leukotriene 1 receptors (cysLT1Rs) and cysteinyl leukotriene 2 receptors (cysLT2Rs). CysLT1Rs are expressed on cells (e.g., eosinophils and mast cells) involved in allergic pathways and on bronchial epithelium and smooth muscles. The activation of cysLT1Rs leads to worsening asthma pathophysiology such as bronchoconstriction, increased mucus production, and vascular permeability [3].

Leukotriene modifiers available commercially work through either blocking the LO pathway upstream via the inhibition of 5-LO, the key enzyme involved in the generation of LTs (LTC4, LTD4, and LTE4) that bind to cysLT1Rs, or by directly blocking cysLT1Rs downstream [Fig. 24.1] [4].

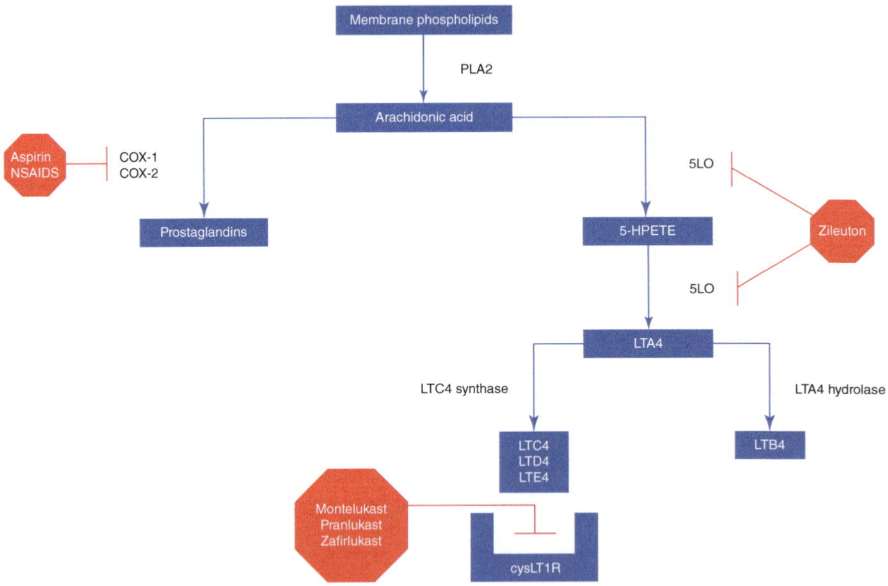

Fig. 24.1 Arachidonic acid metabolism and leukotriene modifiers

The Role of Leukotriene Receptor Agonists in Chronic Rhinosinusitis

In the USA, there are two FDA-approved leukotriene receptor antagonists available: montelukast and zafirlukast. Additionally, there is one FDA-approved lipoxygenase inhibitor: zileuton [5]. Montelukast is currently FDA-approved for asthma, exercise-induced bronchoconstriction, and allergic rhinitis [6]. Zafirlukast and zileuton are FDA-approved for the prophylaxis and chronic treatment of asthma [7, 8].

Outside of the FDA-approved indications, leukotriene modifiers have been specifically studied in chronic rhinosinusitis with nasal polyposis (CRSwNP). The current standard of care in the management of CRSwNP includes intranasal corticosteroids (INC), saline irrigation, a short course of oral corticosteroids, and, in medically refractory cases, endoscopic sinus surgery [9]. Despite these methods, the polyp recurrence rate remains high, with an estimated 40–60% of patients experiencing recurrence [10]. More recently, due to increased research into the underlying inflammatory mechanisms in uncontrolled polypoid disease, biologic therapeutics have emerged as an important targeted treatment option [11].

The majority of sinonasal polyps consist of an abundance of eosinophils, mast cells, and fibroblasts [12]. Produced within these tissues, prostaglandins and leukotrienes can contribute to nasal edema and mucus production as well as signaling eosinophil chemotaxis. High levels of LTC4 in the nasal mucosa have been correlated to a greater risk of polyp recurrence [13]. This characterization suggests a potential benefit of leukotriene modifiers in refractory CRSwNP.

Several studies have investigated the use of leukotriene modifiers as either comparative or add-on therapy in CRSwNP, though high-quality evidence is limited. Table 24.1 presents a summary of these studies using literature review and adaptation from prior systemic reviews [Table 24.1] [14–16]. Multiple studies have investigated the use of montelukast in the postoperative setting for CRSwNP, either alone or as add-on therapy, and have shown an overall reduction in symptom scores and polyposis. Studies that compared montelukast to INC did not show significant differences in symptom score reduction between the patient groups [17–19]. One study showed more polyp recurrence in the montelukast-treated group than the INC group [18]. As such, the current literature provides little evidence that leukotriene antagonists provide benefit in the management of CRSwNP as a monotherapy.

Montelukast was also studied as an add-on therapy to intranasal corticosteroids in CRSwNP with varying results. A randomized controlled trial by Van Gerven et al. did not show significant differences in symptoms, polyps, or Lund-Mackay score with the addition of montelukast [17]. Suri et al. and Stewart et al. showed reduction in certain symptoms with montelukast, such as headache and sneezing, but no difference in obstruction or drainage [20, 21]. Nonaka et al. found a decrease in CT and nasal polyp scores in a prospective case series of 20 patients, while Kieff et al. found symptomatic improvement only in patients with perennial allergies (seasonal allergies were excluded from the case series) [22, 23].

Table 24.1 Summary of studies using leukotriene modifiers in chronic rhinosinusitis with nasal polyposis

Study	Type	Disease	Drug	Intervention	Outcome measures	Conclusion
Dahlen (1998) [29]	DBPCT Crossover $n = 40$	AERD	Zileuton	Zileuton (600 mg) QID + INC and/or PO glucocorticoids × 6 weeks vs. Placebo + INC and/or PO glucocorticoids × 6 weeks	VAS: Loss of sense of smell, rhinorrhea, and nasal congestion	Significant improvement in the sense of smell and rhinorrhea
Ulualp (1999) [30]	Retrospective case series $n = 15$	AERD postoperatively	Zafirlukast or zileuton	Zafirlukast (20 mg) BID or zileuton (600 mg) QID × 1–15 months	Symptom scores, subjective self-reports, and nasal endoscopy	Significant reduction in major and minor symptom scores, subjective overall benefit in 12/15 patients. Endoscopic exams consistent with self-reports.
Parnes (2000) [31]	Prospective case series $n = 36$	CRSwNP	Zafirlukast or zileuton	Zafirlukast (20 mg) BID or zileuton (600 mg) QID × 7.4 months mean duration	Symptom score	Improvement in symptomatology in 72% of patients. Subjective degree of sinonasal polyposis: 50% improvement, 42% no change, 8% worsening
Kutting (2000) [33]	Prospective case series (non-blinded or randomized) $n = 9$	CRSwNP postoperatively	Montelukast and short-term oral steroids	Methylprednisolone (40 mg) daily × 5 days followed by taper until day 12. Then montelukast (10 mg) daily as maintenance treatment up to 1 year	Subjective interviews, serial endoscopic examinations, and MRI	7/9 with subjective improvement of symptoms, with 4 being free of symptoms. Improvement in polyps endoscopically and via MRI. Recurrence of nasal polyps within 4–8 weeks of discontinuing montelukast therapy
Ragab (2001) [24]	Prospective case series $n = 41$	CRSwNP refractory to medical therapy and Asthma: AERD and AT	Montelukast	Montelukast (10 mg) daily × 3 months as add-on therapy to INC and inhaled corticosteroids	VAS, nasal volumes by acoustic rhinometry, NIPF	Significant subjective symptom improvement in AT but not in AERD. No significant change in acoustic rhinometry or NIPF

Mostafa (2005) [19]	RCT: Prospective, double blind $n = 40$	CRSwNP postoperatively	Montelukast	Montelukast (10 mg) daily × 1 year vs. Beclomethasone dipropionate spray (200 ⌠g) BID × 1 year	VAS symptom score	Significant reduction in symptom scores in both groups. Greater improvement in itching, postnasal discharge, and headache in montelukast group. Greater improvement in smell disturbances and obstruction in steroid group
Kieff (2005) [23]	Prospective case series $n = 24$	CRSwNP *(excluded seasonal allergies)*	Montelukast	Montelukast (10 mg) daily × 3 months as add-on therapy to INC	ICSD symptom score, polyp eosinophilia	Significant improvement in symptom score and polyp eosinophilia in the perineal allergies group
Pauli (2007) [28]	DBPCT $n = 30$	CRSwNP	Montelukast	Montelukast (10 mg) daily × 4 weeks vs. Placebo × 4 weeks	Symptom score, polyposis stage	Significant improvement in symptom scores. Significant decrease in polyposis
Stewart (2008) [21]	RCT $n = 35$	CRSwNP	Montelukast	Two-week oral steroid taper plus montelukast (10 mg) daily + INC × 8 weeks vs. Two-week oral steroid taper plus INC × 8 weeks	ICSD	Significantly greater reduction in symptom scores (headache, facial pain, and sneezing) with montelukast. No significant effect on nasal blockage, hyposmia, or nasal discharge b/w groups. Effects were not maintained 4 weeks after stopping montelukast
Nonaka (2010) [22]	Prospective case series $n = 20$	CRSwNP and asthma	Montelukast	Montelukast (10 mg) daily and intranasal fluticasone propionate (200 ⌠g) daily × 1 year	Nasal polyp score, peripheral blood eosinophilia, CT score	Significant decrease in CT score and nasal polyp score at 6 and 12 months

(continued)

Table 24.1 (continued)

Study	Type	Disease	Drug	Intervention	Outcome measures	Conclusion
Vuralkan (2011) [18]	RCT $n = 50$	CRSwNP postoperatively	Montelukast	Montelukast (10 mg) daily × 6 months vs. Intranasal mometasone furoate (400 ⌠g) BID × 6 months	SNOT, polyp grades, CT score, eosinophils in peripheral blood and polyp tissue	Significant reduction in SNOT scores in both groups but no significant difference b/w the groups. Significant reduction in CT score in both groups. Significantly more recurrences with montelukast
Schaper (2011) [25]	SBPCT Crossover $n = 24$	CRSwNP postoperatively and asthma	Montelukast	Montelukast (10 mg) daily × 6 weeks vs. Placebo × 4 weeks	Nasal symptom scores, rhinomanometry, olfactometry, nasal lavage procedure	Significant improvement in nasal symptom score with montelukast. No significant changes in symptoms with placebo. Significant improvement in edema, nasal airflow, inflammatory mediators, and eosinophils in nasal secretion with montelukast
Suri (2015) [20]	RCT: Prospective $n = 40$	CRSwNP	Montelukast	PO steroid taper × 2 weeks + INC × 8 weeks vs. PO steroid taper × 2 weeks + INC and montelukast (10 mg) daily × 8 weeks	ICSD	Significant improvement in the sense of smell, sneezing, headache, and overall score with montelukast. No statistical difference in discharge, facial pain, or nasal blockage between groups

Yelverton (2016) [27]	Retrospective review $n = 52$	CRSwNP postoperatively	Montelukast	Review of patients with a lapse in montelukast therapy for 1 month or longer	Comparison of SNOT-20 and endoscopic scores at the single time point immediately prior to a lapse in therapy with scores at the visit when the patient first reported noncompliance	All patients: SNOT-20 and Lund-Kennedy endoscopy scores with montelukast were significantly lower than the scores without montelukast therapy Hx of AERD: No significant improvement Hx of asthma: Significant improvement in both categories
Van Gerven (2018) [17]	RCT: Prospective, randomized $n = 72$	CRSwNP postoperative	Montelukast	Montelukast (10 mg) daily and intranasal mometasone furoate (200 ∫g) BID × 1 year vs. Intranasal mometasone furoate (200 ∫g) BID × 1 year	Total five-symptom score [T5SS], nasal polyp score [NPS], Lund-Mackay [LMK] score, olfactometry	Significantly reduced T5SS, NPS, and LMK score in both groups without significant differences between the groups
San Nicolo (2020) [26]	Retrospective study $n = 61$	AERD postoperative	Montelukast	Montelukast daily or INS or aspirin desensitization	SNOT, endoscopic exam	Montelukast and aspirin desensitization had significantly less polyp recurrences compared to INS after >12 months. Montelukast showed significant improvement in nasal symptoms

DBPCT double-blind placebo-controlled trial; *AERD* aspirin-exacerbated respiratory disease; *QID* four times per day; *INC* intranasal corticosteroids; *PO* oral; *VAS* visual analog scale; *BID* two times per day; *CRSwNP* chronic rhinosinusitis with nasal polyposis; *NIPF* nasal inspiratory peak flow; *ICSD* International Classification of Sinus Disease; *RCT* randomized controlled trial; *SBPCT* single-blind placebo-controlled trial; *SNOT* Sino-Nasal Outcome Test

Montelukast is a well-known therapeutic in asthma management. Three studies investigated nasal symptoms and polyposis in a cohort with both CRSwNP and asthma. One study reviewed a cohort with just aspirin-exacerbated respiratory disease (AERD) [22, 24–26]. Ragab et al. found significant symptomatic nasal relief in aspirin-tolerant asthma (ATA) but not in AERD, while none of the patients had improvement on objective outcome measures [24]. When accounting for AERD, Yelverton et al. also did not find significant nasal changes with montelukast, although San Nicolo et al. demonstrated symptomatic improvement and less polyp recurrence in a small cohort [26, 27]. Nonak et al. found general improvement in CT and nasal polyp scores with montelukast added to INC, and Schaper et al. found improvement in edema, inflammatory mediators, and symptoms with montelukast alone [22, 25]. In studies that were not fully composed of asthma patients but accounted for the demographic within both treatment arms, there was no significant difference in nasal symptoms or polyp score in those with or without asthma [14].

There are only a few randomized controlled trials studying montelukast for the treatment of nasal polyposis. Two placebo-controlled studies showed significant improvement in symptom score with montelukast alone compared to placebo [25, 28]. Two studies showed similar improvement in symptoms with intranasal corticosteroids when compared to montelukast [18, 19]. A meta-analysis of three RTCs evaluating the addition of montelukast to standard INC therapy found no significant additive benefit [16, 17, 20, 21].

Only three studies examined the alternative leukotriene receptor antagonist zafirlukast or the lipoxygenase inhibitor zileuton in relation to nasal symptoms in CRSwNP and AERD. Dahlen et al. conducted a double-blind, placebo-controlled crossover trial with zileuton in AERD and showed a significant improvement in the sense of smell and rhinorrhea [29]. Ulualp et al. retrospectively examined 15 AERD patients who received zafirlukast or zileuton post-polypectomy, revealing symptomatic and endoscopic improvement [30]. Lastly, Parnes et al. conducted a prospective trial of zafirlukast or zileuton in CRSwNP with similar results as above [31].

Overall, high-quality evidence involving leukotriene modifiers in CRSwNP is lacking. Leukotriene antagonists could potentially benefit patients who have failed or are intolerant to INC as studies have shown superiority to placebo and effects similar to INC [14]. Current evidence suggests that montelukast does not have additive benefit to standard of care with INC.

Additionally, although montelukast is a well-known therapeutic in AERD, there is insufficient evidence to support its use for improving nasal symptoms and polyps; further investigations are necessary. It appears to be more advantageous for the treatment of asthma in AERD. The European EPOS2020 steering group published recommendations based on previous randomized controlled trials, stating that they did not advise the addition of montelukast to INC in CRSwNP but may consider its use in situations where INC have failed or are not tolerated. Further studies are needed to determine the exact benefit in this setting [16].

Side effects should be considered when determining the therapeutic benefit of leukotriene antagonists. In 2020, the FDA released a drug safety communication requiring a boxed warning on montelukast to describe the risk of neuropsychiatric events. Therefore, leukotriene antagonists are only recommended to patients who have suboptimal response or intolerance to alternative therapeutics in asthma and allergic rhinitis [6]. This recommendation should furthermore be applied to its use in CRSwNP. Zileuton requires monitoring of liver function tests due to the risk of hepatotoxicity and monitoring of certain drug plasma concentrations [32].

Conclusions

Leukotriene receptor antagonists may have a role in the management of refractory chronic rhinosinusitis, but current evidence regarding their efficacy is lacking, with the current body of literature demonstrating conflicting data or showing minimal to no benefit from the addition of this class of medications.

References

1. Boyce JA. Mast cells and eicosanoid mediators: a system of reciprocal paracrine and autocrine regulation. Immunol Rev. 2007 Jun;217:168–85.
2. Yokomizo T, Uozumi N, Takahashi T, Kume K, Izumi T, Shimizu T. Leukotriene A4 hydrolase and leukotriene B4 metabolism. J Lipid Mediat Cell Signal. 1995 Oct;12(2–3):321–32.
3. Laidlaw TM, Boyce JA. Lipid mediators of hypersensitivity and inflammation. In: Middleton's allergy: principles and practice. 9th ed. Elsevier; 2020. p. 132–53.
4. Stokes Peebles R. Antileukotriene therapy in asthma. In: Middleton's allergy: principles and practice. 9th ed. Elsevier; 2020. p. 1584–1598.e1.
5. DailyMed [Internet]. [cited 2022 Jun 20]. Available from: https://dailymed.nlm.nih.gov/dailymed/
6. Administration D. FDA Briefing Document Pediatric Advisory Committee meeting neuropsychiatric events with use of Montelukast in pediatric patients. 2019.
7. FDA. ACCOLATE® (zafirlukast) TABLETS DESCRIPTION [Internet]. 2013 [cited 2022 Jun 20]. Available from: https://www.accessdata.fda.gov/drugsatfda_docs/label/2013/020547s033lbl.pdf
8. FDA. ZYFLO® (zileuton tablets) [Internet]. 2012 [cited 2022 Jun 20]. Available from: https://www.accessdata.fda.gov/drugsatfda_docs/label/2012/020471s017lbl.pdf
9. de Corso E, Bilò MB, Matucci A, Seccia V, Braido F, Gelardi M, et al. Personalized management of patients with chronic rhinosinusitis with nasal polyps in clinical practice: a multidisciplinary consensus statement. J Pers Med [Internet]. 2022;12(5):846. [cited 2022 Jun 20]. Available from: https://pubmed.ncbi.nlm.nih.gov/35629268/
10. DeConde AS, Mace JC, Levy JM, Rudmik L, Alt JA, Smith TL. Prevalence of polyp recurrence after endoscopic sinus surgery for chronic rhinosinusitis with nasal polyposis. Laryngoscope [Internet]. 2017;127(3):550–5. [cited 2022 Jun 20]. Available from: https://pubmed.ncbi.nlm.nih.gov/27859303/
11. Tai J, Han M, Kim T. Therapeutic strategies of biologics in chronic rhinosinusitis: current options and future targets. Int J Mol Sci [Internet]. 2022;23(10) [cited 2022 Jun 20]. Available from: https://pubmed.ncbi.nlm.nih.gov/35628333/
12. Arango P, Borish L, Frierson HF, Kountakis SE. Cysteinyl leukotrienes in chronic hyperplastic rhinosinusitis. Otolaryngol Head Neck Surg [Internet]. 2002;127(6):512–5. [cited 2022 Jun 20]. Available from: https://pubmed.ncbi.nlm.nih.gov/12501101/
13. Klapan I, Čulo F, Čulig J, Bukovec Ž, Simović S, Višeslav Ć, et al. Arachidonic acid metabolites and sinonasal polyposis. I. Possible prognostic value. Am J Otolaryngol [Internet].

1995;16(6):396–402. [cited 2022 Jun 20]. Available from: https://pubmed.ncbi.nlm.nih.gov/8572256/
14. Wentzel JL, Soler ZM, DeYoung K, Nguyen SA, Lohia S, Schlosser RJ. Leukotriene antagonists in nasal polyposis: a meta-analysis and systematic review. Am J Rhinol Allergy [Internet]. 2013;27(6):482–9. [cited 2022 Jun 20]. Available from: https://pubmed.ncbi.nlm.nih.gov/24274224/
15. Alobid I, Cardelús S, Picado C, Mullol J. Antileukotrienes in rhinosinusitis and nasal polyposis. Expert Rev Clin Immunol [Internet]. 2008;4(3):331–7. [cited 2022 Jun 20]. Available from: https://pubmed.ncbi.nlm.nih.gov/20476923/
16. Fokkens WJ, Lund VJ, Hopkins C, Hellings PW, Kern R, Reitsma S, et al. European Position Paper on Rhinosinusitis and Nasal Polyps 2020. Rhinology [Internet]. 2020;58(Suppl S29):1–464. [cited 2022 Jun 20]. Available from: https://pubmed.ncbi.nlm.nih.gov/32077450/
17. van Gerven L, Langdon C, Cordero A, Cardelús S, Mullol J, Alobid I. Lack of long-term add-on effect by montelukast in postoperative chronic rhinosinusitis patients with nasal polyps. Laryngoscope [Internet]. 2018;128(8):1743–51. [cited 2022 Jun 20]. Available from: https://pubmed.ncbi.nlm.nih.gov/29114894/
18. Vuralkan E, Saka C, Akin I, Hucumenoglu S, Unal BU, Kuran G, et al. Comparison of montelukast and mometasone furoate in the prevention of recurrent nasal polyps. Ther Adv Respir Dis [Internet]. 2012;6(1):5–10. [cited 2022 Jun 20]. Available from: https://pubmed.ncbi.nlm.nih.gov/22042749/
19. Mostafa BE, Hay HA, Mohammed HE, Yamani M. Role of leukotriene inhibitors in the postoperative management of nasal polyps. ORL J Otorhinolaryngol Relat Spec [Internet]. 2005;67(3):148–53. [cited 2022 Jun 20]. Available from: https://pubmed.ncbi.nlm.nih.gov/15925911/
20. Suri A, Gupta R, Gupta N, Kotwal S. Montelukast as an adjunct to treatment of chronic rhinosinusitis with polyposis: a prospective Randomized Controlled Trial. www.jkscience.org [Internet]. 2015 ;17(1). [cited 2022 Jun 20]. Available from: www.jkscience.org
21. Stewart RA, Ram B, Hamilton G, Weiner J, Kane KJ. Montelukast as an adjunct to oral and inhaled steroid therapy in chronic nasal polyposis. Otolaryngol Head Neck Surg [Internet]. 2008;139(5):682–7. [cited 2022 Jun 20]. Available from: https://pubmed.ncbi.nlm.nih.gov/18984264/
22. Nonaka M, Sakanushi A, Kusama K, Ogihara N, Yagi T. One-year evaluation of combined treatment with an intranasal corticosteroid and montelukast for chronic rhinosinusitis associated with asthma. J Nippon Med Sch [Internet]. 2010;77(1):21–8. [cited 2022 Jun 20]. Available from: https://pubmed.ncbi.nlm.nih.gov/20154454/
23. Kieff DA, Busaba NY. Efficacy of montelukast in the treatment of nasal polyposis. 2005;Ann Otol Rhinol Laryngol [Internet], 114(12):941–5. [cited 2022 Jun 20]. Available from: https://pubmed.ncbi.nlm.nih.gov/16425561/
24. Ragab S, Parikh A, Darby YC, Scadding GK. An open audit of montelukast, a leukotriene receptor antagonist, in nasal polyposis associated with asthma. Clin Exp Allergy [Internet]. 2001;31(9):1385–91. [cited 2022 Jun 20]. Available from: https://pubmed.ncbi.nlm.nih.gov/11591188/
25. Schäper C, Noga O, Koch B, Ewert R, Felix SB, Gläser S, et al. Anti-inflammatory properties of montelukast, a leukotriene receptor antagonist in patients with asthma and nasal polyposis. J Investig Allergol Clin Immunol. 2011;21(1):51–8.
26. San Nicoló M, Habermann N, Havel M. AERD associated nasal polyposis: efficacy of postoperative Antileukotriene therapy in comparison with aspirin desensitization. A retrospective study. Int Arch Allergy Immunol [Internet]. 2020;181(10):790–8. [cited 2022 Jun 21]. Available from: https://pubmed.ncbi.nlm.nih.gov/32777782/
27. Yelverton JC, Holmes TW, Johnson CM, Gelves CR, Kountakis SE. Effectiveness of leukotriene receptor antagonism in the postoperative management of chronic rhinosinusitis. Int Forum Allergy Rhinol [Internet]. 2016;6(3):243–7. [cited 2022 Jun 20]. Available from: https://pubmed.ncbi.nlm.nih.gov/26834076/

28. Pauli C, Fintelmann R, Klemens C, Hilgert E, Jund F, Rasp G, et al. Polyposis nasi--improvement in quality of life by the influence of leukotrien receptor antagonists. Laryngorhinootologie [Internet]. 2007;86(4):282–6. [cited 2022 Jun 20]. Available from: https://pubmed.ncbi.nlm.nih.gov/17286243/
29. Dahlén B, Nizankowska E, Szczeklik A, Zetterström O, Bochenek G, Kumlin M, et al. Benefits from adding the 5-lipoxygenase inhibitor zileuton to conventional therapy in aspirin-intolerant asthmatics. Am J Respir Crit Care Med. 1998;157(4 PART I):1187–94.
30. Ulualp SO, Sterman BM, Toohill Md RJ. Antileukotriene therapy for the relief of sinus symptoms in aspirin triad disease. Ear Nose Throat J [Internet]. 1999;78(8):604–16. [cited 2022 Jun 20]. Available from: https://pubmed.ncbi.nlm.nih.gov/10485156/
31. Parnes SM, Chuma A v. Acute effects of antileukotrienes on sinonasal polyposis and sinusitis. Ear Nose Throat J 2000 Jan;79(1):18–20, 24–5.
32. Bouchette D, Patel P, Preuss CV. Zileuton. xPharm: The Comprehensive Pharmacology Reference [Internet]. 2022;1–3. [cited 2022 Jun 20]. Available from: https://pubmed.ncbi.nlm.nih.gov/28846301/
33. Kutting B, Nieschalk M, Brehler R. A new concept for treatment of sinonasal polyposis. Allergy [Internet]. 2000;55(11):1091–2. [cited 2022 Jun 20]. Available from: https://pubmed.ncbi.nlm.nih.gov/11097323/

Biological Treatment for Chronic Rhinosinusitis with Nasal Polyposis

25

Joseph K. Han and Dafna Gershnabel Milk

Key Points

- Chronic rhinosinusitis with nasal polyposis (CRSwNP) is a challenging, difficult-to-treat disease with a significant impact on the patient's quality of life (QOL) and well-being.
- New insights on chronic rhinosinusitis (CRS) pathophysiology have revealed that it is a heterogeneous condition with several phenotypes and pathophysiological mechanisms. These insights have led to a shift towards endotype-driven management of CRS.
- The common endotype of CRSwNP among Caucasian patients is type 2 inflammation.
- In CRSwNP, the term "biological medications" refers to monoclonal antibodies targeting specific type 2 inflammatory mediators.
- The implementation of biological medications to the treatment scheme of CRSwNP is considered a "game changer" in the management of severe type 2 CRS, with significant improvement in patients' subjective and objective factors.

J. K. Han (✉)
Division of Rhinology & Endoscopic Sinus and Skull Base Surgery,
East Virginia Medical School, Norfolk, VA, USA
e-mail: hanjk@evms.edu

D. G. Milk
Department of Otolaryngology Head and Neck Surgery, Eastern Virginia Medical School,
Norfolk, VA, USA

Department of Otolaryngology Head and Neck Surgery, Meir Medical Center,
Kfar Saba, Israel

J. T. Lee et al. (eds.), *Advances in Surgical and Medical Interventions for Recalcitrant Chronic Rhinosinusitis*,
https://doi.org/10.1007/978-3-031-89191-5_25

Background

In the Western world, most patients with CRSwNP show a type 2 inflammatory signature [1]. Type 2 inflammation is characterized by the activation of both innate and adaptive inflammatory cells: group 2 innate lymphoid cells (ILC2s), mast cells, and T helper 2 lymphocytes. This leads to the release of type 2 cytokines (IL-5, IL-13, and IL-4), eosinophil activation, and IgE formation [2] (Fig. 25.1).

Type 2 CRS is associated with severe sinus disease that is recalcitrant to standard-of-care medical treatment and with prompt polyp recurrence following ESS, leading to multiple operations. It is also associated with comorbidities that share similar inflammatory pathways, such as asthma and aspirin-exacerbated respiratory disease (AERD) [3].

In the last decade, monoclonal antibodies targeting specific type 2 inflammatory mediators were developed to treat type 2 diseases such as asthma and atopic dermatitis. Their success in controlling these diseases has led to further research and

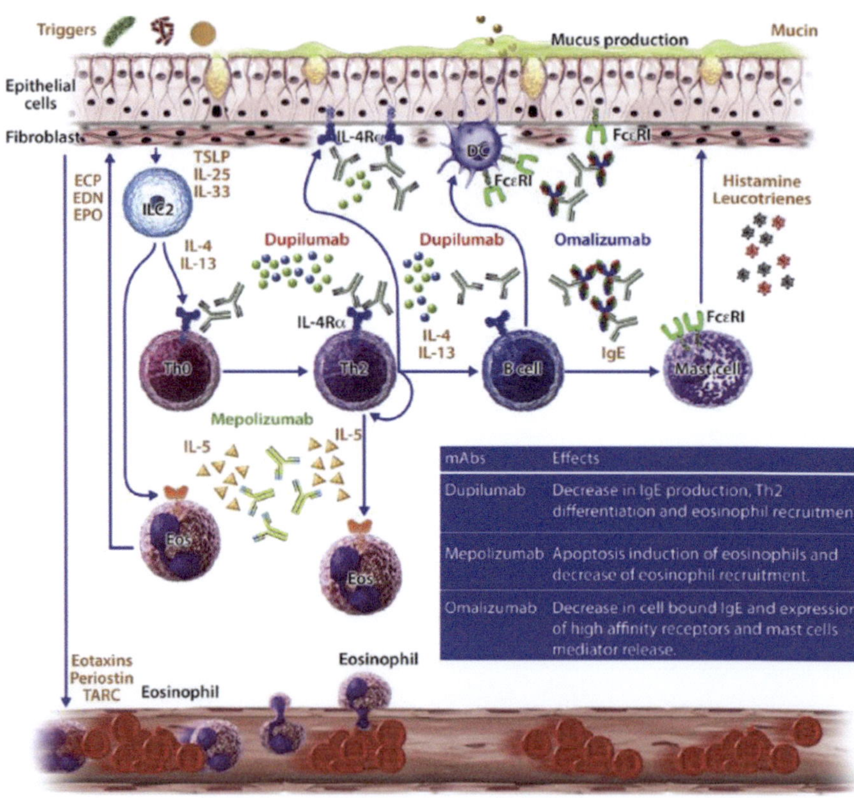

Fig. 25.1 Type 2 inflammatory pathway inside the sinonasal cavity and biological mechanism of action (with permission from Claus Bachert). *DC* Dendritic cell, *ECP* eosinophil cationic protein, *EDN* eosinophil-derived neurotoxin, *Eos* eosinophils, *EPO* eosinophil peroxidase, *IL-4Ra* IL-4 receptor a, *TSLP* thymic stromal lymphopoietin

adaptation of the medications to treat CRSwNP. Three monoclonal antibodies are currently approved by the Food and Drug Administration (FDA) and the European Medicines Agency (EMA) for patients with uncontrolled severe CRSwNP, and more monoclonal antibodies are expected to be approved in the future.

Patient Selection

The currently accepted treatment algorithm, supported by several published guidelines, suggests that biologics are indicated for patients with uncontrolled type 2 CRS, despite appropriate medical treatment and surgical failure [3–5]. The term "appropriate medical treatment" requires further clarification. A recently published international survey among otolaryngologists found that most participants (73%) would prescribe biologics in case of failure of topical steroid therapy postoperatively [6]. Fokkens et al. recommend considering biologics in adult patients with CRSwNP who have a history of previous ESS or in patients who are unfit to undergo surgical intervention, as well as three of the five described characteristics: (1) presence of type 2 eosinophilic inflammation, (2) regular need for systemic corticosteroids or contraindication to systemic steroids, (3) significant impact of CRSwNP on quality of life, (4) loss of sense of smell, and/or (5) comorbid asthma [5]. These criteria are listed in Fig. 25.2.

*Adult patient with CRS with bilateral nasal polyps

and

*History of previous ESS/ patient is not fit for surgery

and

***Three** of the following characteristics:

1. Presence of type 2 inflammation: tissue eosinophils $\geq$10/HPF **or** blood eosinophils $\geq$150 cells/μL **or** total IgE $\geq$100 IU/mL
2. Regular need for systemic corticosteroids ($\geq$2 courses per year OR >3 months low dose steroids) or contraindication to systemic steroids
3. Significant impact on QOL (SNOT-22 score $\geq$40)
4. Loss of smell (anosmic on smell test)
5. Comorbid asthma (asthma needing regular inhaled corticosteroids)

Fig. 25.2 Eligibility criteria for biological therapy [5]

FDA- and EMA-Approved Biological Medications for CRSwNP

A summary of the FDA- and EMA-approved biologics are available in Table 25.1 [7–12]. Three biologics—dupilumab, omalizumab, and mepolizumab—are currently approved by the FDA and the EMA for the treatment of patients with CRSwNP. The drugs' major clinical trials are summarized in Table 25.2. In all the clinical trials, the efficacy of these biologics was tested, while study participants continued the use of intranasal topical steroid spray. Consequently, biologics are considered add-on treatments to intranasal corticosteroids.

For patients with steroid-dependent CRS and/or asthma starting biological treatment, gradual and careful corticosteroid cessation is advised because an abrupt reduction in corticosteroid dosage may be associated with systemic withdrawal symptoms and/or unmask conditions previously suppressed by systemic corticosteroid therapy (e.g., eosinophilic granulomatosis with polyangiitis) [7–12].

Type 2 inflammation plays a significant role in the immune system's defense mechanism against parasitic (helminth) infection. As a result, patients who take biologics might be at an increased risk of acquiring parasitic infection or being unable to clear parasitic infections [10–14]. Further studies are needed to gather additional information. The FDA addressed this issue and summarized that preexisting parasitic (helminth) infection should be treated before initiating biologics. If patients become infected while receiving dupilumab and do not respond to anti-helminth treatment, consider discontinuing the treatment until the infection resolves [10–12].

Table 25.1 Summary of the FDA- and EMA-approved biologicals

Name	Brand name	Mechanism	Administration route	Dose	Common adverse reactions [7–12]
Dupilumab	Dupixent	Anti-IL-4Rα (anti-IL-4, IL-13)	S.C	300 mg every 2 weeks	(Incidence ≥1%) Injection site reactions, temporary eosinophilia, insomnia, toothache, gastritis, arthralgia, and conjunctivitis
Omalizumab	Xolair	Anti-IgE	S.C	75–600 mg every 2 or 4 weeks	(Incidence ≥3%) Headache, injection site reaction, arthralgia, upper abdominal pain, and dizziness
Mepolizumab	Nucala	Anti-IL-5	S.C	750 mg every 4 weeks	(Incidence ≥5%) Headache, injection site reaction, back pain, and fatigue

Table 25.2 Summary of the major studies on biologicals for CRSwNP

Study	Type of study	Medical intervention	Number of patients	Reported outcome
Dupilumab				
LIBERTY NP SINUS 24 [15]	Multicenter, randomized, double-blind, placebo-controlled, parallel-group phase 3 trial	Patients were randomly assigned (1:1) to dupilumab 300 mg or placebo every 2 weeks for 24 weeks	Dupilumab (n = 143) placebo (n = 133)	Least squares mean difference vs placebo (95% CI) at week 24: NPS: −2.06 (−2.43 to −1.69) NCS: −0.89 (−1.07 to −0.71) UPSIT: 10.56 (8.79–12.34) LMS: −7.44 (−8.35 to −6.53) Least squares mean change from baseline at week 24 (SE): SNOT-22: −30.43 (1.54)
LIBERTY NP SINUS 52 [15]	Multicenter, randomized, double-blind, placebo-controlled, parallel-group phase 3 trial	Patients were randomly assigned (1:1:1): dupilumab 300 mg every 2 weeks for 52 weeks/ placebo for 52 weeks/ dupilumab every 2 weeks for 24 weeks and every 4 weeks until week 52	Dupilumab every 2 weeks for 52 weeks (n = 150) Placebo (n = 153) Dupilumab every 2 weeks for 24 weeks and then every 4 weeks until week 52 (n = 145)	Least squares mean difference vs placebo (95% CI) at week 52: NPS: −1.80 (−2.10 to −1.51) NCS: −0.87 (−1.03 to −0.71) UPSIT: 10.52 (8.98–12.07) LMS: −5.13 (−5.80 to −4.46) Least squares mean change from baseline at week 24 (SE): SNOT-22: −29.84 (1.63) Asthma outcomes (pooled SINUS-24 and SINUS-52 [95% CI]): FEV1: 0.21 (0.13–0.29) ACQ-6: −0.82 (−0.98 to −0.67)

(continued)

Table 25.2 (continued)

Study	Type of study	Medical intervention	Number of patients	Reported outcome
NCT01920893 [25, 26]	Multicenter, randomized, double-blind, placebo-controlled, parallel-group phase IIa trial	Patients were randomly assigned: (1:1): dupilumab (a 600 mg loading dose followed by 300 mg) Weekly or placebo for 16 weeks	Dupilumab (n = 30) placebo (n = 30)	Least squares mean difference vs placebo (95% CI) at week 16: NPS: −1.6 (−2.4 to −0.7) UPSIT: 14.8 (10.9–18.7) LMS: −8.8 (−11.1 to −6.6) Least squares mean change from baseline at week 16 (SE): SNOT-22: −27.3 (2.7) The proportion of patients with moderate-to-severe CRSwNP (VAS > 3–10) decreased from 86.2% to 21.4% with dupilumab and 88.0% to 84.2% with placebo Significantly greater improvement in HRQoL, based on SNOT-22, SF-36, and EQ-5D VAS scores Significantly lower adjusted annualized mean number of sick leave days (0.09, vs 4.18 with placebo) and significantly greater improvement (vs placebo) in the SNOT-22 item "reduced productivity"
Omalizumab				
POLYP 1 [21]	Double-blind, multicenter, parallel-group randomized controlled, phase III trial	75–600 mg omalizumab every 2–4 weeks (with dose and frequency determined by serum total IgE level and body weight using a dosing table) or placebo for 24 weeks and 4 weeks of follow-up	Omalizumab (n = 72) Placebo (n = 66)	Treatment arm mean differences (95%CI) at week 24: NPS: −1.14 (−1.59 to −0.69) NCS: −0.55 (−0.84 to −0.25) UPSIT: 3.81 (1.38–6.24) TNSS: –1.91 (–2.85 to –0.96) Loss of smell score: –0.33 (–0.60 to –0.06) Postnasal drip score: –0.56 (–0.84 to –0.28) Runny nose score: –0.43 (–0.70 to –0.16) AQLQ: OR 3.71 (1.0–13.71) of achieving MCID Adjusted mean change from baseline at week 24 (SE): SNOT-22: −24.7 (2.01)

(POLYP 2) [21]	Double-blind, multicenter, parallel-group randomized controlled, phase III trial	75–600 mg omalizumab every 2–4 weeks (with dose and frequency determined by serum total IgE level and body weight using a dosing table) or placebo for 24 weeks and 4 weeks of follow-up	Omalizumab (n = 62) Placebo (n = 65)	Treatment arm mean differences (95%CI) at week 24: NPS: −0.59 (−1.05 to −0.12) NCS: −0.50 (−0.80 to −0.19) UPSIT: 3.86 (1.57–6.15) TNSS: −2.09 (−3.00 to −1.18) Loss of smell score: −0.45 (−0.73 to −0.16) Postnasal drip score: −0.54 (−0.81 to −0.27) Runny nose score: −0.63 (−0.90 to −0.35) Adjusted mean change from baseline at week 24 (SE): SNOT-22: −21.59 (2.25) AQLQ: OR 4.04 (1.07–15.25) of achieving MCID
Open label extension of Polyp 1,2 [27]	Open-label extension study of POLYP 1 and 2	After 24 weeks of omalizumab or placebo in POLYP 1 and 2, patients received omalizumab for 28 weeks and followed for another 24 weeks	(n = 249)	Patients who continued omalizumab experienced further improvements in NPS, NCS, SNOT-22, TNSS, and UPSIT scores through 52 weeks Patients who switched from placebo to omalizumab experienced favorable responses across end points through week 52 that were similar to POLYP 1 and 2 at week 24 After omalizumab discontinuation, scores gradually worsened over the 24-week follow-up but remained improved from pretreatment levels for both groups

(continued)

Table 25.2 (continued)

Study	Type of study	Medical intervention	Number of patients	Reported outcome
Mepolizumab				
SYNAPSE [28]	Randomized, multicenter, double-blind, placebo-controlled, parallel-group, phase 3 trial	Patients were randomly assigned (1:1), to receive either 100 mg mepolizumab subcutaneously or placebo once every 4 weeks for 52 weeks	Mepolizumab ($n = 206$) Placebo ($n = 201$)	Adjusted difference in median (95% CI) at Week 52 NPS: −0.73 (−1.11 to −0.34) Nasal obstruction VAS score: −3.14 (−4.09 to −2.18) Loss of smell VAS score: −0.37 (−0.65 to −0.08) Mean (SD) change from baseline at week 52: SNOT-22: −29·4 (24·67) The proportion of patients having nasal surgery up to week 52 (time-to-first nasal surgery): 0·43 (0·25–0·76) The proportion of patients requiring systemic corticosteroids (≥1 course) for nasal polyps until week 52: 0·58 (0·36–0·92) Changes in UPSIT were not statistically significant
NCT01362244 [29]	Randomized, double-blind, placebo-controlled trial	Patients received intravenous mepolizumab 750 mg or placebo every 4 weeks for a total of six doses (24 weeks)	Mepolizumab ($n = 54$) Placebo ($n = 51$)	Significantly greater proportion of patients no longer required surgery at week 25 (16[30%]) compared to placebo (5[10%]) Significant improvement in nasal polyposis severity VAS score, endoscopic nasal polyp score, VAS symptom scores, and sino-nasal outcome test [SNOT]-22 PRO score No improvement in olfaction testing and lung function tests
Comparison among biologics				
[30]	Systematic review	Included in the SR: 9 RCTs on dupilumab, omalizumab, mepolizumab, and reslizumab. Overall 1236 adults, with follow-up of 20–64 weeks		Dupilumab reduces the need for surgery or OCS use (moderate certainty, improves smell and quality of life (high certainty)) Omalizumab reduces the need for surgery (high certainty), improves smell and quality of life (high certainty) Mepolizumab reduces the need for surgery (low certainty), improving smell and quality of life

[31]	Cochrane Library Intervention Review, systematic review	10 studies. Of 1262 adult participants		Dupilumab improves disease-specific HRQOL compared to placebo. It likely results in a reduction in disease severity (on a 0- to 10-point VAS) and may result in a reduction in the number of serious adverse events Mepolizumab improves disease-specific HRQL. It likely results in the reduction difference of disease severity and the number of serious adverse events Omalizumab probably improves disease-specific HRQOL compared to placebo. It is uncertain if there is a difference in the number of serious adverse events
[32]	Systematic review and network meta-analysis	Twenty-nine randomized controlled trials ($n = 3461$) were included in the network meta-analysis		Dupilumab, omalizumab, mepolizumab, benralizumab, and ASA-D improved patient-important outcomes with clinically important differences in effects and ranking among agents, with dupilumab uniquely ranking among the most beneficial for all outcomes studied

NPS nasal polyp score, *NCS* nasal congestion score, *SNOT-22* sinonasal outcome test-22, *UPSIT* University of Pennsylvania Smell Identification Test, *LMS* Lund-Mackay score, *FEV1* forced expiratory volume in 1 s, *ACQ* asthma control questionnaire, *SF-36* short-form health survey, *TNSS* total nasal symptom score, *AQLQ* asthma quality of life questionnaire, *EQ-5D* 5-dimension EuroQoL general health status VAS, *CI* confidence interval

Dupilumab

Dupilumab is a fully human monoclonal antibody that binds to the IL-4Ra subunit and thereby inhibits the signaling of IL-4 and IL-13 (Fig. 25.1). The effectiveness and safety of dupilumab vs. placebo have been evaluated in several studies. The phase III studies were LIBERTY NP SINUS-24 and SINUS-52 [15] (Table 25.2). These studies found that:

- Dupilumab was found to induce significant improvement in nasal symptoms (nasal congestion, sense of smell), disease-related QOL, nasal polyp score (NPS), sense of smell, and radiologic sinus opacification (LMS).
- Dupilumab also reduced the need for systemic corticosteroids and ESS.
- Stopping the medication after 24 weeks of treatment led to a gradual exacerbation of symptoms, which might indicate that prolonged and even life-long treatment is required.

***Special Considerations**
Transient eosinophilia is a common side effect of dupilumab treatment. The exact pathogenesis is unclear. One hypothesis is that dupilumab blocks eosinophil tissue migration by inhibiting the production of eotaxins mediated by IL-13, thereby increasing circulating blood eosinophils [15]. Another explanation is that the corticosteroid-sparing effect of dupilumab can expose existing cases of eosinophilic granulomatosis with polyangiitis (EGPA) and hypereosinophilic syndrome (HES) that were masked by prolonged treatment with systemic corticosteroids which is eventually weaned when taking the biologic [16]. This eosinophilia is typically transient and asymptomatic, occurring within 2–6 months of treatment. However, a growing number of publications have highlighted a possible correlation between dupilumab treatment and eosinophilic complications such as EGPA and HES [17–20]. An unpublished postmarketing analysis of the FDA Adverse Event Reporting System Public Dashboard found 218 reports of eosinophilic complications of dupilumab treatment, including 92 reports of EGPA and 92 reports of eosinophilic complications of the respiratory tract. The recent EUFOREA guideline addressed this issue and suggested the following algorithm to monitor eosinophil levels during dupilumab treatment [5]. Figure 25.3 details a proposed algorithm for monitoring blood eosinophil levels during dupilumab treatment.

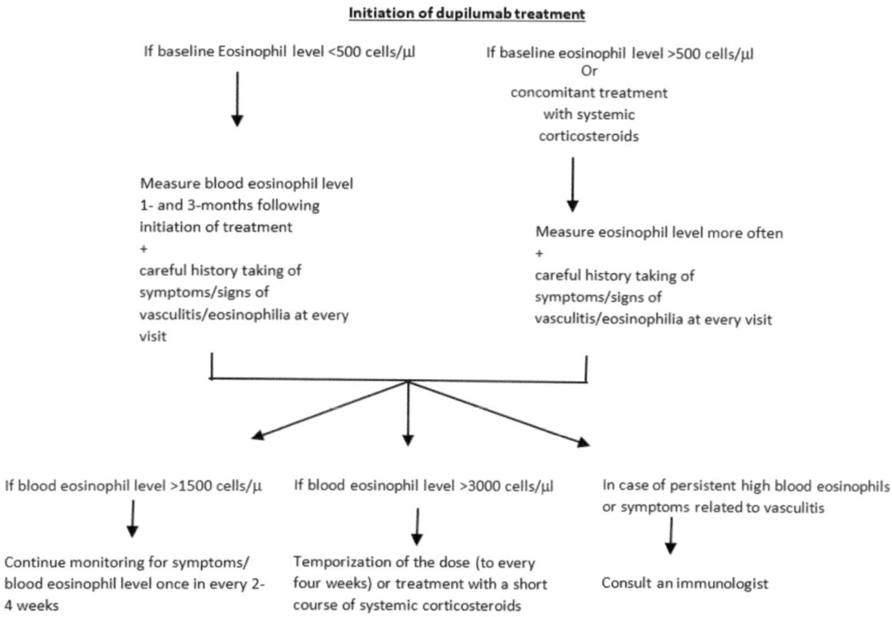

Fig. 25.3 Proposed algorithm to monitor blood eosinophil levels during dupilumab treatment [5]

Omalizumab

Omalizumab is an anti-IgE monoclonal antibody, approved by the FDA in 2020 for the treatment of CRSwNP. POLYP 1 and POLYP 2 were phase III clinical trials (Table 25.2) that studied the effectiveness and safety of omalizumab vs. placebo in participants with CRSwNP [21]. These studies found that:

- Omalizumab improved nasal symptoms, NPS, disease-related QOL, and sense of smell and reduced the need for ESS.
- There was no significant change in the need for rescue treatment with systemic corticosteroids.

***Special Considerations**

IgE is thought to play a vital role in cancer immune surveillance. Some studies have reported a possible link between absent or very low serum IgE levels and malignancy and between omalizumab treatment and an increased risk of malignancy [22, 23]. A recent literature review by the World Allergy Organization addressed this question and summarized that there is no evidence of an increased risk of malignancy in omalizumab-treated patients. They concluded that there was no increase in the number of tumor cases in omalizumab patients compared to the general population based on systematic studies and meta-analyses performed on more than 40,000 patients [24].

Anaphylaxis and other hypersensitivity reactions, such as serum sickness, were described. The FDA advises administering the drug only in a healthcare setting prepared to manage anaphylaxis and stopping treatment in the case of fever, arthralgia, and rash [11].

Mepolizumab

Mepolizumab is an anti-IL-5 monoclonal antibody, and its binding to IL-5 reduces the production and survival of eosinophils. The FDA has approved mepolizumab for treating CRSwNP since 2021. SYNAPSE (summarized in Table 25.2) was the main phase III clinical trial evaluating mepolizumab vs. placebo over a 52-week period [28]. This study found that:

- Mepolizumab demonstrated efficacy in improving nasal symptoms, disease-related QOL, NPS, sense of smell, and sinus opacification.
- It reduced the need for ESS and systemic corticosteroids and reduced the levels of blood eosinophils.
- Half of the patients in the mepolizumab group had an improvement of 1 point or more in nasal polyp scores.

***Special Considerations**
Herpes zoster infections have occurred in patients receiving mepolizumab. Consider vaccination if medically appropriate [12].

Matching the Biologic to the Patient

Thus far, no study has directly compared the efficacy of one biologic to another in treatment of CRSwNP. In addition, no biomarkers have been identified to define a certain group of type 2 CRS patients that will respond best to a certain biological medication. However, indirect treatment analyses have suggested that dupilumab may have a better response than mepolizumab and omalizumab in CRSwNP patients [32–34]. Further studies are required to establish a definitive preference for one biologic over another.

Deciding on the appropriate biologic should be tailored to the individual patient, be based on a multidisciplinary approach, and take into account several factors, including comorbidities (e.g., allergic asthma, atopic dermatitis, and eosinophilic diseases), the option of home administration, cost, local health economics, and patient compliance and preference. One other factor to consider is the duration of treatment response with various biologics. For instance, one study showed that mepolizumab may have a possible sustained effect for a duration of 6 months [35]. Some evidence suggests benefits of switching biological medications or even combining biologics for patients with type 2 comorbidities (e.g., asthma). It is

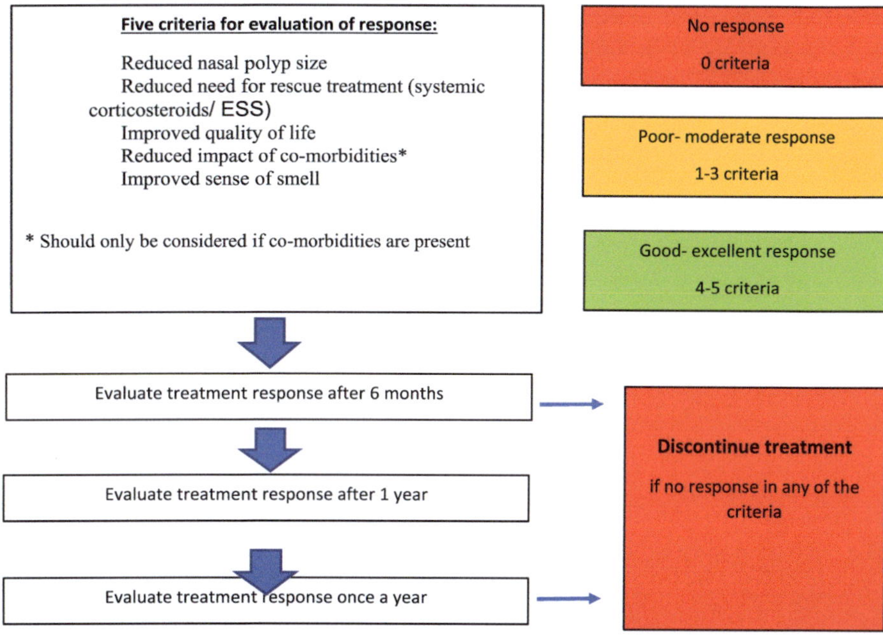

Fig. 25.4 Suggested algorithm to monitor and assess patient's response to treatment

also reasonable to consider transitioning to an alternative biologic when the response is suboptimal or an adverse reaction is encountered. However, further studies are required to establish definitive recommendations. Figure 25.4 is a suggested algorithm to monitor treatment response. It is important to note that the time until medication response is observed can vary significantly from days to months.

Biological Treatment for Aspirin-Exacerbated Respiratory Disease (AERD)

AERD or NERD (nonsteroidal anti-inflammatory drug-exacerbated respiratory disease) is a subgroup of CRSwNP, that is characterized by CRSwNP, asthma, and hypersensitivity reactions to aspirin and NSAIDs. It is also known as "Samter's triad." [36]. Its prevalence is approximately 10% in CRSwNP and 15% in severe asthma [37]. This entity is driven by type 2 inflammation, is associated with severe and difficult-to-treat asthma and rhinosinusitis, and often presents with aggressive and rapid recurrence of nasal polyps following ESS [38]. The integration of biologics into the management of asthma and CRSwNP gave new hope to patients with these frustrating diseases. The current evidence supports the use of biologics in AERD; however, more high-quality studies are needed to further assess the impact of biologics on this specific subgroup of patients and to determine what is the best biological medication for them. The major studies evaluating the role of biological treatment in AERD are summarized in Table 25.3.

Table 25.3 Summary of the major studies on biological treatment in AERD *patients*

Study	Study design	Number of patients	Reported outcome
Dupilumab			
[39]	Post hoc analysis of SINUS-24 and SINUS-52	AERD + dupilumab: *n* = 121 AERD + placebo: *n* = 82 Non-AERD + dupilumab: *n* = 319 Non-AERD + placebo: *n* = 200	*Least squares mean treatment differences between AERD + dupilumab and AERD + placebo at 24 weeks: Significant improvements in: NPS, NCS, Lund-Mackay score, SNOT-22, TSS, rhinosinusitis severity VAS, peak nasal inspiratory flow, ACQS, UPSIT * Comparison between AERD+ dupilumab vs non-AERD+ dupilumab: Significantly greater improvements for AERD at NCS, SNOT-22, and PNIF
Omalizumab			
[40]	Subgroup analysis of POLYP1 and POLYP2	AERD patients = 40	Adjusted mean difference (95% CI) (omalizumab-placebo) in NCS, NPS, SNOT-22, TNSS, and UPSIT change from baseline at week 24 consistently favored omalizumab treatment over placebo, regardless of aspirin sensitivity or asthma status
[41]	Double-blind, randomized, crossover, placebo-controlled, single-center study Patients were randomized (1:1) to a 3-month treatment with omalizumab or placebo, followed by a >18-week washout period (crossover design)	AERD patients = 16	Omalizumab treatment inhibited urinary leukotriene E4 overproduction and upper/lower respiratory tract symptoms during an oral aspirin challenge 62.5% (10 patients) developed oral aspirin tolerance up to cumulative doses of 930 mg in the omalizumab phase
Mepolizumab			
[42]	Post hoc analysis of SYNAPSE	AERD + mepolizumab: *n* = 45 AERD + placebo: *n* = 63 Non-AERD + mepolizumab: *n* = 161 Non-AERD + placebo: *n* = 138	Mepolizumab vs placebo reduced NP size, nasal obstruction, risk of surgery, and use of SCS for NP, while improving nasal symptoms in patients with severe, bilateral CRSwNP, regardless of the presence/absence of asthma or AERD

(continued)

Table 25.3 (continued)

Study	Study design	Number of patients	Reported outcome
Comparison among biologics			
[32]	Systematic review and network meta-analysis	Twenty-nine randomized controlled trials ($n = 3461$) were included in the network meta-analysis	Similar effects among patients with and without asthma and AERD vs non-AERD

Summary

Incorporating biologics into the treatment arsenal of CRSwNP was a turning point in the management of refractory sinusitis. Their excellent efficacy and safety profile make them an extremely attractive treatment option for patients with recalcitrant CRSwNP. Nonetheless, many questions regarding their selection and use remain unanswered. Further research and guidelines are needed. More biological medications, currently used for other type 2 diseases, are under investigation for CRSwNP and are expected to be approved in the near future.

References

1. Wang X, Zhang N, Bo M, Holtappels G, Zheng M, Lou H, et al. Diversity of TH cytokine profiles in patients with chronic rhinosinusitis: a multicenter study in Europe, Asia, and Oceania. J Allergy Clin Immunol [Internet]. 2016. [cited 2023 Jan 25];138(5):1344–53.
2. Han JK. Subclassification of chronic rhinosinusitis. Laryngoscope. 2013;123(Suppl 2):S15–27. https://doi.org/10.1002/lary.23979. Epub 2013 Jan 31. PMID: 23371324
3. Fokkens WJ, Lund VJ, Hopkins C, Hellings PW, Kern R, Reitsma S, et al. Executive summary of EPOS 2020 including integrated care pathways. Rhinology [Internet]. 2020. [cited 2023 Jan 23];58(2):82–111.
4. Roland LT, Smith TL, Schlosser RJ, Soler ZM, Peters AT, Laidlaw TM, et al. Guidance for contemporary use of biologics in management of chronic rhinosinusitis with nasal polyps: discussion from a National Institutes of Health-sponsored workshop. Int Forum Allergy Rhinol [Internet]. 2020. [cited 2023 Jan 26];10(9):1037–42.
5. Fokkens WJ, Viskens AS, Backer V, Conti D, De Corso E, Gevaert P, et al. EPOS/EUFOREA update on indication and evaluation of biologics in chronic rhinosinusitis with nasal polyps 2023. Rhinology [Internet]. 2023. [cited 2023 May 25];0(0):194.
6. Maza-Solano J, Biadsee A, Sowerby LJ, Calvo-Hernández C, Tucciarone M, Rocha T, et al. Chronic rhinosinusitis with nasal polyps management in the biologic therapy era: an international YO-IFOS survey. Eur Arch Otorhinolaryngol [Internet]. 2022; [cited 2023 Jan 26]
7. https://www.ema.europa.eu/en/documents/product-information/dupixent-epar-product-information_en.pdf
8. https://www.ema.europa.eu/en/documents/product-information/xolair-epar-product-information_en.pdf
9. https://www.ema.europa.eu/en/documents/product-information/nucala-epar-product-information_en.pdf
10. https://www.accessdata.fda.gov/drugsatfda_docs/label/2022/761055s042lbl.pdf
11. https://www.accessdata.fda.gov/drugsatfda_docs/label/2021/103976s5238lbl.pdf
12. https://www.accessdata.fda.gov/drugsatfda_docs/label/2022/761122s008,125526s019lbl.pdf

13. Tan LD, Schaeffer B, Alismail A. Parasitic (helminthic) infection while on asthma biologic treatment: not everything is what it seems. J Asthma Allergy [Internet]. 2019. [cited 2023 Jan 25];12:415–20.
14. Cruz AA, Lima F, Sarinho E, Ayre G, Martin C, Fox H, et al. Safety of anti-immunoglobulin E therapy with omalizumab in allergic patients at risk of geohelminth infection. Clin Exp Allergy [Internet]. 2007. [cited 2023 Jan 25];37(2):197–207.
15. Bachert C, Han JK, Desrosiers M, Hellings PW, Amin N, Lee SE, et al. Efficacy and safety of dupilumab in patients with severe chronic rhinosinusitis with nasal polyps (LIBERTY NP SINUS-24 and LIBERTY NP SINUS-52): results from two multicentre, randomised, double-blind, placebo-controlled, parallel-group phase 3 trials. Lancet [Internet]. 2019. [cited 2023 Jan 23];394(10209):1638–50.
16. Rabe KF, Nair P, Brusselle G, Maspero JF, Castro M, Sher L, et al. Efficacy and safety of Dupilumab in glucocorticoid-dependent severe asthma. N Engl J Med [Internet]. 2018. [cited 2022 Nov 16];378(26):2475–85.
17. Caminati M, Olivieri B, Dama A, Micheletto C, Paggiaro P, Pinter P, et al. Dupilumab-induced hypereosinophilia: review of the literature and algorithm proposal for clinical management. Expert Rev Respir Med [Internet]. 2022. [cited 2022 Oct 21];16(7):713–21.
18. Descamps V, Deschamps L, el Khalifa J, Groh M, Gibier JB, Lefèvre G, et al. Eosinophilic vasculitis associated with persistent dupilumab-induced hypereosinophilia in severe asthma. Respir Med Res [Internet]. 2021. [cited 2022 Oct 19];79
19. Persaud P, Karmali R, Sankar P, Majid M. Dupilumab-associated eosinophilic granulomatosis with polyangiitis. Cureus [Internet]. 2022. [cited 2022 Oct 19];14:8.
20. Murag S, Melehani J, Filsoof D, Nadeau K, Sharon Chinthrajah R. Dupilumab Unmasks Eosinophilic Granulomatosis With Polyangiitis. Chest [Internet]. 2021. [cited 2022 Oct 19];160(4):A8–9.
21. Gevaert P, Omachi TA, Corren J, Mullol J, Han J, Lee SE, et al. Efficacy and safety of omalizumab in nasal polyposis: 2 randomized phase 3 trials. J Allergy Clin Immunol [Internet]. 2020. [cited 2023 Jan 24];146(3):595–605.
22. Ferastraoaru D, Bax HJ, Bergmann C, Capron M, Castells M, Dombrowicz D, et al. AllergoOncology: ultra-low IgE, a potential novel biomarker in cancer-a position paper of the European Academy of Allergy and Clinical Immunology (EAACI). Clin Transl Allergy [Internet]. 2020. [cited 2023 Jan 25];10(1):32.
23. Mota D, Rama TA, Severo M, Moreira A. Potential cancer risk with omalizumab? A disproportionality analysis of the WHO's VigiBase pharmacovigilance database. Allergy [Internet]. 2021. [cited 2023 Jan 19];76(10):3209–11.
24. Bagnasco D, Canevari RF, del Giacco S, Ferrucci S, Pigatto P, Castelnuovo P, et al. Omalizumab and cancer risk: current evidence in allergic asthma, chronic urticaria, and chronic rhinosinusitis with nasal polyps. World Allergy Organ J [Internet]. 2022. [cited 2023 Jan 25];15(12):100721.
25. Bachert C, Mannent L, Naclerio RM, Mullol J, Ferguson BJ, Gevaert P, et al. Effect of subcutaneous Dupilumab on nasal polyp burden in patients with chronic sinusitis and nasal polyposis: a randomized clinical trial. JAMA [Internet]. 2016. [cited 2023 Jan 24];315(5):469–79.
26. Bachert C, Hellings PW, Mullol J, Hamilos DL, Gevaert P, Naclerio RM, et al. Dupilumab improves health-related quality of life in patients with chronic rhinosinusitis with nasal polyposis. Allergy [Internet]. 2020. [cited 2023 Jan 24];75(1):148–57.
27. Gevaert P, Saenz R, Corren J, Han JK, Mullol J, Lee SE, et al. Long-term efficacy and safety of omalizumab for nasal polyposis in an open-label extension study. J Allergy Clin Immunol [Internet]. 2022. [cited 2023 Jan 24];149(3):957–965.e3.
28. Han JK, Bachert C, Fokkens W, Desrosiers M, Wagenmann M, Lee SE, et al. Mepolizumab for chronic rhinosinusitis with nasal polyps (SYNAPSE): a randomised, double-blind, placebo-controlled, phase 3 trial. Lancet Respir Med [Internet]. 2021. [cited 2023 Jan 24];9(10):1141–53.
29. Bachert C, Sousa AR, Lund VJ, Scadding GK, Gevaert P, Nasser S, et al. Reduced need for surgery in severe nasal polyposis with mepolizumab: randomized trial. J Allergy Clin Immunol [Internet]. 2017. [cited 2023 Jan 24];140(4):1024–1031.e14.

30. Agache I, Song Y, Alonso-Coello P, Vogel Y, Rocha C, Solà I, et al. Efficacy and safety of treatment with biologicals for severe chronic rhinosinusitis with nasal polyps: a systematic review for the EAACI guidelines. Allergy [Internet]. 2021. [cited 2023 Jan 24];76(8):2337–53.
31. Chong LY, Piromchai P, Sharp S, Snidvongs K, Webster KE, Philpott C, et al. Biologics for chronic rhinosinusitis. Cochrane Database Syst Rev [Internet]. 2021. [cited 2023 Jan 24];3(3)
32. Oykhman P, Paramo FA, Bousquet J, Kennedy DW, Brignardello-Petersen R, Chu DK. Comparative efficacy and safety of monoclonal antibodies and aspirin desensitization for chronic rhinosinusitis with nasal polyposis: a systematic review and network meta-analysis. J Allergy Clin Immunol [Internet]. 2022. [cited 2023 Jan 24];149(4):1286–95.
33. Cai S, Xu S, Lou H, Zhang L. Comparison of different biologics for treating chronic rhinosinusitis with nasal polyps: a network analysis. J Allergy Clin Immunol Pract. 2022;10(7):1876–1886.e7.
34. Peters AT, Han JK, Hellings P, Heffler E, Gevaert P, Bachert C, et al. Indirect treatment comparison of biologics in chronic rhinosinusitis with nasal polyps. J Allergy Clin Immunol Pract [Internet]. 2021. [cited 2023 Jan 18];9(6):2461–2471.e5.
35. Desrosiers M, Diamant Z, Castelnuovo P, Hellings PW, Han JK, Peters AT, Silver J, Smith SG, Fuller A, Sousa AR, Chan RH. Gevaert P; SYNAPSE study investigators. Sustained efficacy of mepolizumab in patients with severe chronic rhinosinusitis with nasal polyps: SYNAPSE 24-week treatment-free follow-up. Int Forum Allergy Rhinol. 2024;14(1):18–31. https://doi.org/10.1002/alr.23219. Epub 2023 Jul 18. PMID: 37345861
36. Xu X, Reitsma S, Wang DY, Fokkens WJ. Updates in biologic therapy for chronic rhinosinusitis with nasal polyps and NSAID-exacerbated respiratory disease. Allergy [Internet]. 2022. [cited 2023 Jan 19];77(12):3593.
37. Rajan JP, Wineinger NE, Stevenson DD, White AA. Prevalence of aspirin-exacerbated respiratory disease among asthmatic patients: a meta-analysis of the literature. J Allergy Clin Immunol [Internet]. 2015. [cited 2023 Jan 26];135(3):676–681.e1.
38. White AA, Stevenson DD. Aspirin-Exacerbated Respiratory Disease. Longo DL, editor. N Engl J Med [Internet]. 2018;379(11):1060–70. [cited 2023 Jan 26]
39. Mullol J, Laidlaw TM, Bachert C, Mannent LP, Canonica GW, Han JK, et al. Efficacy and safety of dupilumab in patients with uncontrolled severe chronic rhinosinusitis with nasal polyps and a clinical diagnosis of NSAID-ERD: results from two randomized placebo-controlled phase 3 trials. Allergy [Internet]. 2022. [cited 2023 Jan 26];77(4):1231–44.
40. Damask C, Chen M, Holweg CTJ, Yoo B, Millette LA, Franzese C. Defining the efficacy of Omalizumab in nasal polyposis: a POLYP 1 and POLYP 2 subgroup analysis. Am J Rhinol Allergy [Internet]. 2022. [cited 2023 Jan 26];36(1):135–41.
41. Hayashi H, Fukutomi Y, Mitsui C, Kajiwara K, Watai K, Kamide Y, et al. Omalizumab for Aspirin Hypersensitivity and Leukotriene Overproduction in Aspirin-exacerbated Respiratory Disease. A Randomized Controlled Trial. Am J Respir Crit Care Med [Internet]. 2020. [cited 2023 Jan 26];201(12):1488–98.
42. Bachert C, Sousa AR, Han JK, Schlosser RJ, Sowerby LJ, Hopkins C, et al. Mepolizumab for chronic rhinosinusitis with nasal polyps: treatment efficacy by comorbidity and blood eosinophil count. J Allergy Clin Immunol [Internet]. 2022. [cited 2023 Jan 26];149(5):1711–1721.e6.

Novel Therapies for Recalcitrant Chronic Rhinosinusitis

26

Juan Carlos Hernaiz-Leonardo, Bader M. Alim, and Amin R. Javer

Key Points

- Recalcitrant chronic rhinosinusitis (rCRS) is a complex disease state with few therapeutic options available.
- Most of the research on rCRS treatment focuses on reducing type 2 inflammation using monoclonal antibodies. However, there is a subgroup of patients whose main problem is bacterial biofilm formation and sinonasal dysbiosis.
- There is an urgent need for novel therapeutic strategies aimed at improving the microbial sinonasal environment.
- Current investigational treatments begin with povidone-iodine, manuka honey, mupirocin irrigations, and colloidal silver, each of which has varying degrees of evidence supporting its use in the management of CRSwNP.

Background

Research into novel therapeutic strategies for recalcitrant chronic rhinosinusitis (rCRS) has grown in the last few years. The biggest breakthrough came with monoclonal antibodies targeting type 2 inflammation (i.e., dupilumab, mepolizumab, and omalizumab), which have shown efficacy for treating CRS with nasal polyps (CRSwNP) in large phase three clinical trials [1–3], followed by several

J. C. Hernaiz-Leonardo · A. R. Javer (✉)
Department of Otolaryngology—Head and Neck Surgery, University of British Columbia, Vancouver, BC, Canada
e-mail: hernaiz@student.ubc.ca

B. M. Alim
Department of Otolaryngology—Head and Neck Surgery, Prince Mohammed Bin Abdul Aziz Hospital, National Guard Health Affairs, Medina, Saudi Arabia

J. T. Lee et al. (eds.), *Advances in Surgical and Medical Interventions for Recalcitrant Chronic Rhinosinusitis*,
https://doi.org/10.1007/978-3-031-89191-5_26

real-life publications indicating efficacy from around the globe [3–6]. With multiple trials currently ongoing for other CRS subtypes such as allergic fungal rhinosinusitis (AFRS) [7] and CRSsNP [8], the use of biologics is likely to significantly change the landscape of CRS management and is destined to increase with time. However, not every patient is a candidate for these medications. In our experience, individuals whose symptoms are primarily due to recalcitrant biofilm formation are unlikely to improve with monoclonal antibodies. Similarly, patients who don't have typical signs of type 2 inflammation, such as elevated tissue or peripheral eosinophils, eosinophilic mucin, or high IgE levels, may have a poor response to these drugs. Consequently, there is still a need for other types of therapeutic strategies that can improve the health of rCRS patients, particularly those that are unlikely to benefit from, or unable to utilize, monoclonals that target type 2 inflammation.

In this chapter, we will discuss a series of emerging treatments for rCRS that are currently being investigated. Our objective is not to give an exhaustive list of experimental therapies for rCRS but to discuss possible therapeutic strategies that are likely to improve the quality of life of these difficult-to-treat individuals. We will focus on treatments that target sinonasal bacterial biofilm and bacterial dysbiosis. Excellent review papers are already available on the topic for those who seek further information on the subject [9, 10]. There are a vast number of molecules under development that target the immune system. The EPOS 2020 guideline gives an excellent review of some of these drugs, and we highly encourage the reader to consult it [11]. A detailed exploration of these drugs as well as further discussion regarding biologics is beyond the scope of this chapter and will not be mentioned further.

Biofilm in rCRS

Bacterial biofilms are common in rCRS individuals and contribute to persistent disease [12, 13]. In about half the cases, *Staphylococcus aureus* (*S. aureus*) is a major contributor to biofilm formation [14]. Evidence shows that *S. aureus* can contribute to persistent inflammation through diverse mechanisms, including superantigen formation, direct damage to the epithelial barrier, stimulation of type 2 inflammation, and intracellular reservoirs in the nasal epithelium and osteitic bone [15–18]. Thus, eradication of *S. aureus* and other bacterial biofilms can significantly improve sinus health among rCRS patients.

Povidone-Iodine (PVP-I) Rinses

Several strategies have been devised to disrupt biofilms in the paranasal sinuses. Saline irrigations by themselves can disrupt biofilms in vitro when applied with enough pressure [19]. Adding topical antiseptics to the saline rinse can potentially improve biofilm eradication. One such example is povidone-iodine (PVP-I). This common antiseptic has been safely used for years in otolaryngology and other surgical specialties. In vitro evidence shows that PVP-I solutions can disrupt *Staphylococcus* spp. biofilms [20–22]. Moreover, PVP-I is active against a broad range of viruses [23, 24]. One trial showed that a single application of PVP-I can effectively eliminate nasal *S. aureus* carriage [25]. Nasal PVP-I irrigations are well tolerated by patients [26] and could serve as adjunct treatment during acute bacterial exacerbations or when chronic biofilm is observed. In a prospective study done at our center, rCRS patients were treated with 0.08% PVP-I rinses for 7 weeks and evaluated for changes in their Modified Lund-Kennedy (MLK) score and investigated for signs of thyroid toxicity or ciliary dysfunction. By the end of the follow-up period, 29 included patients decreased their MLK scores by at least one point, while thyroid and ciliary function remained normal [27]. One randomized controlled trial (RCT) involving 55 CRS patients undergoing primary endoscopic sinus surgery compared endoscopic and SNOT-22 scores of individuals randomized to PVP-I rinses versus those receiving normal saline [28]. After 3 months of follow-up, the authors found no difference in clinical scores between the two groups. Finally, one trial involving 62 postsurgical CRS patients failed to demonstrate significant differences in endoscopic scores between PVP-I rinses, mupirocin rinses, and normal saline during acute bacterial exacerbations [26]. However, all three groups showed improvement at 30 days compared to baseline. To date, there is no RCT evaluating PVP-I rinses in rCRS patients. Further research is needed to determine whether PVP-I can remove bacterial biofilms in vivo and improve endoscopic scores and quality of life in rCRS patients.

Manuka Honey Rinses

Manuka honey (MH), the product of a New Zealand scrub plant, has high concentrations of antibacterial molecules including methylglyoxal (MGO), defensin-1, and hydrogen peroxide [29]. It has shown disruptive properties against *S. aureus* and other bacterial biofilm in vitro [30] and could be a potential alternative for sinonasal biofilm control. The efficacy of MH for rCRS is still debated. In 1 single-blind prospective study of 34 recalcitrant AFRS patients, participants were asked to rinse 1 nostril with 2 mL of a 50/50 mixture of honey-saline solution every day for 30 days and saline on the other. At the end of the follow-up period, differences were seen in endoscopic scores between the two sides [31]. There are three RCTs evaluating MH for treatment of bacterial exacerbations of CRS [32–34]. In all three trials, MH treatment was associated with improvement from baseline at 14, 30, and 60 days, respectively, but was not significantly different compared to saline rinses. Treatment was well tolerated by patients, with no significant adverse events associated with MH use. Similarly, one of the trials showed that smell was unaffected by MH use [32]. Although these results suggest that MH rinses are not superior to saline rinses, the trials were underpowered to detect small differences in endoscopic scores, were subject to varying degrees of confounding by indication (e.g., some participants received oral antibiotics or steroids after randomization at the discretion of the treating clinician), and used different concentrations of MH, which makes comparisons difficult. A large, well-designed RCT evaluating the use of MH as sole treatment or adjunct therapy for rCRS is still needed.

Colloidal Silver

Silver has been used in wound healing for years due to its antibacterial properties. Silver nanoparticles of 10–100 nm—also known as colloidal silver (CS)—have shown good antibacterial activity against a wide range of organisms, including methicillin-resistant *S. aureus* (MRSA) [35, 36]. CS can also reduce bacterial biofilm in vitro and in vivo without causing damage to respiratory epithelial cells [36]. The combination of CS with topical antibiotics could have synergistic effects on bacterial biofilm eradication, as suggested by a recent in vitro study [37]. To date, the only evidence regarding the use of CS for rCRS comes from two small trials [38, 39]. The first study compared a CS nasal spray to normal saline in 20 rCRS patients using a cross-over design [38]. Patients randomly received either the CS nasal spray or saline for 6 weeks and then switched treatments for another 6 weeks. No changes were seen in symptomatic or endoscopic scores at the end of follow-up, and no adverse events were reported. The second trial compared high-volume CS rinses to oral antibiotics in 22 rCRS patients [39]. Participants were randomized to either treatment and evaluated after 10 days of treatment for endoscopic, symptomatic, and microbiological improvement. Both groups improved after 10 days, but no differences were seen among the two treatment arms. Although no serious adverse events were reported in either trial, both studies are underpowered to detect any significant benefit of CS compared to saline rinses alone or oral antibiotic therapy. Similarly, the mode of administration (i.e., nasal spray) and duration of CS therapy (i.e., 10 days) were probably insufficient for complete biofilm eradication. Future studies should investigate whether CS rinses alone or in combination with topical antibiotics can eradicate sinonasal biofilms and improve symptoms and endoscopic scores in rCRS individuals.

Topical Antibiotics

Topical antibiotics are widely used in our daily rhinologic practice. We will discuss this therapy briefly, but a more thorough discussion can be found in Chap. 20 of this text. Among the options for topical antibiotic irrigations, mupirocin rinses are probably the most widely used and studied. There is one double-blind, placebo-controlled RCT that compared mupirocin rinses to oral amoxicillin with clavulanate in rCRS patients [40]. At 30 days, patients allocated to mupirocin rinses had negative cultures more frequently compared to those receiving oral antibiotics (8/9 [88.9%] in the mupirocin group vs 0/13 [0%] in the control group). Similarly, mupirocin-treated individuals had a larger reduction in endoscopic Lund-Kennedy scores from baseline compared to the control arm (7.0 [2.5–7.5] for mupirocin vs 1.0 [1.0–1.0] in the control). However, the average culture positivity and endoscopic scores returned to baseline after three months of follow-up in the mupirocin-treated patients. A recent trial by Lee et al. [26]—which was discussed previously in the PVP-I section—reported a 70% culture negativity rate at 30 days with the use of mupirocin rinses. As mentioned previously, these results were not statistically different compared to PVP-I or saline rinses alone. In a systematic review and meta-analysis of six studies—including the one previously described by Jervis-Brady et al. [40]—mupirocin was found to be superior to saline rinses for treating acute exacerbations of CRS (pooled relative risk 0.13; random effects 95% CI 0.06–0.26) [41]. However, a Cochrane review from the same year found no evidence supporting mupirocin's efficacy for CRS treatment mainly due to a lack of high-quality RCTs [42]. Together, these results suggest that mupirocin rinses are probably useful for short-term *S. aureus* eradication but ineffective for long-term biofilm control.

There is a lack of high-quality evidence for other topical antibiotic regimes. Observational data suggests that topical tobramycin, ofloxacin, levofloxacin, and cephalosporins could improve SNOT-22 and endoscopic scores. Most of these studies are discussed thoroughly in a 2019 review paper by Carlton et al. [10] in case the reader would like to learn more about the subject. On a personal note, the authors of this chapter frequently apply tobramycin combined with budesonide directly into the infected sinuses using endoscopic suctions when we see acutely infected sinus cavities. We then instruct the patient to rinse with saline plus mupirocin or 0.08% PVP-I rinses until the infection is resolved. We have found this regime to be tolerable by most patients and have seen good symptomatic and endoscopic outcomes. However, the level of evidence for this practice is low. The use of these therapeutic regimes is left to the discretion of the treating surgeon.

Photodynamic Therapy

Photodynamic therapy refers to the use of artificial light of varying wavelengths for therapeutic purposes. It can be used directly as mixed visible and ultraviolet (mUV/VIS) light therapy or in combination with photosensitizer molecules such as methylene blue. mUV/VIS can have immunosuppressive effects on the nasal epithelium and has shown efficacy in allergic rhinitis [43, 44]. Its use in CRS has been evaluated in two RCTs. The first trial by Kiricsi et al. [45] randomized 87 subjects with eosinophilic CRS with nasal polyps (CRSwNP) to receive either mUV/VIS three times per week for 12 weeks plus topical steroids or topical steroids alone. Patients treated with mUV/VIS improved their symptomatic and endoscopic scores 1 month after treatment completion and showed a sustained response 3 months after finishing the treatment, while control patients did not show statistical improvement compared to baseline. Although these results suggest the efficacy of mUV/VIS, the authors did not compare both groups directly. The lack of blinding and validated endoscopic scores also undermines the validity of their findings. The second study is a double-blind RCT by Dulguerov et al. [46], where 50 CRS without nasal polyp (CRSsNP) patients were randomized to either mUV/VIS or low-intensity visible light (i.e., placebo) for 3 weeks. Notably, CRSwNP patients with a history of bacterial exacerbations and those with acute viral or bacterial infections were excluded. The authors found no difference in symptomatic scores after 3 weeks of treatment and 1 month follow-up. Unfortunately, the patient population in this trial is not well described, and there is little information on whether any of the participants had undergone ESS in the past, making it difficult for the reader to extrapolate their results. Combined, these studies are insufficient to answer whether mUV/VIS is effective for CRS but suggest a possible anti-inflammatory effect in CRSwNP.

In contrast to mUV/VIS, the combination of phototherapy with methylene blue (MB) or other photosensitizing agents is used for biofilm eradication. The stimulation of MB generates reactive oxygen species that rupture microbial membranes and allow for MB to penetrate the cell, causing further photodamage [47]. One in vitro study using clinical isolates from CRS patients showed that antimicrobial photodynamic therapy (aPDT) using MB was able to eradicate >99% of microbial biofilm with a single application [48]. Its use is not associated with epithelial damage in in vitro studies [49]. To perform the treatment in CRS patients, the affected sinus is first coated with MB, and then light is applied using a flexible catheter at a wavelength of approximately 660 nm. Unfortunately, there are no published RCTs that evaluate the use of aPDT in CRS. Pilot data from our center suggests that aPDT use is associated with improvement in endoscopic scores in about half of the patients without causing a significant change to the sinonasal microbiome composition (pending publication). However, it is unknown whether aPDT can help decolonize rCRS patients with MRSA or other resistant bacterial strains. We believe aPDT can help reduce biofilm formation and improve sinus health in a carefully selected subset of patients, but further research is needed on the subject.

Phage Therapy

Bacteriophages or phages are viruses that infect a small number of related bacteria without damaging mammalian cells [50]. They are effective in the presence of biofilms, are specific to particular bacterial species, and cause little to no damage to the host or the rest of the microbiota, which makes them very attractive for therapeutic use [51]. Given that *S. aureus* frequently causes and contributes to rCRS, the use of *S. aureus* specific phages seems particularly enticing. To date, there is one open-label study that evaluates the safety and tolerability of a three-phage cocktail (AB-SA01) for the treatment of rCRS due to *S. aureus* [52]. The nine recruited patients were equally divided into three cohorts that received increasing doses of intranasal irrigation with the AB-SA01 cocktail: cohort 1 received 3×10^8 phage-forming units (PFU) twice a day for 7 days; cohort 2 received 3×10^8 phage-forming units (PFU) twice a day for 14 days; and cohort 3 received 3×10^9 phage-forming units (PFU) twice a day for 14 days. All patients were able to complete the study, and no serious adverse reactions were noted. Preliminary efficacy data is promising, but no conclusions can be made due to the nature of the study. Phage therapy has the potential to become an important therapeutic modality in the future and needs further research.

Sinonasal Microbiota Transfer (SNMT)

Microbial (bacterial, fungal, and viral) disruptions can cause or contribute to sinus inflammation [53–57]. Specific members of the sinonasal microbiome, like *S. aureus*, can drive maladaptive type 2 inflammation in the sinus mucosa via direct superantigen stimulation of T lymphocytes [58], intracellular infection of immune cells [59, 60], superantigen-specific IgE production [61], epithelial barrier disruptions [62], and biofilm formation [60, 63, 64]. When comparing the microbiome composition (i.e., the genetic material derived from the microbiota of a specific site) of CRS patients to healthy controls, diseased individuals have a lower microbiome diversity compared to healthy subjects [65–68]. Similarly, CRS patients experience more epithelial barrier disruptions when their sinonasal microbiome is less diverse [69]. Microbiota-altering therapies, like fecal microbiota transplantation, can successfully displace pathogens (80–94% cure rate for *Clostridioides difficile*) [58, 59] and effectively treat inflammatory diseases like ulcerative colitis [70] and atopic dermatitis [71]. We believe that a similar treatment strategy can treat rCRS patients who primarily fail due to biofilm formation and colonization by resistant bacterial strains.

Currently, there are three RCTs registered in clinicaltrials.gov that investigate the use of a sinonasal microbiota transfer (SNMT) for treatment of rCRS [72–74]. Two trials evaluate the transfer of a nasal wash from a healthy donor into the diseased sinus cavity, while one trial investigates transferring endoscopically suctioned mucus from a healthy donor into the diseased sinus. One of the trials appears as completed, but the authors have yet to publish any results [73]. Pilot data from our center shows that an endoscopically guided SNMT can improve SNOT-22 and Lund-Kennedy scores at 45 days, with two patients showing sustained improvement after 6 months (case-series manuscript in preparation). We are currently in the recruitment phase of a double-blind, placebo-controlled RCT evaluating SNMT vs placebo (i.e., sham SNMT) for the treatment of rCRS [74]. Results from these trials will answer whether SNMT has any place in the treatment of rCRS.

Conclusion

It is increasingly likely that the treatment strategies for rCRS will continue to evolve in the years to come. Multiple questions remain unanswered regarding experimental treatments for rCRS. Specifically, there is an urgent need for high-quality RCT investigating the efficacy of these therapies. Nonetheless, the available evidence for some of these treatments is very promising and will only improve with time. We strongly believe that therapies that target specific members of the sinonasal microbiome (i.e., phages) or the whole sinonasal community (i.e., SNMT) have the potential to change the way we envision rCRS treatment (Table 26.1).

Table 26.1 Summary of studies that evaluate alternative treatment strategies for recalcitrant chronic rhinosinusitis

Treatment	Study design	N	Sample characteristics	Intervention and comparison	Outcomes
PVP-I rinses	Prospective cohort [27] Single-blind RCT [28] Single-blind RCT [26]	29 55 62	Patients with CRSwNP or CRSsNP with persistent symptoms despite adequate therapy and at least 1 point in the discharge MLK subdomain Patients undergoing primary FESS Postsurgical patients with ongoing signs and symptoms of CRS with a positive culture for *Staphylococcus aureus*	0.08% PVP-I every other day for 7 weeks + 1 mg of budesonide in 240 ml of saline OD 2.4 mL of 10% PVP-I in 240 ml of 0.9% saline or saline alone, twice a day for 3 months postoperatively 1% povidone-iodine (PI) vs 0.05% mupirocin rinses vs saline control sinus irrigations, twice daily for 30 days. Antibiotics indicated as needed by the treating surgeon	Median decrease in MLK scores of 1.50 point (95% CI 1.00–1.50) at 7 weeks. 38% improved posttreatment SNOT-22 scores by 9 or more points. No adverse events reported Both groups improved their SNOT-22 and MLK scores at 3 months without any significant differences between them. No difference in the frequency of culture negativity. No adverse events reported. Culture negativity higher in the mupirocin group (14/20, 70%) compared to the PVP-I (9/21, 43%) and saline (9/19, 47%) groups. MLK and SNOT-22 improvement in all groups, without significant differences. No adverse events reported.
Colloidal silver (CS)	Cross-over RCT [38] Open-label, single-blind RCT [39]	22 22	CRSsNP patients who remained symptomatic despite oral antibiotics, oral or topical steroids, shampoo irrigations, or manuka honey irrigations Postoperative patients with ongoing symptoms of CRS despite at least one round or oral antibiotics and a positive bacterial culture	10 ppm of CS twice daily or saline for 6 weeks before crossing over to the other arm, with a two-week washout CS irrigations vs culture-directed oral antibiotics + saline irrigations	No difference seen in SNOT-22 or MLK scores, but significant period effect was seen between the two treatment periods. Severe nasal obstruction and congestion in one patient using CS. 2/11 patients on the CS arm had negative swabs compared to 1/11 in the control group SNOT-22 and MLK scores tended to improve in the CS arm without being statistically significant.

Manuka honey (MH) rinses	Single-blind RCT [32] Single-blind RCT [33] Double-blind RCT [34]	25 42 53	Postoperative patients with ongoing symptoms of CRS despite at least one round or oral antibiotics and a positive bacterial culture Postoperative CRS patients with purulent discharge on endoscopy Postoperative CRS patients	16.5% MH augmented with 1.3 mg/mL MGO vs saline rinses, both for 14 days and with culture-directed oral antibiotics 10% MH vs saline rinses for 30 days with background oral and topical steroids + culture-directed antibiotics Thyme/honey nasal spray 2 puffs per nostril vs saline sprays. Everyone received oral antibiotics after surgery	No significant differences in SNOT-22, MLK, UPSIT, or culture negativity. No adverse events observed. No significant differences in SNOT-22, MLK, or culture negativity. Those receiving no oral antibiotics and MH rinses reduced their bacterial load significantly. No difference on CT, SNOT-22, or endoscopy scores.
Mupirocin rinses	Double-blind RCT [40] Systematic review and meta-analysis [41] Cochrane systematic review [75]	25	CRSwNP with previous full FESS, ongoing symptoms, and positive culture for *Staphylococcus aureus* Included two RCTs, two prospective studies, and two retrospective studies No studies met inclusion criteria	125 mg of mupirocin in 200 ml of saline + placebo tablets for 28 days vs 200 ml of saline + Augmentin for 28 days Mupirocin ranged from 0.05 to 2% once or twice a day. Included the previous study by Jervis et al. [40]	LK scores improved more in the mupirocin group −4.0 (95% CI -7.0–1.3) compared to Augmentin −3.0 (−1.0–4.0). SNOT-22 and VAS scores improved from baseline but were not significantly different. Culture negativity was better in the mupirocin group. Relative risk for residual infection 0.13 (random effects 95% CI 0.06–0.26). Residual *Staphylococcus aureus* infection after 1 month 0.08 (random effects 95% CI: 0.04–0.16). Low-quality studies precluded any type of recommendation.

(continued)

Table 26.1 (continued)

Treatment	Study design	N	Sample characteristics	Intervention and comparison	Outcomes
Antimicrobial photodynamic therapy	Open-label RCT [45] Double-blind RCT [46]	76 50	CRSwNP with grade II–III nasal polyps with previous FESS and long-standing topical steroid treatment CRS criteria met	Mometasone furoate BID vs mometasone furoate BID + mUV/VIS phototherapy 3 times per week for 12 weeks mUV/VIS vs placebo (low-intensity visible light)	mUV/IVS group improved NOSE, TNSS, and PNIF at 6, 12, and 26 weeks and reduced polyp size at 16 and 26 weeks, Mometasone group did not improve, but no comparative analysis was made between groups. No difference seen in symptom severity, RDSI, olfaction, rhinomanometry, or nitric oxide. Carbon monoxide production increased in mUV/VIS group.
Bacteriophage therapy	Phase I pilot open-label trial [52]	9	Postoperative CRS patients with positive cultures for *Staphylococcus aureus* sensitive to the AB-SA01 phage cocktail	3 × 10^8 phage-forming units (PFU) twice a day for 7 days vs 3 × 10^8 phage-forming units (PFU) twice a day for 17 days vs 3 × 10^9 phage-forming units (PFU) twice a day for seven days	Phage therapy was well tolerated in all cohorts, with no serious adverse events reported. Preliminary efficacy data showed improvement with phage therapy, with 2/9 patients having complete irradiation of their infection.
Sinonasal microbiota transfer	Three RCT registered in clinicaltrials.gov [72–74]	–	All trial focus on rCRS	Two trials [72, 73] compare the transfer of sinus washes from healthy donors to placebo. One trial [74] compares the transfer of endoscopically suctioned mucus from healthy donors against placebo	No published results.

AFRS allergic fungal rhinosinusitis, *CRSsNP* chronic rhinosinusitis without nasal polyps, *CRSwNP* chronic rhinosinusitis with nasal polyps, *FESS* functional endoscopic sinus surgery, *MLK* modified Lund-Kennedy endoscopic score, *PNIF* peak nasal inspiratory flow, *PVP-I* povidone-iodine, *rCRS* recalcitrant chronic rhinosinusitis, *UPSIT* University of Pennsylvania Smell Identification Test, *TNSS* total nasal symptom score

References

1. Bachert C, Han JK, Desrosiers M, Hellings PW, Amin N, Lee SE, et al. Efficacy and safety of dupilumab in patients with severe chronic rhinosinusitis with nasal polyps (LIBERTY NP SINUS-24 and LIBERTY NP SINUS-52): results from two multicentre, randomised, double-blind, placebo-controlled, parallel-group phase 3 trials. Lancet. 2019;394(10209):1638–50.
2. Gevaert P, Omachi TA, Corren J, Mullol J, Han J, Lee SE, et al. Efficacy and safety of omalizumab in nasal polyposis: 2 randomized phase 3 trials. J Allergy Clin Immunol. 2020 Sep;146(3):595–605.
3. Agache I, Beltran J, Akdis C, Akdis M, Canelo-Aybar C, Canonica GW, et al. Efficacy and safety of treatment with biologicals (benralizumab, dupilumab, mepolizumab, omalizumab and reslizumab) for severe eosinophilic asthma. A systematic review for the EAACI guidelines—recommendations on the use of biologicals in severe asthma. Allergy. 2020;75(5):1023–42.
4. Bavaro N, Gakpo D, Mittal A, Bensko J, Laidlaw TM, Buchheit KM. Efficacy of dupilumab in patients with aspirin-exacerbated respiratory disease and previous inadequate response to anti-IL-5 or anti-IL-5Rα in a real-world setting. J Allergy Clin Immunol Pract. 2021;9:2910.
5. Callewaert C, Nakatsuji T, Knight R, Kosciolek T, Vrbanac A, Kotol P, et al. IL-4Rα blockade by Dupilumab decreases Staphylococcus aureus colonization and increases microbial diversity in atopic dermatitis. J Invest Dermatol. 2020;140(1):191–202.e7.
6. Fujieda S, Matsune S, Takeno S, Asako M, Takeuchi M, Fujita H, et al. The effect of Dupilumab on intractable chronic rhinosinusitis with nasal polyps in Japan. Laryngoscope. 2020;
7. Sanofi. A randomized double-blind placebo-controlled Parallel Group Study assessing the efficacy and safety of Dupilumab in patients with Allergic Fungal Rhinosinusitis (AFRS) [Internet]. clinicaltrials.gov; 2022 May [cited 2022 Jul 10]. (In: ClinicalTrials.gov [Internet]. Bethesda: U.S. National Library of Medicine. 2000 -). Report No.: NCT04684524. Available from: https://clinicaltrials.gov/ct2/show/NCT04684524
8. Johns Hopkins University. Efficacy of Dupilumab for Patients With Chronic Rhinosinusitis Without Nasal Polyps (CRSsNP): a Randomized Double Blind Placebo Controlled Phase II Study [Internet]. clinicaltrials.gov; 2021 Oct [cited 2022 Jul 10]. (In: ClinicalTrials.gov [Internet]. Bethesda: U.S. National Library of Medicine. 2000 -). Report No.: NCT04362501. Available from: https://clinicaltrials.gov/ct2/show/NCT04362501
9. Miyake MM, Bleier BS. Future topical medications in chronic rhinosinusitis. Int Forum Allergy Rhinol. 2019;9(S1):S32–46.
10. Carlton DA, Beahm DD, Chiu AG. Topical antibiotic therapy in chronic rhinosinusitis: an update. Int Forum Allergy Rhinol. 2019;9(S1):S27–31.
11. Fokkens WJ, Lund VJ, Hopkins C, Hellings PW, Kern R, Reitsma S, et al. European Position Paper on Rhinosinusitis and Nasal Polyps 2020. Rhinology. 2020;58(Suppl S29):1–464.
12. Singhal D, Psaltis AJ, Foreman A, Wormald PJ. The impact of biofilms on outcomes after endoscopic sinus surgery. Am J Rhinol Allergy. 2010;24(3):169–74.
13. Zhao YC. Biofilm and osteitis in refractory chronic rhinosinusitis. Otolaryngol Clin NA. 2017;50(1):49–60.
14. Foreman A, Psaltis AJ, Tan LW, Wormald PJ. Characterization of bacterial and fungal biofilms in chronic rhinosinusitis. Am J Rhinol Allergy. 2009;23(6):556–61.
15. Wood AJ, Fraser J, Swift S, Amirapu S, Douglas RG. Are biofilms associated with an inflammatory response in chronic rhinosinusitis? Int Forum Allergy Rhinol. 2011;1(5):335–9.
16. Panchatcharam BS, Cooksley CM, Ramezanpour M, Vediappan RS, Bassiouni A, Wormald PJ, et al. Staphylococcus aureus biofilm exoproteins are cytotoxic to human nasal epithelial barrier in chronic rhinosinusitis. Int Forum Allergy Rhinol. 2020;10(7):871–83.
17. Martens K, Seys SF, Alpizar YA, Schrijvers R, Bullens DMA, Breynaert C, et al. Staphylococcus aureus enterotoxin B disrupts nasal epithelial barrier integrity. Clin Exp Allergy J Br Soc Allergy Clin Immunol. 2021;51(1):87–98.
18. Ou J, Wang J, Xu Y, Zhang Tao Z, Gang Kong Y, Ming Chen S, et al. Staphylococcus aureus superantigens are associated with chronic rhinosinusitis with nasal polyps: a meta-analysis. Eur Arch Oto-Rhino-Laryngol Off J Eur Fed Oto-Rhino-Laryngol Soc EUFOS Affil Ger Soc Oto-Rhino-Laryngol - Head Neck Surg. 2014;271(10):2729–36.

19. Desrosiers M, Myntti M, James G. Methods for removing bacterial biofilms: in vitro study using clinical chronic rhinosinusitis specimens. Am J Rhinol. 2007;21(5):527–32.
20. Oduwole KO, Glynn AA, Molony DC, Murray D, Rowe S, Holland LM, et al. Anti-biofilm activity of sub-inhibitory povidone-iodine concentrations against Staphylococcus epidermidis and Staphylococcus aureus. J Orthop Res. 2010;28(9):1252–6.
21. Ngaage LM, Elegbede A, Brao K, Chopra K, Gowda AU, Nam AJ, et al. The efficacy of breast implant irrigant solutions: a comparative analysis using an in vitro model. Plast Reconstr Surg. 2020 Aug;146(2):301–8.
22. Jeronimo LP, Choi MR, Yeon SH, Park SK, Yoon YH, Choi SH, et al. Effects of povidone-iodine composite on the elimination of bacterial biofilm. Int Forum Allergy Rhinol. 2020;10(7):884–92.
23. Eggers M, Eickmann M, Zorn J. Rapid and effective virucidal activity of povidone-iodine products against Middle East Respiratory Syndrome Coronavirus (MERS-CoV) and Modified Vaccinia Virus Ankara (MVA). Infect Dis Ther. 2015;4(4):491–501.
24. Bidra AS, Pelletier JS, Westover JB, Frank S, Brown SM, Tessema B. Rapid in-vitro inactivation of Severe Acute Respiratory Syndrome Coronavirus 2 (SARS-CoV-2) using povidone-iodine oral antiseptic rinse. J Prosthodont Off J Am Coll Prosthodont. 2020;29(6):529–33.
25. Rezapoor M, Nicholson T, Tabatabaee RM, Chen AF, Maltenfort MG, Parvizi J. Povidone-iodine-based solutions for decolonization of nasal Staphylococcus aureus: a randomized, prospective, Placebo-Controlled Study. J Arthroplasty. 2017 Sep;32(9):2815–9.
26. Lee VS, Pottinger PS, Davis GE. Tolerability and effectiveness of povidone-iodine or mupirocin versus saline sinus irrigations for chronic rhinosinusitis. Am J Otolaryngol. 2020 Oct;41(5):102604.
27. Panchmatia R, Payandeh J, Al-Salman R, Kakande E, Habib AR, Mullings W, et al. The efficacy of diluted topical povidone-iodine rinses in the management of recalcitrant chronic rhinosinusitis: a prospective cohort study. Eur Arch Otorrinolaringol. 2019;276(12):3373–81.
28. Wu PH, Cheng PC, Chang CM, Lo WC, Cheng PW. Efficacy of povidone-iodine nasal irrigation solution after sinonasal surgery: a Randomized Controlled Study. Laryngoscope. 2022;132(6):1148–52.
29. Kwakman PHS, te Velde AA, de Boer L, Speijer D, Christina Vandenbroucke-Grauls MJ, Zaat SAJ. How honey kills bacteria. FASEB J. 2010;24(7):2576–82.
30. Lu J, Turnbull L, Burke CM, Liu M, Carter DA, Schlothauer RC, et al. Manuka-type honeys can eradicate biofilms produced by Staphylococcus aureus strains with different biofilm-forming abilities. PeerJ. 2014;2:e326.
31. Thamboo A, Thamboo A, Philpott C, Javer A, Clark A. Single-blind study of manuka honey in allergic fungal rhinosinusitis. J Otolaryngol—Head Neck Surg J Oto-Rhino-Laryngol Chir Cervico-Faciale. 2011;40(3):238–43.
32. Ooi ML, Jothin A, Bennett C, Ooi EH, Vreugde S, Psaltis AJ, et al. Manuka honey sinus irrigations in recalcitrant chronic rhinosinusitis: phase 1 randomized, single-blinded, placebo-controlled trial. Int Forum Allergy Rhinol. 2019;9(12):1470–7.
33. Lee VS, Humphreys IM, Purcell PL, Davis GE. Manuka honey sinus irrigation for the treatment of chronic rhinosinusitis: a randomized controlled trial. Int Forum Allergy Rhinol. 2017;7(4):365–72.
34. Hashemian F, Baghbanian N, Majd Z, Rouini MR, Jahanshahi J, Hashemian F. The effect of thyme honey nasal spray on chronic rhinosinusitis: a double-blind randomized controlled clinical trial. Eur Arch Oto-Rhino-Laryngol Off J Eur Fed Oto-Rhino-Laryngol Soc EUFOS Affil Ger Soc Oto-Rhino-Laryngol—Head Neck Surg. 2015;272(6):1429–35.
35. Das CGA, Kumar VG, Dhas TS, Karthick V, Govindaraju K, Joselin JM, et al. Antibacterial activity of silver nanoparticles (biosynthesis): a short review on recent advances. Biocatal Agric Biotechnol. 2020;27:101593.

36. Feizi S, Cooksley CM, Bouras GS, Prestidge CA, Coenye T, Psaltis AJ, et al. Colloidal silver combating pathogenic Pseudomonas aeruginosa and MRSA in chronic rhinosinusitis. Colloids Surf B Biointerfaces. 2021;202:111675.
37. Feizi S, Cooksley CM, Nepal R, Psaltis AJ, Wormald PJ, Vreugde S. Silver nanoparticles as a bioadjuvant of antibiotics against biofilm-mediated infections with methicillin-resistant Staphylococcus aureus and Pseudomonas aeruginosa in chronic rhinosinusitis patients. Pathology (Phila). 2022;54(4):453–9.
38. Scott JR, Krishnan R, Rotenberg BW, Sowerby LJ. The effectiveness of topical colloidal silver in recalcitrant chronic rhinosinusitis: a randomized crossover control trial. J Otolaryngol—Head Neck Surg. 2017;46(1):64.
39. Ooi ML, Richter K, Bennett C, Macias-Valle L, Vreugde S, Psaltis AJ, et al. Topical colloidal silver for the treatment of recalcitrant chronic rhinosinusitis. Front Microbiol [Internet]. 2018;9. [cited 2022 Jul 3]. Available from: https://www.frontiersin.org/article/10.3389/fmicb.2018.00720
40. Jervis-Bardy J, Boase S, Psaltis A, Foreman A, Wormald PJ. A randomized trial of mupirocin sinonasal rinses versus saline in surgically recalcitrant staphylococcal chronic rhinosinusitis. Laryngoscope. 2012;122(10):2148–53.
41. Kim JS, Kwon SH. Mupirocin in the treatment of staphylococcal infections in chronic rhinosinusitis: a meta-analysis. PLoS One. 2016;11(12):e0167369.
42. Head K, Chong LY, Piromchai P, Hopkins C, Philpott C, Schilder AGM, et al. Systemic and topical antibiotics for chronic rhinosinusitis. Cochrane Database Syst Rev. 2016;4:CD011994.
43. Koreck AI, Csoma Z, Bodai L, Ignacz F, Kenderessy AS, Kadocsa E, et al. Rhinophototherapy: a new therapeutic tool for the management of allergic rhinitis. J Allergy Clin Immunol. 2005;115(3):541–7.
44. Kennedy R, Robertson L. Study on the effect of phototherapy for inhibition of symptoms associated with allergic rhinitis. Eur Ann Allergy Clin Immunol. 2019;52(2):66.
45. Kiricsi Á, Tiszlavicz L, Rázga Z, Krasznai M, Vóna I, Hirschberg A, et al. Prospective, multicenter, randomized clinical study to evaluate the clinical efficacy and tolerability of long term mixed ultraviolet and visible light phototherapy in eosinophil nasal polyps. J Photochem Photobiol B. 2017;176:118–23.
46. Dulguerov N, Guinand N, Courvoisier D, Landis BN, Lacroix JS, Hauser C. Rhinophototherapy in chronic rhinosinusitis: a double blind randomized placebo-controlled trial. Rhinol J. 2017;55(2):106–12.
47. Harris F, Chatfield LK, Phoenix DA. Phenothiazinium based photosensitisers--photodynamic agents with a multiplicity of cellular targets and clinical applications. Curr Drug Targets 2005;6(5):615–627.
48. Biel MA, Sievert C, Usacheva M, Teichert M, Balcom J. Antimicrobial photodynamic therapy treatment of chronic recurrent sinusitis biofilms. Int Forum Allergy Rhinol. 2011;1(5):329–34.
49. Biel MA, Jones JW, Pedigo L, Gibbs A, Loebel N. The effect of antimicrobial photodynamic therapy on human ciliated respiratory mucosa. Laryngoscope. 2012;122(12):2628–31.
50. Sulakvelidze A, Alavidze Z, Morris JG. Bacteriophage therapy. Antimicrob Agents Chemother. 2001;45:11.
51. Harper DR, Parracho HMRT, Walker J, Sharp R, Hughes G, Werthén M, et al. Bacteriophages and biofilms. Antibiotics. 2014;3(3):270–84.
52. Ooi ML, Drilling AJ, Morales S, Fong S, Moraitis S, Macias-Valle L, et al. Safety and tolerability of bacteriophage therapy for chronic rhinosinusitis due to Staphylococcus aureus. JAMA Otolaryngol Neck Surg. 2019;145(8):723–9.
53. Okano M, Fujiwara T, Haruna T, Kariya S, Makihara S, Higaki T, et al. Role of fungal antigens in eosinophilia-associated cellular responses in nasal polyps: a comparison with enterotoxin. Clin Exp Allergy. 2011;41(2):171–8.

54. Hayes SM, Biggs TC, Goldie SP, Harries PG, Walls AF, Allan RN, et al. Staphylococcus aureus internalization in mast cells in nasal polyps: characterization of interactions and potential mechanisms. J Allergy Clin Immunol. 2020;145(1):147–59.
55. Ou J, Drilling A, Singhal D, Tan NCW, Wallis-Hill D, Vreugde S, et al. Association of intracellular Staphylococcus aureus with prognosis in chronic rhinosinusitis. Int Forum Allergy Rhinol. 2016;6(8):792–9.
56. Murphy J, Ramezanpour M, Drilling A, Roscioli E, Psaltis AJ, Wormald PJ, et al. In vitro characteristics of an airway barrier-disrupting factor secreted by Staphylococcus aureus. Int Forum Allergy Rhinol. 2019;9(2):187–96.
57. Foreman A, Holtappels G, Psaltis AJ, Jervis-Bardy J, Field J, Wormald PJ, et al. Adaptive immune responses in Staphylococcus aureus biofilm–associated chronic rhinosinusitis. Allergy. 2011;66(11):1449–56.
58. van Nood E, Vrieze A, Nieuwdrop M, Fuentes S, Zoetendal EG, De VWM, et al. Duodenal infusion of donor feces for recurrent Clostridium difficile. N Engl J Med. 2013;368(5):407–15.
59. Gough E, Shaikh E, Manges A. Systematic review of intestinal microbiota transplantation (fecal bacteriotherapy) for recurrent Clostridium difficile infection. Clin Infect Dis Off Publ Infect Dis Soc Am. 2011;53(10):994–1002.
60. Fokkens W, Lund V, Hopkins C, Hellings P, Kern P, Reitsma S, et al. European Position Paper on Rhinosinusitis and Nasal Polyps 2020. Rhinology. 2020;58(Suppl S29):1–464.
61. Ott S, Waetzig G, Rehman A, Moltzau-Anderson J, Bharti R, Grasis JA, et al. Efficacy of sterile fecal filtrate transfer for treating patients with Clostridium difficile infection. Gastroenterology. 2017;152(4):799–811.e7.
62. Lux CA, Wagner Mackenzie B, Johnston J, Zoing M, Biswas K, Taylor MW, et al. Antibiotic treatment for chronic rhinosinusitis: prescription patterns and associations with patient outcome and the sinus microbiota. Front Microbiol. 2020;11:3251.
63. Baxter M, Colville A. Adverse events in faecal microbiota transplant: a review of the literature. J Hosp Infect. W.B. Saunders Ltd. 2016;92:117–27.
64. Osman M. Safety and efficacy of fecal microbiota transplantation for recurrent *Clostridium difficile* infection from an international public stool bank: results from a 2,050 patient multicenter cohort. Idsa. 2016;
65. Abreu NA, Nagalingam NA, Song Y, Roediger FC, Pletcher SD, Goldberg AN, et al. Sinus microbiome diversity depletion and Corynebacterium tuberculostearicum enrichment mediates rhinosinusitis. Sci Transl Med. 2012;4(151):151ra124.
66. Cope EK, Goldberg AN, Pletcher SD, Lynch SV. Compositionally and functionally distinct sinus microbiota in chronic rhinosinusitis patients have immunological and clinically divergent consequences. Microbiome. 2017;5(1):1–16.
67. Wagner Mackenzie B, Waite DW, Hoggard M, Douglas RG, Taylor MW, Biswas K. Bacterial community collapse: a meta-analysis of the sinonasal microbiota in chronic rhinosinusitis. Environ Microbiol. 2017;19(1):381–92.
68. Gan W, Yang F, Tang Y, Zhou D, Qing D, Hu J, et al. The difference in nasal bacterial microbiome diversity between chronic rhinosinusitis patients with polyps and a control population. Int Forum Allergy Rhinol. 2019;9(6):582–92.
69. Kuhar HN, Tajudeen BA, Mahdavinia M, Heilingoetter A, Ganti A, Gattuso P, et al. Relative abundance of nasal microbiota in chronic rhinosinusitis by structured histopathology. Int Forum Allergy Rhinol. 2018;8(12):1430–7.
70. Allegretti JR, Kao D, Sitko J, Fischer M, Kassam Z. Early antibiotic use after fecal microbiota transplantation increases risk of treatment failure. Clin Infect Dis. 2018;66(1):134–5.
71. Luu K, Sutherland J, Crump T, Liu G, Janjua A. The impact of chronic airway disease on symptom severity and global suffering in Canadian rhinosinusitis patients. J Otolaryngol—Head Neck Surg J Oto-Rhino-Laryngol Chir Cervico-Faciale. 2018;47(1):40.

72. The University of Queensland. Phase-II Randomized Control Trial of Nasal Microbiota Transplant Therapy in Chronic Rhinosinusitis Without Nasal Polyps (CRSsNP) [Internet]. clinicaltrials.gov; 2022 [cited 2022 Jun 30]. (In: ClinicalTrials.gov [Internet]. Bethesda: U.S. National Library of Medicine. 2000 -). Available from: https://clinicaltrials.gov/ct2/show/NCT05400616
73. Region Skane. Sinonasal Microbiome Transplant as a Therapy for Chronic Rhinosinusitis Without Nasal Polyps (CRSsNP) [Internet]. clinicaltrials.gov; 2019 [cited 2022 Jun 30]. (In: ClinicalTrials.gov [Internet]. Bethesda: U.S. National Library of Medicine. 2000 -). Available from: https://clinicaltrials.gov/ct2/show/NCT03122795
74. Javer A. SinoNasal Microbiota Transfer (SNMT) to Treat Chronic Rhinosinusitis: A Randomized, Double-blind, Placebo-controlled Trial [Internet]. clinicaltrials.gov; 2022 Jul [cited 2022 Jul 12]. Report No.: NCT05454072. Available from:. https://clinicaltrials.gov/ct2/show/NCT05454072
75. Head K, Chong L, Piromchai P, Hopkins C, Philpott C, Schilder A, et al. Systemic and topical antibiotics for chronic rhinosinusitis. Cochrane Database Syst Rev. 2016:4.

Index

J. T. Lee et al. (eds.), *Advances in Surgical and Medical Interventions for Recalcitrant Chronic Rhinosinusitis*,
https://doi.org/10.1007/978-3-031-89191-5

T

U

V

W

MIX
Papier aus verantwortungsvollen Quellen
Paper from responsible sources
FSC® C105338

If you have any concerns about our products,
you can contact us on
ProductSafety@springernature.com

In case Publisher is established outside the EU,
the EU authorized representative is:
Springer Nature Customer Service Center GmbH
Europaplatz 3, 69115 Heidelberg, Germany

Printed by Libri Plureos GmbH
in Hamburg, Germany